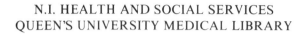

1993
YEAR BOOK OF
VASCULAR SURGERY®

Statement of Purpose

The YEAR BOOK Service

The YEAR BOOK series was devised in 1901 by practicing health professionals who observed that the literature of medicine and related disciplines had become so voluminous that no one individual could read and place in perspective every potential advance in a major specialty. In the final decade of the 20th century, this recognition is more acutely true than it was in 1901.

More than merely a series of books, YEAR BOOK volumes are the tangible results of a unique service designed to accomplish the following:

- to *survey* a wide range of journals of proven value
- to *select* from those journals papers representing significant advances and statements of important clinical principles
- to provide *abstracts* of those articles that are readable, convenient summaries of their key points
- to provide *commentary* about those articles to place them in perspective

These publications grow out of a unique process that calls on the talents of outstanding authorities in clinical and fundamental disciplines, trained literature specialists, and professional writers, all supported by the resources of Mosby, the world's preeminent publisher for the health professions.

The Literature Base

Mosby subscribes to nearly 1,000 journals published worldwide, covering the full range of the health professions. On an annual basis, the publisher examines usage patterns and polls its expert authorities to add new journals to the literature base and to delete journals that are no longer useful as potential YEAR BOOK sources.

The Literature Survey

The publisher's team of literature specialists, all of whom are trained and experienced health professionals, examines every original, peer-reviewed article in each journal issue. More than 250,000 articles per year are scanned systematically, including title, text, illustrations, tables, and references. Each scan is compared, article by article, to the search strategies that the publisher has developed in consultation with the 270 outside experts who form the pool of YEAR BOOK editors. A given article may be reviewed by any number of editors, from one to a dozen or more, regardless of the discipline for which the paper was originally published. In turn, each editor who receives the article reviews it to determine whether or not the article should be included in the YEAR BOOK. This decision is based on the article's inherent quality, its probable usefulness to readers of that YEAR BOOK, and the editor's goal to represent a balanced picture of a given field in each volume of the YEAR BOOK. In addition, the editor indicates when to include figures and tables from the article to help the YEAR BOOK reader better understand the information.

Of the quarter million articles scanned each year, only 5% are selected for detailed analysis within the YEAR BOOK series, thereby assuring readers of the high value of every selection.

The Abstract

The publisher's abstracting staff is headed by a physician-writer and includes individuals with training in the life sciences, medicine, and other areas, plus extensive experience in writing for the health professions and related industries. Each selected article is assigned to a specific writer on this abstracting staff. The abstracter, guided in many cases by notations supplied by the expert editor, writes a structured, condensed summary designed so that the reader can rapidly acquire the essential information contained in the article.

The Commentary

The YEAR BOOK editorial boards, sometimes assisted by guest commentators, write comments that place each article in perspective for the reader. This provides the reader with the equivalent of a personal consultation with a leading international authority—an opportunity to better understand the value of the article and to benefit from the authority's thought processes in assessing the article.

Additional Editorial Features

The editorial boards of each YEAR BOOK organize the abstracts and comments to provide a logical and satisfying sequence of information. To enhance the organization, editors also provide introductions to sections or individual chapters, comments linking a number of abstracts, citations to additional literature, and other features.

The published YEAR BOOK contains enhanced bibliographic citations for each selected article, including extended listings of multiple authors and identification of author affiliations. Each YEAR BOOK contains a Table of Contents specific to that year's volume. From year to year, the Table of Contents for a given YEAR BOOK will vary depending on developments within the field.

Every YEAR BOOK contains a list of the journals from which papers have been selected. The list represents a subset of the nearly 1,000 journals surveyed by the publisher, and occasionally reflects a particularly pertinent article from a journal that is not surveyed on a routine basis.

Finally, each volume contains a comprehensive subject index and an index to authors of each selected paper.

The 1993 Year Book® Series

Year Book of Anesthesia and Pain Management: Drs. Miller, Abram, Kirby, Ostheimer, Roizen, and Stoelting

Year Book of Cardiology®: Drs. Schlant, Collins, Engle, Gersh, Kaplan, and Waldo

Year Book of Chiropractic: Drs. Phillips and Adams

Year Book of Critical Care Medicine®: Drs. Rogers and Parrillo

Year Book of Dentistry®: Drs. Meskin, Currier, Kennedy, Leinfelder, Berry, Roser, and Zakariasen

Year Book of Dermatologic Surgery: Drs. Swanson, Salasche, and Glogau

Year Book of Dermatology®: Drs. Sober and Fitzpatrick

Year Book of Diagnostic Radiology®: Drs. Federle, Clark, Gross, Madewell, Maynard, Sackett, and Young

Year Book of Digestive Diseases®: Drs. Greenberger and Moody

Year Book of Drug Therapy®: Drs. Lasagna and Weintraub

Year Book of Emergency Medicine®: Drs. Wagner, Burdick, Davidson, Roberts, and Spivey

Year Book of Endocrinology®: Drs. Bagdade, Braverman, Horton, Kannan, Landsberg, Molitch, Morley, Odell, Rogol, Ryan, and Sherwin

Year Book of Family Practice®: Drs. Berg, Bowman, Davidson, Dietrich, and Scherger

Year Book of Geriatrics and Gerontology®: Drs. Beck, Reuben, Burton, Small, Whitehouse, and Goldstein

Year Book of Hand Surgery®: Drs. Amadio and Hentz

Year Book of Health Care Management: Drs. Heyssel, Brock, Moses, and Steinberg, Ms. Avakian, and Messrs. Berman, Kues, and Rosenberg

Year Book of Hematology®: Drs. Spivak, Bell, Ness, Quesenberry, and Wiernik

Year Book of Infectious Diseases®: Drs. Wolff, Barza, Keusch, Klempner, and Snydman

Year Book of Infertility: Drs. Mishell, Paulsen, and Lobo

Year Book of Medicine®: Drs. Rogers, Bone, Cline, O'Rourke, Greenberger, Utiger, Epstein, and Malawista

Year Book of Neonatal and Perinatal Medicine®: Drs. Klaus and Fanaroff

Year Book of Nephrology: Drs. Coe, Favus, Henderson, Kashgarian, Luke, Myers, and Curtis

Year Book of Neurology and Neurosurgery®: Drs. Bradley and Crowell

Year Book of Neuroradiology: Drs. Osborn, Eskridge, Harnsberger, and Grossman

Year Book of Nuclear Medicine®: Drs. Hoffer, Gore, Gottschalk, Zaret, and Zubal

Year Book of Obstetrics and Gynecology®: Drs. Mishell, Kirschbaum, and Morrow

Year Book of Occupational and Environmental Medicine: Drs. Emmett, Brooks, Frank, and Hammad

Year Book of Oncology®: Drs. Young, Longo, Ozols, Simone, Steele, and Glatstein

Year Book of Ophthalmology®: Drs. Laibson, Adams, Augsburger, Benson, Cohen, Eagle, Flanagan, Nelson, Rapuano, Reinecke, Sergott, and Wilson

Year Book of Orthopedics®: Drs. Sledge, Poss, Cofield, Frymoyer, Griffin, Hansen, Johnson, Simmons, and Springfield

Year Book of Otolaryngology–Head and Neck Surgery®: Drs. Holt and Paparella

Year Book of Pathology and Clinical Pathology®: Drs. Gardner, Bennett, Cousar, Garvin, and Worsham

Year Book of Pediatrics®: Dr. Stockman

Year Book of Plastic, Reconstructive, and Aesthetic Surgery: Drs. Miller, Cohen, McKinney, Robson, Ruberg, and Whitaker

Year Book of Podiatric Medicine and Surgery®: Dr. Kominsky

Year Book of Psychiatry and Applied Mental Health®: Drs. Talbott, Frances, Freedman, Meltzer, Perry, Schowalter, and Yudofsky

Year Book of Pulmonary Disease®: Drs. Bone and Petty

Year Book of Sports Medicine®: Drs. Shephard, Eichner, Sutton, and Torg, Col. Anderson, and Mr. George

Year Book of Surgery®: Drs. Copeland, Deitch, Eberlein, Howard, Ritchie, Robson, Souba, and Sugarbaker

Year Book of Transplantation®: Drs. Ascher, Hansen, and Strom

Year Book of Ultrasound: Drs. Merritt, Mittelstaedt, Carroll, Babcock, and Goldstein

Year Book of Urology®: Drs. Gillenwater and Howards

Year Book of Vascular Surgery®: Dr. Porter

Roundsmanship® '93–'94: A Student's Survival Guide to Clinical Medicine Using Current Literature: Drs. Dan, Feigin, Quilligan, Schrock, Stein, and Talbott

1993

The Year Book of VASCULAR SURGERY®

Editor

John M. Porter, M.D.

Professor of Surgery; Head, Division of Vascular Surgery, Oregon Health Sciences University School of Medicine, Portland, Oregon

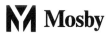 **Mosby**

St. Louis   Baltimore   Boston   Chicago   London   Philadelphia   Sydney   Toronto

Editor-in-Chief, Year Book Publishing: Kenneth H. Killion
Associate Acquisitions Editor: Gretchen C. Templeton
Sponsoring Editor: Linda Steiner
Manager, Literature Services: Edith M. Podrazik
Senior Information Specialist: Terri Santo
Senior Medical Writer: David A. Cramer, M.D.
Assistant Director, Manuscript Services: Frances M. Perveiler
Assistant Managing Editor, Year Book Editing Services: Tamara L. Smith
Senior Production/Desktop Publishing Manager: Max F. Perez
Proofroom Manager: Barbara M. Kelly

Editorial Office:
Mosby, Inc.
200 North LaSalle St.
Chicago, IL 60601

International Standard Serial Number: 0749-4041
International Standard Book Number: 0-8151-0682-3

Contributing Editors

Alexander W. Clowes, M.D.
Professor and Acting Chairman, School of Medicine, Department of Surgery, University of Washington, Seattle, Washington

Ronald Dalman, M.D.
Chief, Vascular Surgery, Surgical Services, Veterans Affairs Medical Center, Stanford University School of Medicine, Palo Alto, California

George Johnson, Jr., M.D.
Professor of Surgery; Coordinator, General Surgery Services, School of Medicine, The University of North Carolina, Chapel Hill, North Carolina

Frank W. LoGerfo, M.D.
Professor of Surgery, Harvard Medical School; Chief, Division of Vascular Surgery, New England Deaconess Hospital, Boston Massachusetts

Joseph Mills, M.D.
Associate Professor of Surgery, Division of Vascular Surgery, University of South Florida College of Medicine, Tampa, Florida

Gregory L. Moneta, M.D.
Associate Professor of Surgery, Division of Vascular Surgery, Oregon Health Sciences University and Veterans Administration Medical Center, Portland, Oregon

Chris Zarins, M.D.
Professor of Surgery; Chief, Section of Vascular Surgery, University of Chicago School of Medicine, Chicago, Illinois

Table of Contents

Journals Represented

Mosby subscribes to and surveys nearly 1,000 U.S. and foreign medical and allied health journals. From these journals, the Editors select the articles to be abstracted. Journals represented in this YEAR BOOK are listed below.

Acta Endocrinologica
Acta Neurologica Scandinavica
American Heart Journal
American Journal of Clinical Pathology
American Journal of Epidemiology
American Journal of Medicine
American Journal of Roentgenology
American Journal of Surgery
Anesthesia and Analgesia
Anesthesiology
Angiology
Annals of Internal Medicine
Annals of Rheumatic Diseases
Annals of Surgery
Annals of Thoracic Surgery
Annals of Vascular Surgery
Archives of Internal Medicine
Archives of Otolaryngology-Head and Neck Surgery
Archives of Surgery
Arteriosclerosis and Thrombosis
Arthritis and Rheumatism
Atherosclerosis
Blood
British Heart Journal
British Journal of Radiology
British Journal of Surgery
British Journal of Urology
British Medical Journal
Catheterization and Cardiovascular Diagnosis
Circulation
Clinical Infectious Diseases
Clinical Nuclear Medicine
Clinical Orthopaedics and Related Research
Clinical Physiology
Clinical Radiology
Clinical Science
Digestive Diseases and Sciences
Diseases of the Colon and Rectum
European Heart Journal
European Journal of Plastic Surgery
European Journal of Surgery
European Journal of Vascular Surgery
Gastroenterology
Hypertension
Israel Journal of Medical Sciences
Journal of Arthroplasty
Journal of Cardiovascular Surgery
Journal of Computer Assisted Tomography
Journal of Internal Medicine
Journal of Interventional Radiology

Journal of Laboratory and Clinical Medicine
Journal of Neurosurgery
Journal of Nuclear Medicine
Journal of Orthopaedic Trauma
Journal of Pediatric Surgery
Journal of Rheumatology
Journal of Thoracic and Cardiovascular Surgery
Journal of Trauma
Journal of Vascular Surgery
Journal of the American Medical Association
Journal of the American Osteopathic Association
Journal of the Royal College of Surgeons of Edinburgh
Journal of the Royal Society of Medicine
Lancet
Magnetic Resonance Imaging
Nephrology, Dialysis, Transplantation
Neurology
Neurosurgery
New England Journal of Medicine
Nuclear Medicine Communications
Ophthalmic Surgery
Ophthalmology
Proceedings of the National Academy of Sciences
Prostaglandins
Radiology
Reviews of Infectious Diseases
S.A.M.J./S.A.M.T – South African Medical Journal
Seminars in Hematology
Seminars in Thrombosis and Hemostasis
Stroke
Surgery
Transplantation
Ultrasound in Medicine and Biology

STANDARD ABBREVIATIONS

The following terms are abbreviated in this edition: acquired immunodeficiency syndrome (AIDS), central nervous system (CNS), cerebrospinal fluid (CSF), computed tomography (CT), electrocardiography (ECG), human immunodeficiency virus (HIV), and magnetic resonance (MR) imaging (MRI).

Introduction

I am honored to be your new editor of the YEAR BOOK OF VASCULAR SURGERY. From the outset, I acknowledge the high standards established by the founding editors, Dr. John Bergan and Dr. James Yao, who served as co-editors from the publication of the YEAR BOOK OF VASCULAR SURGERY in 1986 through the 1991 edition. Dr. Bergan served as the solo editor for the 1992 edition.

Readers will notice that there has been a change in the topic headings for the 1993 YEAR BOOK. The current table of contents is one that I believe represents the best compromise. It is clear that one can never have a group of headings sufficiently long enough to accommodate every article precisely. I have had to make some arbitrary decisions as to the category in which a certain article is placed, and there clearly are occasional inconsistencies. These inconsistencies have been deliberately left in the manuscript to reward the careful examination of the discerning reader. The essence of this book is in its editing. I reviewed thousands of articles before selecting the ones abstracted herein. The selections obviously reflect the bias of the editor. As I believe the future of vascular surgery resides significantly in the area of research, the reader will note that the section on basic considerations (Chapter 1) is rather large. If this is not to your liking, be assured that the remainder of the volume is focused almost exclusively on clinical topics. I have given relatively low priority to case reports and review articles, as these do not readily lend themselves to the abstract format. An occasional case report is included if it makes an especially important point.

I express my appreciation to the physicians who provided guest commentaries for this volume, to the officials of the Mosby, Inc. for their cooperation, courtesy, and professionalism during the period of transition of YEAR BOOK editorship, and especially to Dr. John Bergan for his many kindnesses. I gratefully acknowledge the invaluable assistance of our office manager, Ms. Barbara McNamee, in maintaining a generally peaceful sense of order, despite the enormous amount of material related to this endeavor that passed through our office. This has been an exciting project for me, and I hope this sense of excitement will be perceived by the reader.

John M. Porter, M.D.

1 Basic Considerations

A Prospective Study of Aspirin Use and Primary Prevention of Cardiovascular Disease in Women
Manson JE, Stampfer MJ, Colditz GA, Willett WC, Rosner B, Speizer FE, Hennekens CH (Harvard Med School; Harvard School of Public Health, Boston)
JAMA 266:521–527, 1991   1–1

Background.—Both men and women have shown clear benefit from aspirin therapy in a number of secondary prevention trials involving myocardial infarction, unstable angina, or stroke. However, statistical data in women has been insufficient to determine any sex differences in aspirin efficacy. Only 2 primary prevention trials have been performed, and both included men only. A prospective cohort study was done in women to investigate the association between regular aspirin use and the risk of first myocardial infarction and other cardiovascular events.

Methods.—The sample consisted of participants in the Nurse's Health Study who responded to a 1980 questionnaire. The 87,678 women in 11 states ranged in age from 34 to 65 years. Approximately 98% of the sample were white. Follow-up included 475,265 person-years, representing 96.7% of the total potential follow-up. The main outcome measures were myocardial infarction, stroke, cardiovascular death, and important vascular events.

Results.—A total of 40% of the women reported taking aspirin regularly. There were 240 nonfatal myocardial infarctions, 146 nonfatal strokes, and 130 deaths from cardiovascular disease. The age-adjusted relative risk (RR) of a first myocardial infarction was .68 (95% CI, .52 to .89) among women who took 1–6 aspirin per week compared with those who took no aspirin. An RR of .75 (95% CI, .58 to .99) was obtained after simultaneous adjustment for coronary disease risk factors. The age-adjusted RR was .61 (95% CI, .45 to .84) and the multivariate RR was .68 (95% CI, .5 to .93) among women aged 50 years and older. The risk of stroke appeared to be unaffected. For cardiovascular death and important vascular events, the multivariate RRs were .89 (95% CI, .59 to 1.33) and .85 (95% CI, .69 to 1.04), respectively. Very similar results were seen when subgroups of women taking 1–3 and 4–6 aspirin per week were examined separately; no reductions in risk were seen in those who took 7 or more aspirin per week. The main reasons for taking aspirin were headache, arthritis, and musculoskeletal pain.

Conclusion.—The risk of having a first myocardial infarction appears to be decreased in women who take 1-6 aspirin per week. Conclusive data must await a randomized trial in women. Aspirin should be considered for female patients only on the basis of clinical judgment, based on the patient's cardiovascular risk status, the side effects, and the possible benefits.

▶ One must be very careful in the interpretation of prevention trials, both in respect to the primary vs. secondary nature of the trial as well as the gender of the patient. Although secondary prevention trials have shown benefit in men and women, the only 2 primary prevention trials done before this one included men only. This study, which was based on a survey, indicates statistical benefit in the prevention of primary myocardial infarction in those women taking aspirin. In the absence of contraindications, I believe that all our vascular patients should be taking aspirin, probably at the low dose of one 60-mg tablet per day.—J.M. Porter, M.D.

Antiplatelet Therapy is Effective in the Prevention of Stroke or Death in Women: Subgroup Analysis of the European Stroke Prevention Study (ESPS)
Sivenius J, Riekkinen PJ, Kilpeläinen H, Laakso M, Penttilä I (Univ of Kuopio, Kuopio, Finland)
Acta Neurol Scand 84:286–290, 1991   1–2

Background.—Previous studies have indicated that antiplatelet therapy may be less effective in preventing vascular events and deaths in women than in men; however, the trials have included too few women to be certain of this outcome. The European Stroke Prevention Study is a multicenter trial designed to compare combined treatment with dipyridamole and aspirin with placebo in subjects who have a history of transient ischemic attack, reversible ischemic neurologic deficit, or atherothrombotic stroke.

End Points (Stroke or Death) by Sex and Treatment Group

	Intention-to-treat		Explanatory	
	Male	Female	Male	Female
DP-ASA	61/363	25/290	39/266	15/231
(%)	(16.8)	(8.6)	(14.7)	(6.5)
Placebo	90/354	50/300	61/274	31/243
(%)	(25.4)	(16.6)	(22.3)	(12.8)
End-point reduction (%)	34.9	47.3	39.6	46.4
Statistical significance	P=0.006	P=0.003	P=0.041	P=0.022

Abbreviation: DP-ASA, dipyridamole + aspirin.
(Courtesy of Sivenius J, Riekkinen PJ, Kilpeläinen H, et al: *Acta Neurol Scand* 84:286–290, 1991.)

Methods.—Dipyridamole was given in a dosage of 75 mg administered 3 times daily, and acetylsalicylic acid was given in a dosage of 333 mg given 3 times daily. A total of 45% of the 2,500 subjects were women.

Results.—Women had significantly fewer strokes and deaths than men (table). Compared with placebo recipients, women who received active treatment had nearly 50% fewer strokes and deaths, and men had almost 40% fewer end points. All analytic methods suggested a more marked reduction in end points in women after 2 years.

Conclusion.—Antiplatelet treatment appeared to be effective from the start of the European Stroke Prevention Study. Combined administration of aspirin and dipyridamole appears to be as effective in women as in men for preventing strokes and deaths from any cause.

▶ This important subgroup analysis of 1 center of the European Stroke Prevention Study clearly indicates that antiplatelet therapy is as effective in women as it is in men in the prevention of stroke or death. See also Abstract 1–1.—J.M. Porter, M.D.

Suppression of Thromboxane A$_2$ But Not of Systemic Prostacyclin by Controlled-Release Aspirin

Clarke RJ, Mayo G, Price P, FitzGerald GA (Vanderbilt Univ, Nashville)
N Engl J Med 325:1137–1141, 1991   1–3

Background.—Aspirin reduces the risk of death from unstable coronary artery disease, presumably through inhibiting the production of thromboxane A$_2$. Its efficacy, however, may be limited by inhibition of prostacyclin, which has effects on vascular tone and platelet function opposite those of thromboxane A$_2$. If the rate of drug delivery were below the hepatic threshold for extraction of aspirin, it might be possible to inhibit thromboxane A$_2$ production while limiting exposure of the systemic vascular endothelium to aspirin.

Methods.—A controlled-release preparation containing 75 mg of aspirin, releasing 10 mg per hour, was developed to inhibit platelet prostaglandin synthase activity in the prehepatic circulation. Its effects were compared with those of immediate-release aspirin (162.5 mg, followed by 75 mg daily of controlled-release aspirin for the next 4 days) in 45 normal male volunteers.

Results.—Serum levels of thromboxane B$_2$ were suppressed more rapidly with immediate-release aspirin but, during a month-long period, controlled-release aspirin suppressed thromboxane A$_2$ as effectively as intermediate-release aspirin (given in a dosage of either 162.5 mg daily or 325 mg given every other day) (Fig 1–1). All regimens increased bleeding time to a similar degree. Only immediate-release aspirin prevented the increase in prostacyclin metabolite induced by bradykinin.

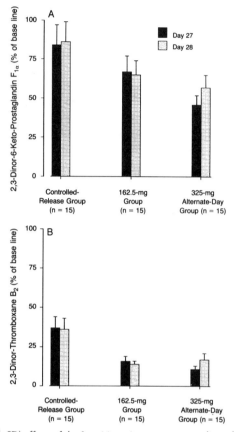

Fig 1–1.—Mean (± SD) effects of the 3 aspirin regimens on prostacyclin and thromboxane biosynthesis in the final 2 days of the dosing period. The levels of excretion of the metabolites of prostacyclin (**A**) and thromboxane (**B**) in aliquots of urine collected for 6 hours after dosing on days 27 and 28, respectively, are shown as a percentage of baseline values. Suppression of thromboxane A_2 and prostacyclin biosynthesis on day 27 was greater in the 325-mg alternate-day group (P < .05) than in either of the other groups. The difference between groups was no longer significant 24 hours after dosing, although prostacyclin remained below baseline levels in all groups. (Courtesy of Clarke, RJ, Mayo G, Price P, et al: *N Engl J Med* 325:1137–1141, 1991.)

Conclusion.—Controlled-release aspirin may allow controlled assessment of the clinical value of preserving the synthesis of prostacyclin during platelet inhibition.

▶ The search continues for a method of aspirin administration that will selectively inhibit thromboxane, but not prostacyclin, synthesis. This very-low-dose controlled-release aspirin product appears promising. Of course, any benefits from selective thromboxane inhibition remain to be proven.—J.M. Porter, M.D.

Aspirin-Induced Decline in Prostacyclin Production in Patients With Coronary Artery Disease Is Due to Decreased Endoperoxide Shift: Analysis of the Effects of a Combination of Aspirin and n-3 Fatty Acids on the Eicosanoid Profile

Force T, Milani R, Hibberd P, Lorenz R, Uedelhoven W, Leaf A, Weber P (Massachusetts Gen Hosp, Boston; Harvard Med School, Boston; Universitat Munchen, Munich)

Circulation 84:2286–2293, 1991   1–4

Introduction.—The effects of aspirin plus fish oil, which is rich in n-3 polyunsaturated fatty acids, on the eicosanoid profile of patients with coronary artery disease were studied. Whether aspirin-induced reduction in prostacyclin (PGI_2) production is the result of inhibition of endothelial cell cyclooxygenase or a reduced endoperoxide shift from the platelets, and whether aspirin negates the potentially beneficial effects of fish oil on the eicosanoid profile were determined.

Methods.—The study included 14 patients with clinically stable but advanced coronary artery disease; for 6 weeks, 8 patients were given 12 g and 6 were given 16 g of fish oil concentrate containing 6 or 8 g of n-3 fatty acids. The patients also received increasing daily doses of aspirin; each dose was taken for 2 weeks.

Results.—Serum thromboxane (TBX) B_2, which represents the production of TXA_2 by maximally stimulated platelets, was suppressed by 38% on fish oil only and by 97% or more on all aspirin doses. Excretion of PGI_2-M, the main urinary metabolite of PGI_2, decreased from a mean of 50 ng/g of creatinine to 42 ng/g on fish oil alone. The main urinary metabolite of PGI_3, PGI_3-M, increased from .2 ng/g of creatinine to 4.9 ng/g on fish oil alone. Excretion of PGI_3-M was unaffected by the addition of aspirin, even at higher doses.

Conclusion.—A moderate dose of aspirin taken once daily does not affect PGI_3 production, despite significant reductions in PGI_2 production. Endothelial cell cyclooxygenase may therefore be minimally inhibited by such doses and aspirin. Furthermore, a large percentage of the PGI_2 produced in patients with advanced coronary artery disease may derive from the transfer of prostaglandin endoperoxides from activated platelets to endothelial cells. These substrate losses explain the reduction in PGI_2 with moderate doses of aspirin. Therefore, aspirin-induced reductions in PGI_2 may largely be part of an unavoidable consequence of aspirin-induced platelet cyclooxygenase inhibition. Aspirin does not negate the potentially beneficial effects of n-3 fatty acids on the eicosanoid profile.

▶ This remarkable study indicates that the primary effect of low-dose aspirin in decreasing PGI_2 synthesis results from the decrease in the transfer of endoperoxide metabolites from activated platelets to the endothelial cells. If so, there may be no dose of aspirin that can differentiate between thromboxane and prostacyclin inhibition. See Abstract 1–3.—J.M. Porter, M.D.

Aspirin Use and Reduced Risk of Fatal Colon Cancer

Thun MJ, Namboodiri MM, Heath CW Jr (American Cancer Society, Atlanta)
N Engl J Med 325:1593–1596, 1991   1–5

Background.—There is growing evidence from animal and human epidemiologic studies indicating that nonsteroidal anti-inflammatory drugs (e.g., aspirin) may have a protective effect against colon cancer. Data from an ongoing prospective cancer mortality study were used to test this hypothesis.

Methods.—The analysis included data on 662,424 adults enrolled since 1982 in the American Cancer Society's Cancer Prevention Study II. The average age at enrollment was 57 years. The study sample included all white subjects who specified their frequency and duration of aspirin use at entry into the study. Mortality data were complete through 1988. Multivariate analysis was done on 598 patients and 3,058 matched controls to address the potential effects of other risk factors for colon cancer.

Results.—Deaths from colon cancer decreased with more frequent aspirin use among both men and women (table). For patients who took aspirin at least 16 times per month for at least 1 year, the relative risks were .60 for men and .58 for women. These risks were unchanged after exclusion of factors that might affect aspirin use and mortality, including arthritis, cancer, heart disease, and stroke at entry. Neither were the re-

Rates of Death From Colon Cancer

ASPIRIN USE (TIMES/MO)	NO. OF DEATHS	PERSON-YEARS AT RISK	AGE-ADJUSTED DEATH RATE PER 100,000	RELATIVE RISK (95% CI)*	P VALUE†
Men					
0	378	646,346	58.3	1.00	
<1	184	486,620	44.8	0.77 (0.61–0.97)	
1–15	127	389,083	40.5	0.69 (0.52–0.93)	0.0004
≥16	85	201,636	34.8	0.60 (0.40–0.89)	
Women					
0	284	705,064	40.8	1.00	
<1	157	671,927	29.8	0.73 (0.56–0.96)	
1–15	100	505,854	26.5	0.65 (0.46–0.93)	0.0022
≥16	73	265,424	23.5	0.58 (0.37–0.90)	

Note: According to frequency of aspirin use, in the cohort before patients with illness at enrollment were excluded.
* In the analysis of risk, the groups with no aspirin use were the referent category. CI denotes confidence interval.
† P values indicate the trend across categories of aspirin use.
(Courtesy of Thun MJ, Namboodiri MM, Heath CW Jr: N Engl J Med 325:1593–1596, 1991.)

sults significantly affected by adjustment for diet, obesity, physical activity, or family history. Acetaminophen use had no significant effect on risk.

Conclusion.—Frequent use of low doses of aspirin might reduce the risk of fatal colon cancer. No conclusions can be drawn as to the mechanism of this effect—whether direct, such as by inhibition of prostaglandin synthesis, or indirect, such as by inducing bleeding in subjects with polyps or early cancer leading to early diagnosis. Controlled trials in high-risk patients may be useful.

▶ The prospective data presented in this study indicate that regular use of low-dose aspirin may decrease the risk of fatal colon cancer. Although additional controlled trials will be required to confirm the apparent association, these results are encouraging. There appears to be an increasing number of reasons to maintain our elderly vascular surgery patients with daily doses of aspirin.—J. M. Porter, M.D.

Effects of Calcitonin Gene-Related Peptide on Normal and Atheromatous Vessels and on Resistance Vessels in the Coronary Circulation in Humans
Ludman PF, Maseri A, Clark P, Davies GJ (Hammersmith Hosp, London)
Circulation 84:1993–2000, 1991   1–6

Background.—Calcitonin gene-related peptide (CGRP) is a potent dilator of normal epicardial coronary arteries in humans, but its effects on myocardial blood flow and atheromatous coronary artery diameter are unknown. The effects of CGRP on coronary circulation in humans were investigated.

Methods.—The study included 15 men and 1 woman (age, 41–70 years) who were undergoing routine coronary arteriography to investigate chest pain. In the first 7 patients, 3 of whom had normal coronary arteries, the diameter of the left anterior descending artery (LAD) at an angiographically normal site, coronary sinus oxygen saturation (CSO_2S), systemic blood pressure, and heart rate were measured during intracoronary infusion of increasing concentrations of CGRP, and during subsequent intracoronary infusions of adenosine and glyceryl trinitrate (GTN). In 13 patients with atheromatous coronary artery disease (CAD), the effects of a single dose of intracoronary CGRP followed by intracoronary GTN infusion were measured at angiographically normal sites, stenoses, angiographically normal sites immediately adjacent to stenoses, and at sites of coronary artery wall irregularity.

Results.—In the first 7 patients, CGRP dilated the normal LAD segment by a mean of 22.6%, with only a small increase in mean CSO_2S, from 40.1% to 47.3%. Adenosine caused no further increase in LAD diameter, but it caused the mean level of CSO_2S to increase further to

76%. Subsequent GTN infusion did not further increase the LAD diameter. Because the heart rate-blood pressure product remained unchanged throughout the study, the increase in CSO_2S represented only a small increase in myocardial blood flow after infusion of CGRP. In the 13 patients with atheromatous CAD, infusion of CGRP dilated the LAD by a mean of 17% at angiographically normal sites, 15.3% at stenoses, 7.6% at angiographically normal sites adjacent to stenoses, and 15.9% at sites of coronary artery wall irregularity. Subsequent GTN infusion did not result in significant further dilatation at any of these sites.

Conclusion.—In humans at rest, CGRP has little effect on coronary resistance vessels in the nonischemic myocardium, but it causes marked dilatation of normal arteries and variable dilatation of atheromatous epicardial arteries.

▶ We have been inundated in recent years with reports of the discovery of numerous vasoactive agents, all of which appear to have important roles in vascular homeostasis. Some of these agents include thromboxane, prostacyclin, endothelial-derived relaxing factor, endothelin and, now, calcitonin gene-related peptide. The latter appears to be a potent dilator of normal epicardial vessels in humans. Definitive information is eagerly awaited.—J.M. Porter, M.D.

Splanchnic and Cerebral Vasodilatory Effects of Calcitonin Gene-Related Peptide I in Humans
Mulholland MW, Sarpa MS, Delvalle J, Messina LM (Univ of Michigan, Ann Arbor)
Ann Surg 214:440–446, 1991   1–7

Background.—Calcitonin gene-related peptide (CGRP) is distributed widely in neuronal tissues, particularly the perivascular peripheral nerves, and it is closely associated with cerebral and splanchnic vessels in a num-

Percentage Increase Over Baseline in Carotid Artery
Parameters During Infusion of CGRP at 8 ng/min
Per km

Parameter	% of Basal Value
Peak systolic velocity	139 ± 13
End diastolic velocity	156 ± 18
Mean velocity	140 ± 10
Volume flow	135 ± 15

Note: For each parameter $P < .05$ vs. control, and $P < .05$ vs. 2 ng/kg/min.
(Courtesy of Mulholland MW, Sarpa MS, Delvalle J, et al: *Ann Surg* 214:440–446, 1991.)

ber of species. Early reports have suggested that the peptide may be a vasodilator in humans.

Methods.—Duplex ultrasonography was used to assess the effects of synthetic human CGRP I on regional arterial flow in 8 healthy young men. The peptide was infused via a forearm vein at rates of 2, 4, and 8 ng/kg/min for 30-minute periods; vasoactivity was studied in the splanchnic, cerebral, and extremity arterial beds.

Results.—When CGRP was infused at a rate of 2ng/kg/min, the calculated volume flow increased by 140% of the baseline in the superior mesenteric artery. Carotid arterial volume flow increased in a dose-dependent manner (table). The flow at both sites remained significantly increased for 30 minutes after the end of steady-state peptide infusion. Although the pulse increased in a dose-dependent manner, but blood pressure did not change. Arterial diameter did not change when CGRP was infused.

Conclusion.—It appears that CGRP-I is a potent arterial vasodilator, which may be useful in the treatment of a variety of conditions characterized by arterial vasoconstrictions.

▶ Calcitonin gene-related peptide appears to be a potent vasodilator of peripheral arteries as well as coronary arteries. The potential usefulness of this compound in the treatment of a variety of vasospastic conditions is intriguing. See the comments after Abstract 1–6.—J.M. Porter, M.D.

Circadian Variation in Vascular Tone and its Relation to α-Sympathetic Vasoconstrictor Activity
Panza JA, Epstein SE, Quyyumi AA (Natl Heart, Lung, and Blood Inst, Bethesda, Md)
N Engl J Med 325:986–990, 1991   1–8

Background.—Studies in both dogs and patients with variant angina suggest that circadian rhythms can affect coronary arterial vasoconstrictor tone. The vasoconstrictor actions are more evident in the morning than at any other time of the day.

Methods.—Blood flow and vascular resistance were measured at baseline and after administration of the vasodilator sodium nitroprusside and the α-adrenergic antagonist phentolamine in 12 normal subjects. The studies were carried out at 7 AM, 2 PM, and 9 PM. The drugs were infused into the brachial artery, and responses were recorded by strain-gauge plethysmography.

Results.—Baseline forearm vascular resistance was significantly higher in the morning than in the afternoon or evening, and blood flow was significantly lower (Fig 1–2). The vasodilator effect of phentolamine also was significantly greater in the morning (Fig 1–3), eliminating the circa-

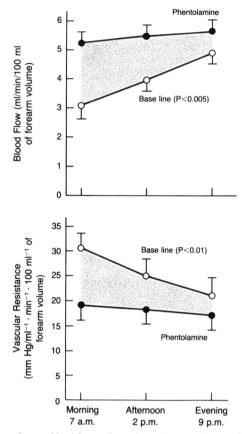

Fig 1–2.—The mean forearm blood flow and vascular resistance at 3 times of day in 12 healthy subjects. Values shown were obtained at baseline (*open circles*) and after α-sympathetic blockade with the infusion of phentolamine (*filled circles*). The *stippled areas* indicate the vascular tone contributed by α-sympathetic vasoconstrictor forces. The P values refer to the slope of the curve and were obtained by analysis of variance. The *vertical bars* indicate standard errors. (Courtesy of Panza JA, Epstein SE, Quyyumi AA: *N Engl J Med* 325:986–990, 1991.)

dian variation in vascular resistance and blood flow. The vasodilatory responses to sodium nitroprusside were similar at all times of the day.

Conclusion.—The circadian rhythm in vascular tone is caused at least in part by increased α-sympathetic vasoconstrictor activity in the morning. This may contribute to the higher blood pressure and greater prevalence of cardiovascular events occurring at this time of the day.

▶ Circadian rhythms may eventually prove to have a dominant effect on human physiology. In this study, the increased forearm resistance seen in the morning hours brings to mind the observation that most myocardial infarctions occur in the morning hours. The probable relationship of melatonin to such circadian variations in vascular tone must be considered.—J.M. Porter, M.D.

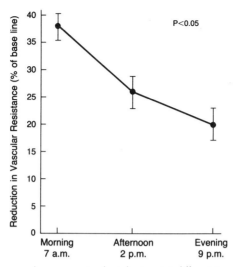

Fig 1–3.—The mean vascular response to phentolamine at 3 different times of day in 12 healthy subjects. The P value refers to the slope of the curve and was obtained by analysis of variance. The *vertical bars* indicate standard errors. (Courtesy of Panza JA, Epstein SE, Quyyumi AA: N *Engl J Med* 325:986–990, 1991.)

Effects of Sympathetic Nerves on Collateral Vessels in the Limb of Atherosclerotic Primates

Lopez JAG, Piegors DJ, Armstrong ML, Heistad D (VA Med Ctr, Iowa City; Univ of Iowa)
Atherosclerosis 90:183–188, 1991   1–9

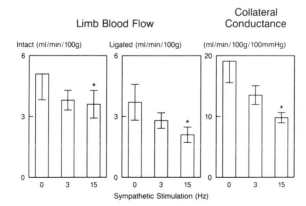

Fig 1–4.—Blood flow and collateral conductance in 7 normal monkeys. The values are mean ± SE under control conditions and during sympathetic stimulation. *Asterisk* indicates P < .05. (Courtesy of Lopez JAG, Piegors DJ, Armstrong ML, et al: *Atheroscleorosis* 90:183–188, 1991.)

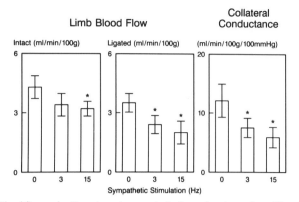

Fig 1-5.—Blood flow and collateral conductance in 8 atherosclerotic monkeys. The values are mean ± SE under control conditions and during sympathetic stimulation. *Asterisk* indicates $P < .05$. (Courtesy of Lopez JAG, Piegors DJ, Armstrong ML, et al: *Atherosclerosis* 90:183–188, 1991.)

Introduction.—Whether the collateral vessels of normal and atherosclerotic monkeys have a sympathetic innervation, and whether they are responsive to sympathetic nerve stimulation were determined.

Methods.—For a mean of almost 20 months, experimental cynomolgus monkeys were fed a diet containing 1 mg of cholesterol per calorie and 43% of total calories as fat. The left common iliac artery was ligated close to the bifurcation, and the collateral flow was measured approximately 13 months later using the labeled microsphere technique. The peripheral end of the cut lumbar sympathetic chain was stimulated electrically.

Results.—Histofluorescence microscopy demonstrated a plexus of noradrenergic nerves in the adventitia of the collateral vessels. Conductance of the collateral vessels was reduced during sympathetic stimulation in normal animals and also in those animals with atherosclerosis (Figs 1–4 and 1–5).

Conclusion.—The collateral vessels of the monkey extremity have a sympathetic innervation, and sympathetic stimulation leads to prolonged constriction in both normal and atherosclerotic animals. The value of collateral vessels for maintaining blood flow after atherothrombotic occlusion may be impaired by increased sympathetic nerve activity.

▶ Do thin-walled, dilated, arterial collaterals possess the potential for sympathetically induced vasoconstriction and, by implication, for drug-mediated vasorelaxation? Many of us have presumed that thin-walled collaterals do not have the potential for meaningful vasoconstriction, and that vasodilator drugs accordingly have no role in the treatment of patients with extremity blood flow maintained through collaterals. This study indicates that we may have to reassess this point of view.—J.M. Porter, M.D.

Muscle Carnitine Deficiency in Patients With Severe Peripheral Vascular Disease

Brevetti G, Angelini C, Rosa M, Carrozzo R, Perna S, Corsi M, Matarazzo A, Marcialis A (Univ of Naples; Univ of Padua, Italy)

Circulation 84:1490–1495, 1991   1–10

Introduction.—Carnitine is a quaternary amine that helps regulate substrate flux and energy balance across the cell membranes. It functions as a co-factor for the transformation of long-chain fatty acids into acylcarnitine derivatives. Ischemia may lead to carnitine deficiency. Supplemental carnitine after coronary ischemia has improved myocardial function and walking ability in patients with peripheral arterial insufficiency.

Methods.—Nine biopsy specimens of ischemic muscle were obtained from 5 patients undergoing reconstructive vascular surgery. The total and free carnitine levels were estimated in these samples and in biopsy specimens obtained from 35 normal individuals.

Results.—Total carnitine levels were significantly reduced in ischemic muscle. Both free carnitine and the acylcarnitine content were significantly reduced (table). Carnintine acetyltransferase activity also was reduced in ischemic muscle, but carnitine palmitoyltransferase activity was unaffected. Treatment with L-propionylcarnitine restored normal levels of carnitine and its esters in 4 patients, but it did not alter enzyme activities.

Conclusion.—These findings warrant clinical trials evaluating L-propionylcarnitine as a treatment for patients with peripheral vascular disease.

▶ This important study from Naples documents a reduced level of total carnitine and carnitine acetyltransferase activity in ischemic skeletal muscle

Muscle Levels of Carnitine and Its Fractions in Normal Persons and Patients With Peripheral Vascular Disease

	Normal subjects		PVD patients	
	Untreated	Treated	Untreated	Treated
Total carnitine	20.9±5.2	18.0±5.0	11.6±6.2*	20.4±5.7‡
Free carnitine	16.3±4.8	13.3±2.0	9.2±5.4*	15.4±2.5‡
Short-chain acylcarnitines	3.4±1.6	4.1±2.0	2.0±1.6†	4.3±3.2
Long-chain acylcarnitines	0.9±0.6	0.6±0.4	0.4±0.2†	0.7±0.2

Note: Values are expressed in nanomoles per milligram of noncollagen protein.
Abbreviation: PVD, peripheral vascular disease.
* Significantly lower than untreated normal subjects ($P < .01$).
† Significantly lower than untreated normal persons ($P < .05$).
‡ Significantly higher than untreated patients with PVD ($P < .05$).
(Courtesy of Brevetti G, Angelini C, Rosa M, et al: *Circulation* 84:1490–1495, 1991.)

specimens obtained from patients undergoing revascularization surgery; it also documents their restoration after intravenous L-propionylcarnitine infusion. Although the numbers are small, this study provides the necessary metabolic underpinning to support the authors' previous clinical observation that carnitine improved walking distance in a controlled claudication trial (1). Carnitine supplementation may well have a role in the pharmacologic management of ischemic syndromes, but confirmatory documentation by other investigators remains to be obtained. Carnitine and its derivatives appear to be the most exciting prospect for new drug development in the treatment of claudication.—R. Dalman, M.D.

Reference

1. Brevetti G, et al: *Circulation* 77:767, 1988.

Effects of Routine Heparin Therapy on Plasma Aldosterone Concentration

Kageyama Y, Suzuki H, Saruta T (Tochigi Natl Hosp, Utsunomiya, Japan; Keio Univ, Tokyo)
Acta Endocrinol (Copenh) 124:267–270, 1991   1–11

Background.—Recent studies have shown that heparin decreases aldosterone production both in humans and in experimental animals; however, the mechanism(s) by which heparin decreases aldosterone production remains controversial. The effect of routine heparin therapy on aldosterone production was determined, and the mechanism of this effect was examined.

Methods.—Six men and 3 women (mean age, 68 years) were treated with heparin for thromboembolic diseases. An initial loading dose of 500 units was given as a bolus injection, followed by 700–1,000 units/hr, given intravenously for 7 to 10 days. The infusion was adjusted to maintain activated partial thromboplastin times at less than 60 seconds. Changes in plasma aldosterone, plasma renin activity, plasma cortisol, sodium, and potassium concentrations were studied. In addition, 5 patients received ACTH and had a low sodium intake during and for 2 weeks after heparin therapy.

Results.—During heparin therapy, plasma aldosterone decreased from 239 to 114 pmol/L. Two weeks after heparin was discontinued, the aldosterone returned to basal levels. Minimal increases in plasma aldosterone were seen in response to low sodium intake, despite an increase in plasma renin activity. The increases were 124% during heparin therapy and 148% 2 weeks thereafter. Plasma aldosterone responses to ACTH were similar during and after heparin therapy, increasing by 190% and 193%, respectively. Serum sodium and potassium were unchanged, despite heparin administration.

Conclusion.—Heparin probably decreases plasma aldosterone by attenuation of angiotensin II-induced aldosterone production. The potential of heparin to produce hyperkalemia is probably of clinical significance in patients with compromised renal potassium excretions. When administering heparin to these patients, the electrolyte balance should be followed carefully.

▶ I was unaware that heparin decreases the plasma aldosterone concentration and attenuates the low sodium-induced increase in plasma aldosterone. These results indicate that heparin may potentiate hyperkalemia in patients with compromised renal potassium excretion. This is another effect of heparin that vascular surgeons must consider.—J.M. Porter, M.D.

Usefulness of Antiplatelet Drugs in the Management of Heparin-Associated Thrombocytopenia and Thrombosis
Gruel Y, Lermusiaux P, Lang M, Darnige L, Rupin A, Delahousse B, Guilmot J-L, Leroy J (Centre Hospitalier Universitaire, Tours, France)
Ann Vasc Surg 5:552–555, 1991   1–12

Background.—Systemic heparin treatment may be complicated by thrombocytopenia and thrombosis. Heparin generally is withdrawn, but some patients who require emergency cardiac or vascular surgery may be reexposed to heparin.

Patients.—Two such patients were treated with antiplatelet drugs during vascular procedures. The combination of Iloprost, a stable prostacyclin analogue, with aspirin and dipyridamole inhibited heparin-induced platelet aggregation in vitro and was administered at operation. The patients underwent surgery with full heparinization and did not have thrombocytopenia. Neither of them had thrombotic or hemorrhagic complications. One of the patients had occlusions of the common and external iliac arteries, which necessitated bypass surgery; the other had thrombus removed from both common iliac arteries and the abdominal aorta.

Conclusion.—Patients who have thrombocytopenia and thrombosis in relation to heparin treatment can safely receive heparin during subsequent surgery as long as antiplatelet therapy also is provided.

▶ The harder you look for heparin-associated thrombocytopenia and thrombosis (HAT), the more you find. If a patient with HAT must be reexposed to heparin, antiplatelet drugs—including Iloprost—appear to convey significant protection (1).—J.M. Porter, M.D.

Reference

1. Kappa JR, et al: *J Vasc Surg* 5:693, 1987.

Coagulation Factors X, Xa, and Protein S as Potent Mitogens of Cultured Aortic Smooth Muscle Cells

Gasic GP, Arenas CP, Gasic TB, Gasic GJ (Salk Inst, La Jolla, Calif; Pennsylvania Hosp, Philadelphia)

Proc Natl Acad Sci USA 89:2317–2320, 1992   1–13

Introduction.—Smooth-muscle cells of the rat carotid artery begin to proliferate after injury from a balloon catheter. The mechanisms involved in this angiogenic response are uncertain. Platelet-derived growth factor (PDGF) is a potent mitogen for smooth-muscle cells and is released from damaged endothelium, macrophages, and activated platelets; however, it cannot be the sole cause of the proliferative response.

Methods.—Using cultures of smooth-muscle cells from rat aorta, several proteins participating in coagulation were examined to identify smooth-muscle cell growth factors other than PDGF.

Results.—Factors X, Xa, and protein S promoted mitosis in cultured aortic smooth-muscle cells at nanomolar concentrations. Factor IX was only weakly mitogenic, and factor VII and protein C had no stimulatory effect. Protein S stimulated DNA synthesis in culture cells in a temporal pattern resembling that seen with PDGF. Specific inhibitors of factor Xa suppressed mitogenesis in response to factor Xa and protein S.

Conclusion.—Coagulation factors that have mitogenic activity may contribute to the proliferation of intimal smooth-muscle cells after vascular injury, whether caused by angioplasty or atherogenic disease.

▶ The number and complexity of factors putatively affecting arterial smooth muscle proliferation continue to increase. If coagulation factors prove important in smooth muscle cell proliferation, the therapeutic use of selected coagulation inhibitors may be a means of preventing restenosis after intervention.—J.M. Porter, M.D.

Intravenous Recombinant Soluble Human Thrombomodulin Prevents Venous Thrombosis in a Rat Model

Solis MM, Cook C, Cook J, Glaser C, Light D, Morser J, Yu S, Fink L, Eidt JF (Univ of Arkansas for Med Sciences; John L McClellan VA Med Ctr, Little Rock; Berlex Biosciences Inc, South San Francisco)

J Vasc Surg 14:599–604, 1991   1–14

Background.—Thrombomodulin is a thrombin receptor on the endothelial cell surface. Bound thrombin loses its procoagulant activity, including the ability to activate platelets, and it becomes able to activate protein C, an endogenous anticoagulant. Recombinant thrombomodulin might be an effective antithrombotic agent because of its ability to convert the procoagulant properties of thrombin into the anticoagulant effects of protein C.

Methods.—A recombinant thrombomodulin analog was compared with sodium heparin and with hirudin (a leech salivary anticoagulant) in rats having thrombosis induced mechanically in the inferior vena cava.

Results.—Thrombus was consistently present in rats given saline, but it was absent in those given recombinant thrombomodulin. Heparin was comparably effective, and 1 of 6 animals given hirudin had thrombosis develop. Bleeding time was approximately doubled in thrombomodulin-treated animals compared with controls. The activated partial thromboplastin time was only slightly longer than in control rats, whereas it was markedly prolonged in rats given heparin or hirudin.

Conclusion.—Recombinant thrombomodulin inhibited venous thrombosis in this rat-model study. Standard hemostatic parameters were only minimally altered, but it remains to be seen whether hemorrhagic side effects can be prevented by using thrombomodulin rather than standard heparin or other anticoagulants.

▶ We are faced with an explosion of new anticoagulant, antithrombotic, and antiplatelet products, many of which appear to have real promise in clinical practice. We shall await with interest more information on recombinant soluble human thrombomodulin.—J.M. Porter, M.D.

New RGD Analogue Inhibits Human Platelet Adhesion and Aggregation and Eliminates Platelet Deposition on Canine Vascular Grafts

Rubin BG, McGraw DJ, Sicard GA, Santoro SA (Washington Univ, St Louis)
J Vasc Surg 15:683–692, 1992   1–15

Background.—Platelet adhesion and aggregation are mediated by fibrinogen via the receptor glycoprotein IIb/IIIa, which recognizes the arginine-glycine-aspartic (RGD) amino acid sequence. A stable RGD analogue, 8-guanidino-octanoyl-Asp-Phe (SC-49992), was studied to determine its ability to inhibit the function of human platelets and counter platelet deposition on prosthetic grafts.

Methods.—In vitro studies involved the aggregation of human platelets by ADP, with and without exposure to SC-49992. Polytetrafluoroethylene grafts were placed in the femoral artery of thrombosis-prone dogs, which received the RGD analogue or normal saline by infusion during the graft procedure. A contralateral graft was placed a week later in a crossover design.

In Vitro Findings.—Adenosine diphosphate-induced platelet aggregation was inhibited by SC-49992 in a concentration-dependent manner. Adenosine diphosphate-induced secretion also was reduced; however, thrombin-induced secretion, which is independent of fibrinogen binding, was unaltered. Activation-dependent platelet adhesion to fibrinogen substrates was reduced by the analogue, which also eluted glycoprotein IIb/IIIa bound to RGD-derivatized sepharose.

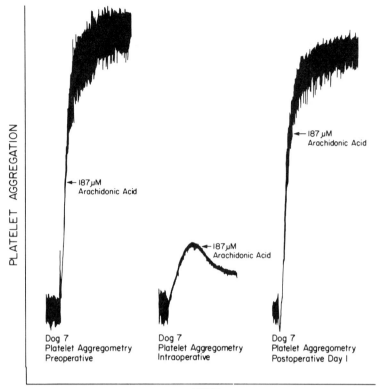

Fig 1–6.—Aggregometry tracings of 1 dog. Preoperative aggregometry demonstrates prompt irreversible aggregation to arachidonic acid. Intraoperative aggregometry during infusion of RGD analogue demonstrates reduced and reversible aggregation to same agonist. Twelve hours after termination of the SC-49992 infusion, full arachidonic acid-induced aggregation is seen. (Courtesy of Rubin BG, McGraw DJ, Sicard GA, et al: *J Vasc Surg* 15:683-692, 1992.)

In Vivo Findings.—Infusion of the RGD analogue in dogs inhibited induced platelet aggregation (Fig 1-6); saline had no such effect. Platelet deposition on the grafts was reduced by more than 90%, and this was confirmed histologically.

Conclusion.—It is possible that RGD inhibition can benefit patients with a wide range of platelet-mediated thromboembolic disorders.

▶ These stable platelet receptor analogues may ultimately prove to be potent and effective antiplatelet drugs. Before this occurs, however, their toxicity in humans must be carefully assessed.—J.M. Porter, M.D.

Predictors of Thromboembolism in Atrial Fibrillation: I. Clinical Features of Patients at Risk

Pearce LA, for the Stroke Prevention in Atrial Fibrillation Investigators (Statistics & Epidemiology Research Corp, Seattle, Wash)
Ann Intern Med 116:1–5, 1992   1–16

Objective.—The development of thromboembolism was examined in 568 patients with atrial fibrillation of nonrheumatic origin, all of whom were assigned to receive placebo when participating in the Stroke Prevention in Atrial Fibrillation Study. The mean follow-up was 1.3 years.

Findings.—The factors significantly (and independently) associated with a greater than 7% annual risk of thromboembolism included congestive heart failure in the past 3 months, a history of hypertension, and previous arterial thromboembolism (Table 1). The risk of thromboembolism correlated well with the number of risk factors present (Table 2). Patients who were nondiabetic and lacking risk factors had a low risk of having thromboembolism, and no thromboembolic events occurred in patients without risk factors who were younger than 60 years of age.

Conclusion.—Simple clinical variables can accurately indicate which patients with nonrheumatic atrial fibrillation are most likely to have thromboembolic complications.

▶ In the past year, there has been a tremendous amount of interest in attempting to determine precisely which atrial fibrillation patients are at highest risk for thromboembolism, and which are most likely to benefit from anticoagulation. These authors conclude that a recent history of congestive heart failure, hypertension, or previous arterial thromboembolism greatly increases the risk of thromboembolism, and that a combination of these factors increases the risk additively. This information will doubtless be of considerable importance in the optimal selection of patients for long-term anticoagulant therapy.—J.M. Porter, M.D.

TABLE 1.—Multivariate Analyses of Prospectively Selected
Features and Thromboembolism

Variable	Relative Risk	95% CI	*P* Value
Age*	1.2	0.9 to 1.6	> 0.2
History of hypertension	2.2	1.1 to 4.3	0.02
Previous thromboembolism	2.1	1.0 to 4.2	0.04
Recent congestive heart failure	2.6	1.2 to 5.4	0.01

* Risk by decade; age forced into the Cox proportional hazards model.
(Courtesy of Pearce LA, for the Stroke Prevention in Atrial Fibrillation Investigators: *Ann Intern Med* 116:1–5, 1992.)

TABLE 2.—Event Rates by Clinical Risk Factors

Clinical Risk Group	Number of Patients	Number of Events	Thrombo-embolism Rate (% per year)	95% CI†
No risk factors	241	8	2.5	1.3 to 5.0
One risk factor	259	24	7.2	4.8 to 10.8
Two or three risk factors	68	14	17.6	10.5 to 29.9

Note: The risk factors are a history of hypertension, recent congestive heart failure, and previous thromboembolism.
† Poisson regression.
(Courtesy of Pearce LA, for the Stroke Prevention in Atrial Fibrillation Investigators: *Ann Intern Med* 116:1–5, 1992.)

Predictors of Thromboembolism in Atrial Fibrillation: II. Echocardiographic Features of Patients at Risk
Pearce LA, for the Stroke Prevention in Atrial Fibrillation Investigators (Statistics and Epidemiology Research Corp, Seattle, Wash)
Ann Intern Med 116:6–12, 1992   1–17

Background.—Patients younger than 60 years of age with "lone" atrial fibrillation are at low risk of thromboembolism; however, for those patients with atrial fibrillation who have a history of hypertension, previous thromboembolism, or recent congestive heart failure, the risk exceeds 7% per year.

Methods.—The echocardiographic findings predictive of thromboembolism were sought in 568 patients enrolled in the Stroke Prevention in Atrial Fibrillation Study who were assigned to receive placebo. Both M-mode and 2-dimensional echocardiograms were acquired.

Results.—The strongest independent predictors of later thromboembolism were a 2-D echocardiographic finding of left ventricular dysfunction and the size of the left atrium on M-mode studies. When the clinical risk factors were taken into account, left ventricular dysfunction of moderate to severe degree had added predictive value. Left atrial enlargement aided risk stratification (table). Fully 38% of the patients who were classified as low risk by clinical variables alone were found to be at higher risk after echocardiography.

Conclusion.—Echocardiography is of value in assessing the risk of thromboembolism in patients with atrial fibrillation, and in identifying those patients who may require antithrombotic prophylaxis.

▶ It is clear that young patients with atrial fibrillation and no risk factors have a very low annual percentage for arterial thromboembolism, whereas pa-

Risk Stratification Using Clinical and
Echocardiographic Predictors

Predictor	Number	Percent of Cohort	Thrombo-embolism Rate (% per year)	95% CI
Clinical predictors alone*				
No risk factors	241	42	2.5	1.3 to 5.0
1 risk factor	259	46	7.2	4.8 to 10.8
≥ 2 risk factors	68	12	17.6	10.5 to 29.9
Clinical plus echo-cardiographic predictors†				
No risk factors	147	26	1.0	0.2 to 4.0
1 or 2 risk factors	336	60	6.0	4.1 to 8.8
≥ 3 risk factors	78	14	18.6	11.6 to 30.1

Note: The independent clinical risk factors are a history of hypertension, recent congestive heart failure, and previous thromboembolism.

† Independent echocardiographic predictors are global left ventricular dysfunction and left atrial size > 2.5 cm/m² by M-mode echocardiography. The analysis excludes 7 patients in whom neither echocardiographic variable was available.

(Courtesy of Pearce LA, for the Stroke Prevention in Atrial Fibrillation Investigators: *Ann Intern Med* 116:6–12, 1992.)

tients with a history of hypertension, recent congestive heart failure, or previous thromboembolism may have as great as a 7% yearly risk for arterial thromboembolism. This study indicates that both left ventricular dysfunction and left atrial enlargement are independent echocardiographic predictors of increased embolism risk. Those patients in the high-risk group probably warrant prophylactic anticoagulation (1).—J.M. Porter, M.D.

Reference

1. Stroke Prevention in Atrial Fibrillation Investigators: *Circulation* 84:527, 1991.

Anastomotic Intimal Hyperplasia: Mechanical Injury or Flow Induced
Bassiouny HS, White S, Glagov S, Choi E, Giddens DP, Zarins CK (Univ of Chicago; Georgia Inst of Technology, Atlanta)
J Vasc Surg 15:708–717, 1992   1–18

Introduction. —Intimal thickening is a normal part of the arterial healing response at sites of graft anastomosis. Its progression to a hyperplastic, occluding lesion at distal end-to-side anastomosis is a major cause of bypass graft failure. The localization of anastomotic intimal thickening in relation to biomechanical and hemodynamic factors was investigated in dogs.

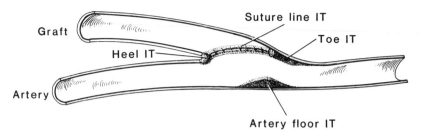

Fig 1–7.—Illustration of sagittal section of end-to-side anastomosis depicts sites of localization of intimal thickening at suture line and artery floor. (Courtesy of Bassiouny HS, White S, Glagov S, et al: *J Vasc Surg* 15:708–717, 1992.)

Methods.—Bilateral iliofemoral saphenous vein and polytetrafluoroethylene (PTFE) grafts were placed in 13 dogs, using a standardized geometry for the distal end-to-side anastomoses. Animals with patent grafts were killed after 8 weeks and the anastomoses were fixed by perfusion to identify regions of intimal thickening and quantify them by oculomicrometry. Transparent silicone models were made from castings of some distal anastomoses, and flow was visualized using helium-neon laser-illuminated particles under conditions simulating pulsatile flow.

Results.—Intimal thickening was seen at the suture line, especially in PTFE anastomoses, as well as on the arterial floor (Fig 1–7). Using the flow model, a point of stagnant flow was seen along the arterial floor, producing an area of low and oscillating shear at which intimal thickening developed. At the hood of the graft, where intimal thickening did not develop, there was high shear and the particle residence time was brief.

Conclusion.—There appears to be at least 2 different types of anastomotic intimal thickening. At the suture line, this change represents vascular healing; the fact that it is more prominent in prosthetic grafts may reflect a mismatch of compliance. Intimal thickening on the arterial floor develops in areas of oscillating flow and low shear, and it is unrelated to the type of graft.

▶ Using innovative modeling techniques and flow visualization studies, these authors conclude that all anastomotic intimal thickening may not be the same. The entire field of fibrointimal hyperplasia becomes more and more complex.—J.M. Porter, M.D.

Inhibition of Cellular Proliferation After Experimental Balloon Angioplasty by Low-Molecular-Weight Heparin

Hanke H, Oberhoff M, Hanke S, Hassenstein S, Kamenz J, Schmid KM, Betz E, Karsch KR (Univ of Tübingen, Germany)

Circulation 85:1548–1556, 1992   1–19

Introduction.—Proliferative changes induced by balloon angioplasty are an important factor in restenosis after successful coronary angioplasty. The effects of low-molecular-weight heparin (LMWH) on cellular proliferation after balloon angioplasty were investigated in rabbits.

Methods.—Intimal fibromuscular plaque formation was induced by electrical stimulation in the carotid artery, and LMWH (3.9 kd, 400 anti-Xa units/kg/day) was given for the next week. Other animals underwent angioplasty without LMWH. Bromodeoxyuridine was administered before the vessels were excised, 3–28 days after angioplasty.

Results.—Intimal thickness increased much less in LMWH-treated animals than in control animals. Immunohistologic study showed a significant increase in the cells undergoing DNA synthesis in control animals and a substantially lesser increase in the heparin-treated animals. The difference was significant 3 and 7 days after angioplasty, but not at 2 weeks.

Conclusion.—Intimal proliferation after balloon angioplasty can be suppressed by early administration of LMWH.

▶ Heparin continues to be one of the most exciting agents available for inhibition of cellular proliferation in intimal thickening after vascular injury, an observation which was first made by a vascular surgeon (1). This study indicates that LMWH has retained the activity of the parent compound. See also Abstract 1–24.—J.M. Porter, M.D.

Reference

1. Clowes AW, Karnowsky MJ: *Nature* 265:625, 1977.

Effects of Angiotensin Converting Enzyme Inhibition With Cilazapril on Intimal Hyperplasia in Injured Arteries and Vascular Grafts in the Baboon

Hanson SR, Powell JS, Dodson T, Lumsden A, Kelly AB, Anderson JS, Clowes AW, Harker LA (Emory Univ, Atlanta; F Hoffmann-La Roche Ltd, Basel, Switzerland; Univ of Washington, Seattle)
Hypertension 18(suppl II):70–76, 1991   1–20

Introduction.—Restenosis resulting from smooth muscle cell proliferation is an important complication of interventional procedures done to improve blood flow in patients with symptomatic atherosclerotic vascular disease. Previous attempts to reduce intimal thickening with drug therapy have had limited success. It was recently reported that inhibition of angiotensin converting enzyme (ACE) activity using the oral ACE inhibitor cilazapril significantly reduced the intimal proliferative response to carotid artery balloon catheter injury in the rat. The effects of cilazapril were examined in a primate model of arterial injury.

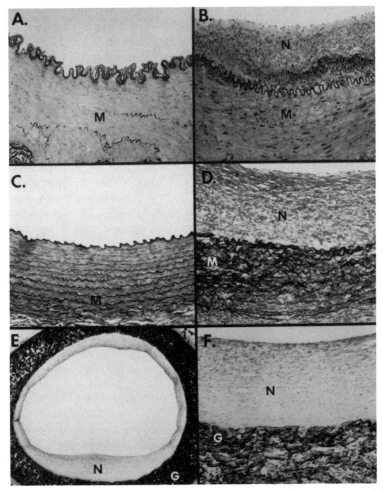

Fig 1–8.—Histological cross sections of arterial injury sites from untreated animals. Uninjured (control) femoral artery (**A**) is compared with balloon catheter-injured vessel (**B**) showing significant intimal thickening after 3 months. Epoxy resin-embedded sections stained with toluidine blue and basic fuchsin. Uninjured carotid artery (**C**) and vessel taken 3 months after carotid endarterectomy (**D**). Paraffin embedding and elastic stain (Verhoeff-van Gieson). Whole graft cross section showing typical eccentric lesion (**E**) and neointima overlying graft matrix (**F**). Paraffin embedding with hematoxylin and eosin stain. *Abbreviations:* M, media; N, neointima; G, graft matrix. (Courtesy of Hanson SR, Powell JS, Dodson T, et al: *Hypertension* 18(suppl II):70–76, 1991.)

Methods.—The intimal response to vascular injury was studied in 5 baboons treated with oral cilazapril, 20 mg/kg/day, and in 5 untreated controls. Each animal underwent carotid artery endarterectomy, balloon catheter deendothelialization of the superficial femoral artery, and surgical placement of bilateral aorto-iliac expanded polytetrafluoroethylene grafts. Cilazapril therapy was begun 1 week before operation and was continued throughout the study interval. The animals were killed at approximately 3 months. The injured vessel and graft segments were evaluated by morphometry using a photoscope with computer-assisted display.

Results.—At 1 and 3 weeks postoperatively, plasma ACE activity was inhibited by more than 96% compared with control values. Although the response between animals was variable, there was no significant difference between cilazapril-treated animals and controls with respect to average cross-sectional areas of neointima at the sites of carotid endarterectomy, femoral artery ballooning, or graft anastomoses (Fig 1–8). Thus, cilazapril did not reduce intimal proliferative lesion formation over 3 months in this primate model of arterial injury.

Discussion.—The lack of benefit in baboons as opposed to rats may be the result of species-specific effects. It has been suggested that the beneficial effects of ACE inhibition are caused by inhibition of local tissue-associated converting enzyme systems that may vary considerably between species with respect to the actions of specific antagonists. Thus, there may be important differences in tissue penetration, metabolism, and drug clearance between the rat and the baboon. Consequently, the measurement of converting enzyme inhibition in plasma may not represent the actual degree of converting enzyme inhibition in tissue. Such species-related differences should be taken into account in future studies.

▶ In this study, angiotensin converting enzyme inhibitor did not reduce intimal thickening as assessed during a 3-month period in the primate arterial injury model. This is different from previously reported results with this agent. Is the primate model more relevant to the human? Probably so, but unfortunately we do not know.—J.M. Porter, M.D.

Evidence Implicating Nonmuscle Myosin in Restenosis: Use of In Situ Hybridization to Analyze Human Vascular Lesions Obtained by Directional Atherectomy
Leclerc G, Isner JM, Kearney M, Simons M, Safian RD, Baim DS, Weir L
(Tufts Univ; Harvard Med School, Boston)
Circulation 85:543–553, 1992   1–21

Introduction.—If those genes that are specifically activated in restenosis after transluminal angioplasty can be identified, then it may be possible to inhibit the cellular proliferation that causes the lesions by means of molecular manipulation. Quiescent smooth muscle cells preferentially express smooth muscle myosin, whereas proliferating cells preferentially express nonmuscle myosin in vitro.

Methods.—The expression of a recently cloned isoform of human nonmuscle myosin heavy chain (MHC-B) was examined in 6 primary lesions of the superficial femoral or coronary artery and in 4 lesions of re-

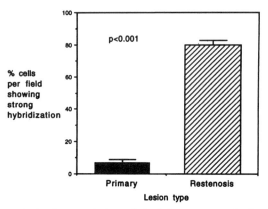

Fig 1-9.—Bar graph showing quantitative analysis of the percentage of cells per high-power field (×250) showing strong hybridization (clustering of more than 20 grains per cell nucleus). The results are expressed as means ± SEM. For primary lesions, 7% of the cells in the ×250 field showed strong hybridization to the antisense nonmuscle myosin heavy chain-B messenger RNA probe. In contrast, 80% of the cells per field of restenosis lesion showed a strong hybridization signal ($P < .001$). (Courtesy of Leclerc G, Isner JM, Kearney M, et al: *Circulation* 85:543–553, 1992.)

stenosis (3 from the superficial femoral artery and 1 from a saphenous vein bypass). Those lesions obtained percutaneously by directional atherectomy were processed for analysis by in situ hybridization with the MHC-B probe.

Results.—Restenotic lesions exhibited intense hybridization to the nonmuscle MHC-B cRNA probe (Fig 1-9). Equivalent hybridization was seen in only 7% of the cells from primary lesions, whereas 80% of the cells in restenosis lesions were positive. Immunocytochemical study using a monoclonal antibody to smooth muscle actin confirmed that the cells exhibiting strong hybridization were of smooth muscle origin.

Conclusion.—These findings provide a rational basis for investigating restenotic lesions on a larger scale to establish potential targets for gene therapy.

▶ Many think that molecular biology is the future of clinical medicine. This fascinating study indicates a clear alteration in gene expression in restenotic vs. primary vascular stenoses; it also identifies possible targets for future gene therapy. The future promises to be exciting.—J.M. Porter, M.D.

Circulating and Tissue Endothelin Immunoreactivity in Advanced Atherosclerosis

Lerman A, Edwards BS, Hallett JW, Heublein DM, Sandberg SM, Burnett JC Jr (Mayo Clinic and Found, Rochester, Minn)
N Engl J Med 325:997–1001, 1991   1-22

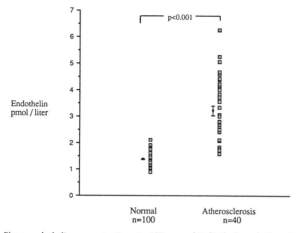

Fig 1–10.—Plasma edothelin concentrations in 100 normal individuals and 40 patients with symptomatic atherosclerosis. The mean (± SD) values are shown to the left of each column of data points. (Courtesy of Lerman A, Edwards BS, Hallett JW, et al: *N Engl J Med* 325:997–1001, 1991.)

Introduction.—Endothelin is an endothelium-derived contracting peptide that can constrict the systemic, coronary, and renal vessels. In addition, it exhibits mitogenic properties in vitro and may be a growth factor. Endothelial-cell injury, hypertension, and congestive heart failure are associated with increased plasma endothelin levels.

Methods.—Plasma endothelin levels were estimated by radioimmunoassay in 40 patients with atherosclerotic disease at various sites and also in 100 normal individuals. Endothelin was sought immunohistochemically in the walls of the atherosclerotic vessels.

Results.—The mean plasma endothelin level was significantly higher in the patients with atherosclerosis than in normal subjects (Fig 1–10) even when participants were matched for age. The endothelin levels did not correlate with age, mean arterial pressure, or the serum creatinine level. Endothelin-1–like immunoreactivity was identified in endothelial cells, vascular smooth muscle cells in aortic-wall vessels, and the medial smooth muscle of the aorta itself.

Conclusion.—These findings support a possible role for endothelin in the development of atherosclerotic disease, presumably based on the mitogenic properties of the factor. An increased local concentration of endothelin might promote the proliferation of vascular smooth-muscle cells.

▶ Endothelin, a potent endothelium-derived vasoconstrictor, has been documented to be increased in conditions of endothelial cell injury, essential hypertension, and congestive heart failure. This study indicates that endothelin is significantly increased in patients with symptomatic atherosclerosis, independent of age. Endothelin also appears to have mitogenic activity and may participate in the atherosclerotic process. Perhaps plasma endothelin will become a marker for the existence of significant arterial disease.—J.M. Porter, M.D.

Regression of Coronary Atherosclerosis: An Achievable Goal? Review of Results From Recent Clinical Trials

Waters D, Lespérance J (Montreal Heart Inst; Univ of Montreal)
Am J Med 91:10S–17S, 1991   1–23

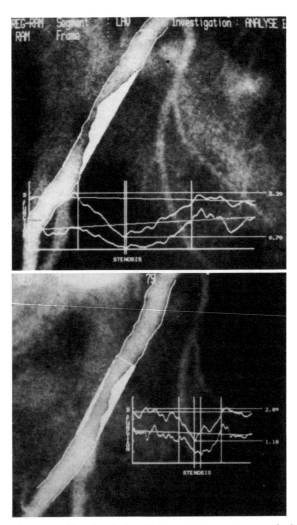

Fig 1–11.—An illustration of "true" regression. The quantitative measurements of a distal circumflex artery stenosis (C) were .70 mm for minimum diameter and 76% for diameter stenosis. At the second study (D), the minimum diameter had increased to 1.18 mm, and the diameter stenosis had improved to 56%. (Courtesy of Waters D, Lespérance J: Am J Med 91: 10S–17S, 1991.)

Introduction.—Coronary mortality has decreased steadily in the United States since 1968, but coronary atherosclerotic disease continues to exact a high toll. It has long been recognized that atherosclerosis is reversible in experimental animals, and increasing evidence from clinical trials indicates that reducing cholesterol can improve the course of coronary atherosclerotic disease and reduce the risk of coronary events.

Trials.—Evidence from large, placebo-controlled, randomized trials suggests that coronary events are less frequent when hyperlipidemia is treated. A marked reduction in total and LDL cholesterol levels, with a concomitant increase in HDL cholesterol, lessens the progression of coronary disease and promotes regression (Fig 1–11). Treatment prevented atherosclerosis in coronary bypass grafts in the Cholesterol-Lowering Atherosclerosis Study, and it clearly induced regression of coronary disease in the Familial Atherosclerosis Treatment Study. Benefit appears to be proportional to the degree of reduction in lipid levels.

Interventions.—In addition to reducing lipid levels, recent evidence suggests that use of aspirin and calcium antagonists may prevent early coronary lesions. Angiotensin converting enzyme inhibitors have exhibited antiatherogenic activity in animals.

▶ There is a great deal of interest and enthusiasm in treating hyperlipidemia to arrest the progression of and induce the regression of coronary atherosclerosis. During the past 30 years, there has been a 30% reduction in mortality caused by coronary artery disease; this reduction began long before it became popular to control serum cholesterol. This reduction has mainly been a result of improved methods of treatment of coronary artery disease rather than a reduction in coronary atherosclerosis. Recent Framingham data reveal no change in the incidence of coronary artery disease during the past 30 years. A number of controlled clinical trials of cholesterol reduction have demonstrated a small reduction in the number of coronary events but, interestingly, none has demonstrated an increase in survival.

Although some angiographic trials have demonstrated statistically significant changes suggestive of regression on serial coronary angiography, a significant number of plaques simultaneously progress in the same patients. The demonstrated clinical benefits of cholesterol reduction are small, and the costs of screening, measuring, and drug treatment are high. Furthermore, all of the trials have been focused on predominantly white, middle-aged, severely hypercholesterolemic men. These data have been extrapolated to women, all races and all age groups. For low-risk individuals with moderate lipid abnormalities, therapeutic recommendations are being made on the basis of faith rather than scientific evidence. There is no evidence that aspirin will prevent coronary atherosclerosis; however, it does appear to reduce coronary thrombosis.—C. Zarins, M.D.

Effect of Low Molecular Weight Heparin on Intimal Hyperplasia

Wilson NV, Salisbury JR, Kakkar VV (King's College Hosp, London)
Br J Surg 78:1381–1383, 1991   1–24

Background.—Intimal hyperplasia is an important reason why vascular grafts fail. The potential for using low-molecular-weight heparins (LMWHs) to prevent graft thrombosis was examined in the clinical setting.

Methods.—Groups of rabbits had aortic intimal hyperplasia induced by endothelial denudation using an embolectomy balloon catheter. Experimental animals received LMWH subcutaneously once or twice a day for 4 weeks, after which the aortas were harvested and intimal hyperplasia was quantified using a computerized image analysis system.

Results.—A 60% reduction in intimal hyperplasia was noted after administration of LMWH (Figs 1–12 and 1–13). Morphometric analysis revealed considerably less reduction in the luminal area after either daily or twice-daily heparin treatment than in control specimens. The ratio of intimal to medial area also decreased with treatment (table).

Conclusion.—Subcutaneous LMWH effectively inhibited intimal hyperplasia in this experimental model.

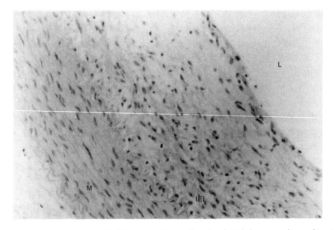

Fig 1–12.—A transverse section of rabbit aorta (control) stained with hematoxylin and eosin, showing the lumen (*L*), thick intimal layer (*I*), internal elastic lamina (*IEL*), and media (*M*) (Original magnification, × 100). (Courtesy of Wilson NV, Salisbury JR, Kakkar VV: *Br J Surg* 78:1381–1383, 1991.)

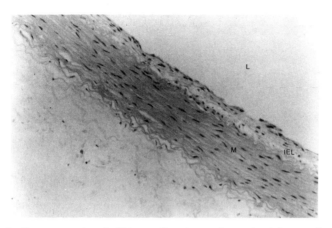

Fig 1–13.—Transverse section of rabbit aorta (heparin group) stained with hematoxylin and eosin, showing the lumen (*L*), thick intimal layer (*I*), internal elastic lamina (*IEL*), and media (*M*) (Original magnification, × 100). (Courtesy of Wilson NV, Salisbury JR, Kakkar VV: *Br J Surg* 78:1381–1383, 1991.)

▶ Stenosis occurring on account of intimal hyperplasia is an important cause of graft failure. At present, further vascular reconstruction offers the only hope of preserving patency. The study by Wilson et al. provides evidence that LMWH is an effective pharmacologic inhibitor of injury-induced arterial intimal hyperplasia. Whether heparin will inhibit vein graft stenosis in the same fashion is not known. The experimental data of Kohler et al. suggest that there may be differences in healing vein grafts and damaged arteries treated with heparin (1). Clinical trials designed to test the effect of heparin on restenosis after coronary angioplasty are in progress.—A.W. Clowes, M.D.

Reference

1. Kohler TR, et al: *Arteriosclerosis* 9:523, 1989.

Morphometric Analysis of Intimal Hyperplasia

	Vessel diameter (mm)	Medial area (mm²)	Intima:media area ratio	Percentage luminal reduction
Control	2·71(0·31)	0·65(0·15)	1·11 (0·96–1·17)	26 (18–31)
Daily LMWH	2·81(0·14)	0·69(0·13)	0·38 (0·24–0·61)	8 (5–12)
Twice-daily LMWH	2·65(0·20)	0·59(0·11)	0·44 (0·32–0·61)	10 (6–11)

The values for the diameter and medial area are mean (s.d.); the values for intimal hyperplasia are medians, with the interquartile range in parentheses. *Abbreviation:* LMWH, low-molecular-weight heparin. Controls vs. LMWH, $P < .001$; daily LMWH vs. twice-daily LMWH, $P > .05$ (Mann-Whitney U test).
(Courtesy of Wilson NV, Salisbury JR, Kakkar VV: *Br J Surg* 78:1381–1383, 1991.)

Peptide Inhibition of Neointimal Hyperplasia in Vein Grafts

Calcagno D, Conte JV, Howell MH, Foegh ML (Georgetown Univ, Washington, DC)

J Vasc Surg 13:475–479, 1991   1–25

Background.—Thickening of vein grafts at arterial sites may result in graft failure. Laboratory work has demonstrated effective inhibition of arterial neointimal hyperplasia using a novel octapeptide, angiopeptin.

Methods.—Carotid artery interposition bypass grafts of reversed autologous jugular vein were carried out in rabbits, some of which received angiopeptin in a daily dose of 20 μg/kg by subcutaneous injection. Treatment began a day before grafting and continued for 3 weeks, when the animals were killed.

Results.—Computerized morphometric analysis revealed that neointimal hyperplasia in angiopeptin-treated animals was .0, whereas that in control rabbits was .08.

Conclusion.—Angiopeptin inhibits neointimal hyperplasia in vein grafts, as it does in models of arterial neointimal hyperplasia. Its inhibitory effect may prove useful in maintaining vein graft patency in the clinical setting.

▶ These investigators document that the somastostatin analog, angiopeptin, is an effective inhibitor of wall thickening in vein grafts inserted into the carotid circulation. Although the mechanism of action is not clear, the drug has been used in a number of animal models, and it is currently being tested in clinical trials in patients undergoing coronary angioplasty.—A.W. Clowes, M.D.

Oral Contraceptives, Sex Steroid-Induced Antibodies and Vascular Thrombosis: Results From 1,318 Cases

Beaumont V, Lemort N, Beaumont JL (INSERM U 32; Centre de Recherches sur les Maladies des Arteres de l'Association Claude Bernard, Creteil, France)

Eur Heart J 12:1219–1224, 1991   1–26

Background.—Although the dose of estrogen has been progressively reduced in oral contraceptives (OCs), there remains a risk for arterial thrombosis and death in OC users, even those without factors known to be associated with thrombotic complications. Previous studies have shown that OCs may induce antibodies to the synthetic hormones contained in the pill. The prevalence of antiethinyl-estradiol antibodies (anti-EE Ab) was evaluated in OC users hospitalized for thrombosis.

Methods.—The multicenter investigation yielded 1,318 eligible patients treated from 1976 to 1988 (Table 1). They were compared with a group of women without thrombosis: 61 who had never used OCs or other sex steroid hormones and 124 symptom-free current users of OCs.

TABLE 1.—Thrombosis in Users of Oral Contraceptives

Uncomplicated deep vein thrombosis		264
legs	244	
arms	20	
Pulmonary embolism		159
with venous thrombosis	88	
without venous thrombosis	71	
Coronary artery thrombosis		37
Systemic arterial thrombosis		53
in the legs	40	
in the arms	13	
Cerebrovascular thrombosis		763
transient ischemic attack	136	
permanent neurological deficit	541	
cerebral thrombophlebitis	86	
Hepatic vein thrombosis		10
Miscellaneous		32
	Total cases	1318

(Courtesy of Beaumont V, Lemort N, Beaumont JL: *Eur Heart J* 12:1219-1224, 1991.)

TABLE 2.—Comparison of Arterial and Venous Thrombosis

	Arterial n = 773		Venous n = 545
Age (years)	34 ± 10	*	29 ± 9
Duration of OC use (months)	66 ± 56	*	53 ± 52
Predisposing conditions (%)			
none	91·8		80·7
surgery	1·0	*	9·7
childbirth	1·4		4·0
others	5·8		5·5
Arterial risk factors (%)			
hyperlipidaemia	5·3	*	1·8
hypertension	5·8	*	1·3
smoking‡	64·3	†	53·2
Anti EE Ab (c . min^{-1})	307 ± 371		333 ± 398
> 150 c . min^{-1} (%)	72·3		72·1

Note: Chi-square test.
* $P < .001$.
† $P < .001$.
‡ Information available on 313 arterial and 259 venous thromboses.
(Courtesy of Beaumont V, Lemort N, Beaumont JL: *Eur Heart J* 12:1219-1224, 1991.)

In all cases and controls, radioimmunoassay with tritiated ethinylestradiol was used to determine anti-EE Ab. The role of the associated risk factors was also examined.

Results.—The vast majority of women (87.2%) who had a thrombotic event had no history of a predisposing illness. Most (87.9%) were current OC users, although some were ex-users who had stopped more than 3 months before (8.3%) or were women who had just resumed the use of OCs (3.7%). The Anti-EE Ab were present in 33% of healthy users and in 72% of those with thrombosis, either arterial or venous (Table 2). No anti-EE Ab were found in the 61 women who had never used OCs. The risk factors of increased age, longer duration of use, hyperlipidemia, and smoking were associated with thrombosis only in women with arterial disease. Nearly half of the women with thrombosis (47.7%) had a combination of the 2 predominant factors: anti-EE Ab and smoking.

Conclusion.—The apparent thrombogenic effect of the antibodies may result from damage to the vascular endothelium and interference with clotting factors and platelet aggregation. Determination of anti-EE Ab may identify which healthy OC users are at risk for thrombosis.

▶ It is interesting to note that the role, if any, of OCs in the production of vascular thrombosis remains unproven. Modern OCs containing very low doses of estrogen certainly appear to have a low likelihood of inducing thrombosis. Perhaps a small number of patients who are taking OCs and who also have the combination of smoking and antiestrogen antibodies are at increased risk for thrombosis. This information may lead to the recommendation of alternate methods of birth control in susceptible patients.—J.M. Porter, M.D.

Prospective Study of Alcohol Consumption and Risk of Coronary Disease in Men

Rimm EB, Giovannucci EL, Willett WC, Colditz GA, Ascherio A, Rosner B, Stampfer MJ (Harvard Univ, Boston; Brigham and Women's Hosp, Boston)
Lancet 338:464–468, 1991   1–27

Introduction.—Several different types of studies have reported an inverse association between alcohol consumption and the risk of coronary artery disease (CAD). However, some studies suggest that the inverse association is an artifact resulting from preexisting disease or the inclusion of heavy drinkers in reference groups of nondrinkers who are lying about their alcohol intake. Few studies of alcohol intake and CAD have taken dietary intake into consideration. The relationship between alcohol consumption and the risk of CAD was examined prospectively, with control for diet and other risk factors.

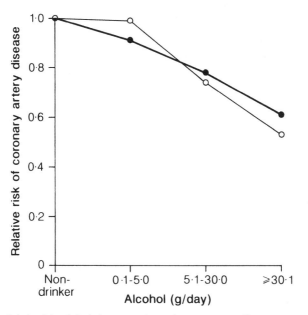

Fig 1–14.—Relative risks of alcohol consumption and coronary artery disease among men from the health Professionals Follow-up Study. *Open circles* indicate 44,059 men free of myocardial infarction, angina CABG or PCTA, stroke, and cancer (except nonmelanoma skin cancer.) *Filled circles* indicate cohort without 16,242 men who, at baseline, reported myocardial infarction, angina, CABG, PCTA, stroke, cancer (except nonmelanoma skin cancer), gout, diabetes, high cholesterol, high triglycerides, hypertension, tachycardia, heart rhythm disturbances, or other heart disturbances. (Courtesy of Rimm EB, Giovannucci EL, Willett WC, et al: *Lancet* 338:464-468, 1991.)

Methods.—A 131-item semiquantitive food frequency questionnaire including questions about alcoholic beverage consumption was mailed to a cohort of 51,529 men (age, 40-75 years) who were enrolled in an on-going study of the dietary etiologies of heart disease and cancer. All the men were health professionals. Questions concerning medical history, heart disease risk factors, and dietary changes during the past 10 years were also included in the survey. The data from 44,059 men were evaluable.

Results.—Analysis of the replies revealed that 23.4% of the men consumed alcohol either never or less than once per month; 26.4% drank more than 15 g of alcohol (or 1 drink) per day; and 3.5% drank more than 50 g of alcohol (or 3-4 drinks) per day. There were 350 confirmed new cases of CAD. After adjustment for coronary risk factors, including dietary intake of cholesterol, fat, and dietary fiber, increasing alcohol consumption was inversely related to the incidence of CAD (Fig 1-14). The exclusion of current nondrinkers or of those with disorders potentially related to CAD, which might have led them to reduce their alcohol intake, did not substantially affect the relative risks.

Conclusion.—The findings provide additional support for the hypothesis that moderate alcohol intake reduces the risk of CAD. The inverse association between moderate alcohol consumption and risk of CAD is not an artifact caused by preexisting disease or differences in dietary habits; however, it is causal.

▶ Isn't it a pleasure to learn that moderate alcohol intake reduces the risk of CAD? This is one of the few truly gratifying results that we have realized from our expenditure of hundreds of millions of dollars to investigate the relationship between diet and human disease.—J.M. Porter, M.D.

Effects of Tamoxifen on Cardiovascular Risk Factors in Postmenopausal Women
Love RR, Wiebe DA, Newcomb PA, Cameron L, Leventhal H, Jordan VC, Feyzi J, DeMets DL (Univ of Wisconsin Clinical Cancer Ctr, Madison)
Ann Intern Med 115:860–864, 1991   1–28

Introduction.—Tamoxifen is a synthetic antiestrogen used in the treatment of breast cancer that has been associated with disease-free survival in many studies; however, the optimal duration of adjuvant therapy remains to be determined.

Methods.—The effects of tamoxifen on cardiovascular risk factors were examined in a double-blind, placebo-controlled, 2-year trial in postmenopausal women who had breast cancer not involving the axillary nodes, and who were free of disease at the time of treatment.

Results.—Tamoxifen-treated women had a decrease in total cholesterol levels, which differed significantly from the stable levels found in placebo recipients (Fig 1-15). The mean decrease in total cholesterol

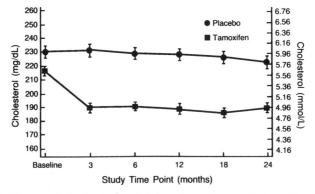

Fig 1–15.—The mean fasting levels of total cholesterol over time in patients receiving tamoxifen or placebo. *Circles* indicate control patients; $n = 70$ at baseline and $n = 70, 68, 67, 64$, and 62 patients at 3, 6, 12, 18, and 24 months respectively. *Squares* indicate patients receiving tamoxifen; $n = 70$ at baseline and $n = 66, 66, 65, 64$, and 64 patients at 3, 6, 12, 18, and 24 months respectively. *Bars* indicate 95% confidence intervals. Cholesterol levels decreased significantly at all time points in patients receiving tamoxifen ($P < .001$). (Courtesy of Love RR, Wiebe DA, Newcomb PA, et al: *Ann Intern Med* 115:860-864, 1991.)

from baseline levels was approximately 12%. Low-density-lipoprotein cholesterol levels also decreased, whereas apolipoprotein A-I levels increased significantly in women who were given tamoxifen. The apolipoprotein B levels decreased significantly in this group.

Conclusion.—A persistent reduction in cholesterol was found in this trial of tamoxifen in postmenopausal women. There is preliminary evidence suggesting reduced cardiovascular mortality in patients with breast cancer undergoing long-term tamoxifen therapy.

▶ Tamoxifen is a widely used agent in the treatment of breast cancer of all stages, and it is frequently continued for very long periods of time. This important study concludes that long-term administration of tamoxifen results in a significant decrease in total cholesterol and low-density lipoprotein cholesterol levels. This unexpectedly favorable effect may partially explain the decrease in coronary heart disease mortality reported in patients receiving tamoxifen.—J.M. Porter, M.D.

Hyperhomocyst(e)inaemia: An Independent Risk Factor for Intermittent Claudication
Mölgaard J, Malinow MR, Lassvik C, Holm A-C, Upson B, Olsson AG (University Hosp, Linköping, Sweden; Oregon Regional Primate Research Ctr)
J Intern Med 231:273–279, 1992   1–29

Objective.—Whether hyperhomocyst(e)inemia is a risk factor for intermittent claudication (IC) independent of such factors as smoking, hypertension, diabetes, high levels of cholesterol and triglycerides, and low levels of high-density lipoprotein cholesterol was determined.

Method.—A group of 78 subjects with confirmed IC were taken from an epidemiologic study of middle-aged Swedish men; they were compared with 98 healthy subjects matched for age and gender.

Results.—Plasma homocyst(e)ine levels, including free and bound forms of homocysteine and their disulfide oxidation products, were significantly higher in the subjects with IC than in control (Fig 1–16). The difference was independent of other risk factors, and it was seen chiefly in those with serum folate levels equal to or greater than 11 nmol/L.

Conclusion.—It may be worthwhile to provide supplemental folic acid to subjects with IC who have hyperhomocyst(e)inemia.

▶ Confirmatory evidence from all over the world indicates that, as a group, patients with symptomatic peripheral vascular disease have significantly higher blood levels of homocyst(e)ine than age-matched controls. In every study, nearly 30% of patients with peripheral vascular disease have marked increases. We eagerly await evidence that treatment with folic acid or vitamin B_{12}, which can return homocys(e)tine levels to near normal, will retard the rate of atherosclerosis progression.—J.M. Porter, M.D.

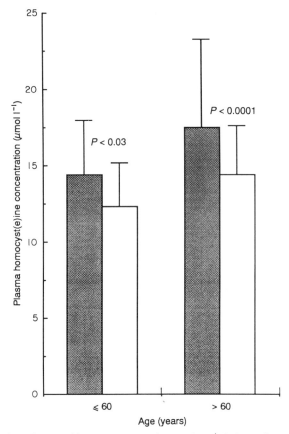

Fig 1–16.—Plasma homocyst(e)ine concentration (mean values ± SD) in male patients with intermittent claudication (IC) (*filled bars*), and in sex- and age-matched controls (*open bars*), grouped according to age > 60 years (*n* = 119) and ≤ 60 years (*n* = 57). The mean plasma homocyst(e)ine concentration is significantly increased in patients, and it also increases with age. (Courtesy of Mölgaard J, Malinow MR, Lassvik C, et al: *J Intern Med* 231:273–279, 1992.)

Prevalence of Familial Hyperhomocyst(e)inemia in Men With Premature Coronary Artery Disease

Genest JJ Jr, McNamara JR, Upson B, Salem DN, Ordovas JM, Schaefer EJ, Malinow MR (Tufts Univ, Boston; New England Med Ctr Hosp, Boston; Oregon Regional Primate Research Ctr, Beaverton)
Arterioscler Thromb 11:1129–1136, 1991 1–30

Introduction.—Because increased plasma homocysteine levels have been found in patients with coronary artery disease, an attempt was made to determine whether this increase is genetic in origin. Homocysteine levels were determined in 176 men who had at least 50% stenosis of a major coronary artery before 60 years of age, and in 255 controls without cardiovascular disease.

Results.—Significantly higher plasma homocysteine levels were found in the patients with premature coronary artery disease. More than one fourth of these patients had levels above the 90th percentile of controls. Genetic studies in the relatives of 71 coronary patients suggested that homocysteine levels are in part determined genetically. Familial hyper-homocysteinemia was identified in 14% of the patients with coronary disease.

Implications.—Increased plasma homocysteine appears to be a risk factor for premature coronary artery disease. Whether homocysteine is toxic to the endothelial cells remains to be established.

▶ Not only is symptomatic peripheral vascular disease independently related to increased homocyst(e)ine levels, but coronary artery disease also appears to be so related. The association between coronary disease peripheral vascular disease and increased plasma homocyst(e)ine is incontrovertible. Now we are eagerly awaiting a description of pathophysiology and data on response to treatment.—J.M. Porter, M.D.

Interleukin-1α as a Factor in Occlusive Vascular Disease
Brody JI, Pickering NJ, Capuzzi DM, Fink GB, Can CA, Gomez F (Med College of Pennsylvania; Thomas Jefferson Univ, Philadelphia)
Am J Clin Pathol 97:8–13, 1992   1–31

Introduction.—Interleukin-1 alpha (IL-1α) is able to alter endothelial cells functionally and induce the replication of smooth muscle cells and fibroblasts. These changes might implicate IL-1α in the development of myointimal proliferation and vascular sclerosis.

Methods.—A peroxidase-immunoperoxidase technique was used to detect IL-1α in samples of saphenous veins and internal mammary arteries before they were implanted as aortocoronary bypass grafts. Occluded vein grafts obtained from patients with recurrent angina also were examined.

Results.—Deposits of IL-1α were seen on the luminal surface, in the subintima, and on spindle cells and infiltrating macrophages in the media of sclerotic veins. Normal-appearing veins and arteries that appeared structurally intact contained no deposits. Bypass grafts that exhibited histopathologic abnormalities such as reduced lumina patency, myointimal proliferation, mural collagenization, luminal-mural hemorrhage, and mononuclear-cell infiltration contained widely distributed deposits of IL-1α.

Conclusion.—These findings may help explain why internal mammary arteries tend to remain patent and survive better than vein grafts when used for coronary revascularization. The presence of IL-1α may be an important marker of vascular injury, and the cytokine may actually participate in the processes leading to vascular occlusion.

▶ The cytokine IL-1α apparently acts as both an autocrine and a paracrine, and it has a wide range of biological actions, including promotion of monocyte chemothraxis, smooth muscle proliferation, suppression of fibrinolysis, and activation of endothelial cells in a prothrombotic fashion. This study suggests that IL-1α may be a marker of vascular injury.—J.M. Porter, M.D.

Transdermal Nicotine for Smoking Cessation: Six-Month Results From Two Multicenter Controlled Clinical Trials
Rennard S, for the Transdermal Nicotine Study Group (Univ of Nebraska, Omaha)
JAMA 266:3133–3138, 1991   1–32

Objective.—A new transdermal nicotine system was evaluated in 2 6-week double-blind, placebo-controlled parallel group trials. A total of 935 patients were enrolled.

Methods.—Healthy subjects who smoked a pack or more of cigarettes each day were assigned either to the nicotine system, which delivered nicotine at a rate of 7, 14, or 21 mg in 24 hours, or to a placebo condition. All participants received group counseling. Those who abstained participated in a trial for blind down-titration from medication and in a 12-week off-drug follow-up.

Results.—The cessation rate in the last 4 weeks of the trials was 61% for 21 mg of nicotine, 48% for 14 mg of nicotine, and 27% for placebo. The 6-month abstinence rate was 26% for patients given 21 mg of nicotine and 12% for placebo recipients. All doses of nicotine lessened nicotine withdrawal symptoms; they also reduced cigarette use by those who did not abstain. There were no serious systemic side effects.

Conclusion.—Transdermal nicotine is a promising aid to smoking cessation.

▶ I continue to be concerned with the widespread willingness of physicians to prescribe exogenous nicotine to assist in cigarette withdrawal among their addicted patients. The 2 obvious questions are: Does it work and does it do harm? I still do not know, but neither does anyone else.—J.M. Porter, M.D.

Arteriographic Findings in EDTA Chelation Therapy on Peripheral Arteriosclerosis
Sloth-Nielsen J, Guldager B, Mouritzen C, Lund EB, Egeblad M, Nørregaard O, Jørgensen SJ, Jelnes R (Skejby Hosp, Aarhus, Denmark; Hillerød Hosp,

Hillerød, Denmark; Alborg Hosp, Alborg, Denmark)
Am J Surg 162:122–125, 1991   1–33

Background.—Because many patients with coronary or peripheral arteriosclerotic disease spend much money on ethylenediaminetetraacetic acid (EDTA) treatment in hope of improvement, it is appropriate to assess the efficacy of this treatment objectively.

Methods.—A randomized double-blind study was undertaken in 153 patients with stable intermittent claudication. The patients, all older than 40 years of age, had walking ranges of 50–200 meters and ankle/brachial indices less than .8. They received 20 infusions of either 3 g Na$_2$EDTA or saline. The analyses of the 30 patients entered from Aarhus were examined.

Results.—There were no significant clinical differences between the EDTA-treated and control groups. The ankle/brachial indices were comparable before and after treatment. Only 2 of 30 arteriographic studies showed improvement. Transcutaneous oxygen tensions did not differ significantly between the treatment and control groups.

Conclusion.—Chelation therapy with EDTA has no apparent effect on patients with intermittent claudication secondary to arteriosclerotic disease.

▶ I suspect that every vascular surgeon in America has encountered patients who have received EDTA chelation therapy in an effort to improve symptomatic atherosclerosis. Proponents of this therapy have traditionally cited anecdotal improvement, and they have challenged the rest of us to produce negative results. This randomized double-blind study does just that. For anyone who is interested, the same authors published a slightly different version of this same data in the May 1992 *Journal of Internal Medicine.*—J.M. Porter, M.D.

Long-Term Mortality After 5-Year Multifactorial Primary Prevention of Cardiovascular Diseases in Middle-Aged Men

Strandberg TE, Salomaa VV, Naukkarinen VA, Vanhanen HT, Sarna SJ, Miettinen TA (Univ of Helsinki, Natl Public Health Inst, Helsinki; Jorvi Hosp, Espoo, Finland)
JAMA 266:1225–1229, 1991   1–34

Background.—A randomized primary prevention trial was undertaken from 1974 to 1980 to assess the value of intensive hypolipidemic therapy with clofibrate and/or probucol, and antihypertensive therapy (chiefly with BETA-blockers and diuretics). The 10-year follow-up data on the 612 initially healthy men who were assigned to primary prevention and the 610 control subjects were examined.

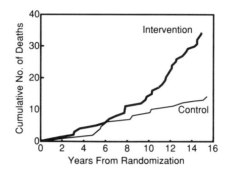

Fig 1–17.—The cumulative incidence of cardiac deaths in the intervention and control groups during the 15-year follow-up. P = .0035 for the difference between the groups. (Courtesy of Strandberg TE, Salomaa VV, Naukkarinen VA, et al: JAMA 266:1225–1229, 1991.)

Findings.—Half the subjects in the intervention group received antihypertensive medication, and 45% were given hypolipidemic medication. The overall mortality was 10.9% in the intervention group and 7.5% in the control group. The respective rates of mortality from coronary heart disease were 5.6% and 2.3% (Fig 1–17). Multiple logistic regression analysis failed to explain the excess cardiac mortality.

Implications.—Coronary mortality increased in the intervention group, despite effective reduction of cardiovascular risk factors. The findings may relate only to this particular population. They do, however, mean that ongoing research is needed to select methods for primary prevention of cardiovascular disease.

▶ Aren't intervention trials amazing? In this study, 1,222 clinically healthy men with risk factors were entered into a primary prevention trial; half were randomized to blood pressure and lipid intervention, and half were randomized to a control group. Critical analyses done 15 years after the start of the study and 10 years after the completion of the intervention phase, have revealed the remarkable fact that, after 10 years, there were significantly more cardiac deaths in the intervention group than in the control group. The proponents of multiple risk factor intervention continue to have great difficulty proving the value of their increasingly expensive interventions.—J.M. Porter, M.D.

Variability of Body Weight and Health Outcomes in the Framingham Population
Lissner L, Odell PM, D'Agostino RB, Stokes J III, Kreger BE, Belanger AJ, Brownell KD (Göteborg, Sweden; Bryant College, Smithfield, RI; Boston Univ; Yale Univ, New Haven, Conn)
N Engl J Med 324:1839–1844, 1991   1–35

Objective.—Fluctuations in body weight are frequent, partly because of the popularity of dieting.

Methods.—An attempt was made to relate variation in body weight to health end points in the Framingham Heart Study population, which was followed at 2-year intervals.

Findings.—A review of 32-year follow-up data indicated that individuals with considerable variation in body weight had higher overall mortality, higher mortality from coronary disease, and higher morbidity from this cause. The relationship could not be ascribed to obesity or indicators of cardiovascular risk. The relative risk estimates for end points in individuals whose body weight varied substantially ranged from 1.27 to 1.93 compared with those of individuals with relatively stable weight.

Implication.—If, as the findings suggest, fluctuating body weight has adverse effects on health independent of obesity, it may be necessary to critically assess the public health effects of current weight loss practices.

▶ As the authors of this study observed, continuous fluctuations in body weight may have significantly adverse health consequences that are independent of obesity or any trends in changes net body weight over time. The ingrained prejudice that lean is healthy should be periodically reevaluated.—J.M. Porter, M.D.

Changes in Lipid and Lipoprotein Levels and Body Weight in Tarahumara Indians After Consumption of an Affluent Diet
McMurry MP, Cerqueira MT, Connor SL, Connor WE (Oregon Health Sciences Univ, Portland)
N Engl J Med 325:1704–1708, 1991   1–36

Background.—The consequences of changing from a traditional to a modern diet are potentially significant as developing countries become increasingly affluent. Changes in blood lipid levels were investigated in a group of Tarahumara Indians—a Mexican people who partake of a low-fat, high-fiber diet—who began consuming a diet typical of affluent societies.

Methods.—Thirteen Indians took their traditional diet, containing 2,700 kcal/day, for 1 week; they were then fed a diet containing 4,100 kcal/day. The latter diet included excessive total fat, saturated fat, and cholesterol; it was consumed for 5 weeks.

Results.—The mean plasma cholesterol increased by 31% after 5 weeks of the "affluent" diet, chiefly reflecting an increase in the low-density lipoprotein (LDL) fraction (Fig 1–18). The high-density lipoprotein (HDL) fraction, which is low in this population, also increased substantially, and the LDL:HDL ratio showed little change. Body weight increased by an average of 3.8 kg.

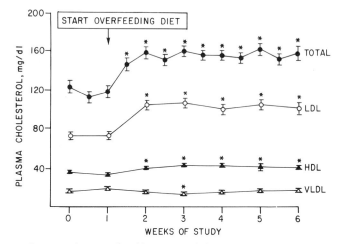

Fig 1–18.—The mean plasma total and lipoprotein cholesterol concentrations in 10 Tarahumara Indians. Values are included for the 10 subjects who completed the entire 6-week study. Plasma total, LDL, and HDL cholesterol levels increased rapidly when the affluent diet was introduced after 1 week of the baseline Tarahumara diet. The *asterisks* indicate values significantly different from the baseline by paired *t*-test. To convert cholesterol values to millimoles per liter, multiply by .02586. (Courtesy of McMurry MP, Cerqueira MT, Connor SL, et al: N Engl J Med 325:1704–1708, 1991.)

Conclusion.—Dramatic increases in plasma lipids and greater body weight result when a typical Tarahumara Indian diet is replaced by a modern affluent diet. Such changes, if sustained, could increase the risk of coronary heart disease.

▶ What will be the health consequences in developing countries as increasing wealth and urbanization leads the population to adopt more affluent dietary habits? In this study of an Indian population in Mexico, the individuals had a dramatic increase in plasma lipid, lipoproteins, and body weight when consuming the new diet. Interestingly, they also appeared to enjoy the new diet. Is this going to be harmful? I am sure the nut-and-berry crowd will think so.—J.M. Porter, M.D.

2 Endovascular

Standards for Evaluating and Reporting the Results of Surgical and Percutaneous Therapy for Peripheral Arterial Disease
Rutherford RB, Becker GJ (Univ of Colorado, Denver; Baptist Hosp, Miami)
Radiology 181:277–281, 1991   2–1

Introduction.—Proper management of peripheral vascular disease requires adherence to uniform standards of evaluating and reporting therapeutic interventions. Standard reporting practices for arterial and venous disease have been recommended by the joint council of the Society for Vascular Surgery and the North American Chapter of the International Society for Cardiovascular Surgery, but they are only gradually being adopted.

Standards.—When reporting treatment for peripheral vascular disease, physicians should not exclude failures to complete treatment successfully, immediate technical failures, or failures to produce improvement. Acute ischemic limbs should be categorized before treatment as viable, threatened, or irreversible; chronic ischemic limbs should also be stratified with the aid of objective, noninvasive criteria (table). Changes in limb status should be graded on a scale of +3, indicating marked improvement, to −3, indicating marked worsening. All initial failures should be categorized as aborted, completed but technically unsuccessful, or technically successful but no improvement. The overall success rate should be reported when the results are divided into initial success and late patency. The standards specify objective means to be used in determining patency. Primary patency is defined as uninterrupted patency with no procedures either on or at the margins of the treated segment; primary patency is lost when any procedure that might prevent eventual failure is performed before thrombosis. In treated segments, assisted primary patency may be used in measuring success. Patency should be analyzed by the life-table method. The 30-day limit should be used in reporting procedural mortality, unless death occurs during the same, but longer, hospitalization. Pertinent local nonvascular complications and systemic remote complications must be listed and graded along with vascular complications. Finally, risk factors that may affect outcome should be recorded, graded, and compared.

Conclusion.—Standards for published reports of revascularization for lower extremity ischemia were examined. Observation of the standards

Clinical Categories of Chronic Limb Ischemia

Grade	Category	Clinical Description	Objective Criteria
	0	Asymptomatic, no hemodynamically significant occlusive disease	Normal results of treadmill*/stress test
I	1	Mild claudication	Treadmill exercise completed, postexercise AP is greater than 50 mm Hg but more than 25 mm Hg less than normal
	2	Moderate claudication	Symptoms between those of categories 1 and 3
	3	Severe claudication	Treadmill exercise cannot be completed, postexercise AP is less than 50 mm Hg
II	4	Ischemic rest pain	Resting AP of 40 mm Hg or less, flat or barely pulsatile ankle or metatarsal plethysmographic tracing, toe pressure less than 30 mm Hg
III	5	Minor tissue loss, nonhealing ulcer, focal gangrene with diffuse pedal ischemia	Resting AP of 60 mm Hg or less, ankle or metatarsal plethysmographic tracing flat or barely pulsatile, toe pressure less than 40 mm Hg
	6	Major tissue loss, extending above transmetatarsal level, functional foot no longer salvageable	Same as for category 5

Abbreviation: AP, ankle pressure.
* Five minutes at 2 mph on a 12-degree incline.
(Courtesy of Rutherford RB, Becker GJ: *Radiology* 181:277–281, 1991.)

will improve the quality of reports, allowing comparative analysis of different modalities.

▶ Interventional radiologists have been appropriately chastised by vascular surgeons for their failure to adhere to widely accepted standards of outcome reporting in patients with vascular disease. To their eternal credit, members of the newly formed Society for Interventional Radiology have recognized this deficiency and have adopted for their journal the same strict set of reporting standards that we use for vascular surgery (1).—J.M. Porter, M.D.

Reference

1. Rutherford RB, et al: *J Vasc Surg* 4:80, 1986.

Outcome Predictors in Selection of Balloon Angioplasty or Surgery for Peripheral Arterial Occlusive Disease
Dalsing MC, Cockerill E, Deupree R, Wolf G, Wilson S (Indiana Univ Med Ctr, Dept of Veterans Affairs, West Haven, Conn)
Surgery 110:636-644, 1991   2-2

Background.—Surgical bypass and percutaneous balloon angioplasty (PTA) are equally effective measures for ileofemoropopliteal occlusive disease in selected men, excluding immediate failures of angioplasty. Whether those patients who are likely to have immediate PTA failure can be identified, and whether pretreatment factors can predict whether angioplasty or surgery will be best in the remaining cases are relevant questions.

Methods.—A total of 263 patients treated at 9 Veterans Administration hospitals included 19 who immediately failed after PTA, 17 others who failed within 2 years after PTA, and 24 who failed within 2 years of surgical bypass. A total of 130 patients were assigned to PTA, and 133 were assigned to surgery.

Results.—On univariate analysis, the site and degree of stenosis and systolic and diastolic blood pressure predicted immediate PTA failures. Multivariate analysis, however, indicated that only percent stenosis and diastolic blood pressure predicted immediate failures. No factors were found to predict delayed PTA failure, and no pretreatment patient features that predicted failure after surgical bypass were identified.

Conclusion.—Some patients with a severely stenotic or occluded lower limb artery and diastolic hypertension are poor candidates for PTA. Others are adequately managed by either PTA or surgical bypass.

The situation may change when improved PTA adjunctive measures become available.

▶ This is a follow-up to an important, previously published study describing the prospective randomized outcome of balloon angioplasty vs. bypass surgery (1). Multivariant analysis now indicates that both diastolic hypertension and severe stenosis predict immediate PTA failure.—J.M. Porter, M.D.

Reference

1. Wilson SE, et al: *J Vasc Surg* 9:1, 1989.

Chronic Lower Limb Ischaemia. A Prospective Randomised Controlled Study Comparing the 1-Year Results of Vascular Surgery and Percutaneous Transluminal Angioplasty (PTA)
Holm J, Arfvidsson B, Jivegård L, Lundgren F, Lundholm K, Scherstén T, Stenberg B, Tylén U, Zachrisson BF, Lindberg H, Mattsson E, Persson B, Spangen L, Jonsson E (Univ of Göteborg; Karlstad Central Hosp, Karlstad; Karolinska Inst, Stockholm, Sweden)
Eur J Vasc Surg 5:517–522, 1991   2–3

Objective.—The early results of angioplasty were compared with those of conventional reconstructive surgery in a prospective series of 102 patients seen during a 6-year period. The patients had severe lower limb ischemia or claudication resistant to exercise training, and all were deemed appropriate for angioplasty or vascular surgery. Only 5% of patients seen during this time were eligible for randomization. The 2 groups were similar in age, severity of symptoms, and the presence of diabetes. The patients were prospectively randomized to angioplasty or surgery.

Results.—The primary patency rates were 60% in the angioplasty group and 62% in the surgery group at 1 year. The respective secondary patency rates were 77% and 67%. A total of 5 patients in the angioplasty group required surgery for complications; 5 in the vascular surgery group required early reoperation. Ten repeat procedures were necessary after angioplasty; 9 of these patients did well subsequently. Three patients who underwent angioplasty and 8 who were treated operatively later required amputation. A total of 6 angioplasty patients and 4 vascular surgery patients died.

Conclusions.—If angiography demonstrates a stenosis of occlusion that is 6 cm or less in length and is amenable to both angioplasty and surgery, the former treatment is initially indicated. However, angioplasty should be done only if facilities for vascular surgery are immediately available.

▶ Do not be deceived by this paper. All it indicates is that good angioplasty is as good as mediocre vascular surgery. I cannot imagine a 1-year vascular surgery primary patency rate of only 62%, especially when almost 40% of the vascular surgery patients underwent aortofemoral procedures, which by themselves should have produced a 1-year patency rate of 95%.—J.M. Porter, M.D.

Recurrence of Stenoses Following Balloon Angioplasty and Simpson Atherectomy of the Femoro-Popliteal Segment: A Randomised Comparative 1-Year Follow-Up Study Using Colour Flow Duplex

Vroegindeweij D, Kemper FJM, Tielbeek AV, Buth J, Landman G (Catharina Hosp, Eindhoven, The Netherlands)
Eur J Vasc Surg 6:164–171, 1992 2-4

Objective.—The early and late outcomes after balloon angioplasty and atherectomy with the Simpson atherocath were compared in patients with symptomatic stenosis or occlusion in the superficial femoral and popliteal arteries.

Methods.—All 30 patients in the randomized, prospective study had intermittent claudication. Balloon angioplasty was performed in 14 extremities, and atherectomy was performed in 16. Color flow duplex scanning was carried out 6 weeks after treatment, every 3 months for the first year, and then at 6-month intervals. The average follow-up was 10 months. Digital subtraction angiography was done a year after treatment if a patient was symptomatic or the duplex study showed 50% or greater stenosis.

Results.—Two patients in each group had residual stenosis exceeding 20%. All but 1 patient in each treatment group improved clinically. Significantly more patients who had balloon angioplasty remained free of restenosis and new atherosclerotic lesions (Fig 2–1).

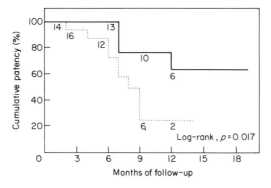

Fig 2–1.—Cumulative patency (no restenosis greater than 49%) in patients with balloon angioplasty (*solid line*) and atherectomy (*dotted line*). (Courtesy of Vroegindeweij D, Kemper FJM, Tielbeek AV, et al: *Eur J Vasc Surg* 6:164–171, 1992.)

Conclusion.—In patients who are treated for femoropopliteal atherosclerotic disease, restenosis is more likely in those who have atherectomy than in those who have balloon angioplasty.

▶ A small number of patients with lesions of the superficial femoral artery were randomized to balloon angioplasty or Simpson atherectomy. Although the initial results were quite satisfactory in both groups, by the end of 1 year, only 25% of patients in the atherectomy group had no recurrent stenosis. The atherectomy devices appear to be fading rapidly away.—J.M. Porter, M.D.

Palmaz Stent in Atherosclerotic Stenoses Involving the Ostia of the Renal Arteries: Preliminary Report of a Multicenter Study
Rees CR, Palmaz JC, Becker GJ, Ehrman KO, Richter GM, Noeldge G, Katzen BT, Dake MD, Schwarten DE (Univ of Texas Health Science Ctr, San Antonio; Indiana Univ, Indianapolis; Univ of Freiburg, Germany; Baptist Mem Hosp, Miami; St Vincent's Hosp, Indianapolis)
Radiology 181:507–514, 1991   2–5

Background.—Percutaneous transluminal angioplasty (PTA) has a limited role in treating ostial atheromatous renal artery lesions, with early success in only 20% to 24% of patients. The Palmaz renal stent was evaluated in 28 hypertensive patients who had atherosclerosis involving the ostia of the renal arteries.

Methods.—Twenty patients had stents placed to treat elastic recoil immediately after conventional angioplasty. Eight others had stents placed for treatment of restenosis after PTA.

Results.—In all but 1 patient, there was less than 30% residual stenosis after stenting. Five serious complications, including 1 death, occurred in this small group of patients. Hypertension was absent in 3 patients at follow-up 1–25 months after treatment, and 15 other patients had improvement. Renal function improved in 5, stabilized in 5, and deteriorated in 4 patients with an initial serum creatinine level of 1.5 mg/dL or higher. Follow-up angiography (Fig 2–2) demonstrated restenosis in 7 of 18 patients.

Conclusion.—Renal stenting appears to benefit some patients with renal ostial atheromatous disease who respond poorly to conventional angioplasty, but it is associated with a very high rate of serious complications.

▶ I have never understood the rationale for using stents after arterial dilatation. I have not been impressed that elastic recoil is a primary cause of recurrent stenosis in dilated arteries. This is another example of the widespread use of a very expensive endovascular device without any convincing proof of its efficacy.—J.M. Porter, M.D.

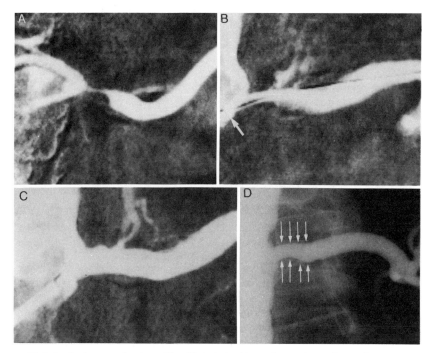

Fig 2–2.—Angiograms of patient with mild myointimal hyperplasia without substantial restenosis. **A,** there is 85% stenosis before renal PTA. **B,** residual stenosis is 55% after renal PTA. The stent is being positioned. The proximal edge of the stent (*arrow*) corresponds to the proximal radiopaque marker on the angioplasty balloon. **C,** after placement was complete, the stent was not dilated beyond 7 mm in diameter, because the patient experienced excruciating pain at that level. The renal artery measured approximately 9.5 mm in diameter distal to the lesion. **D,** there was 25% stenosis 5 months after stent placement. The stent struts are faintly seen (*arrows*). A layer of myointimal tissue covers the stent without resulting in a substantial restenosis. Hypertension remains under markedly better control than before renal PTA and stent placement. (Courtesy of Rees CR, Palmaz JC, Becker GJ, et el: *Radiology* 181:507–514, 1991.)

Intravascular Stents in the Management of Superior Vena Cava Syndrome

Solomon N, Wholey MH, Jarmolowski CR (Shadyside Hosp, Pittsburgh)

Cathet Cardiovasc Diagn 23:245–252, 1991   2–6

Introduction.—The signs and symptoms of superior vena cava (SVC) syndrome include edema of the head, neck, and upper extremities; headache; cyanosis of the upper body; dyspnea; pleural effusions; and the development of numerous superficial venous collateral vessels. Malignancy is the most common cause of SVC syndrome, whereas benign masses, mediastinal fibrosis, aortic aneurysm, and iatrogenic consequences of indwelling central venous lines are less common etiologies. Superior vena cava syndrome can be effectively palliated by placement of intravas-

Clinical Response

Patient	Resolved	Recurrence	SVC syndrome at death	Survival post-stent (days)
1	Partial (1)[a]	No	Partial	17
2	Yes	No	No	73
3	Yes	Yes (twice) (2)[b]	No	103
4	Yes	Yes (3)[c]	No	54
5	Yes	No	No	22
6	Yes	No	Alive	18

[a] Improved but persistent head and neck edema.
[b] Thrombosis of stent requiring percutaneous thrombectomy and PTA.
[c] SVC compression below stent requiring repeat PTA.
(Courtesy of Solomon N, Wholey MH, Jarmolowski CR: *Cathet Cardiovasc Diagn* 23:245–252, 1991.)

cular stents, but thrombolytic therapy and balloon angioplasty may be tried before stent placement.

Patients.—Intravascular stent placement for palliation was carried out in 6 patients with SVC syndrome caused by an underlying malignancy. All 6 patients had been evaluated with a venogram from the femoral or the basilic vein approach. Four patients were given 100,000 units of urokinase per hour for 15–24 hours. During urokinase infusion, systemic fibrinolysis was monitored by serial measurement of fibrinogen, fibrin degradation products, prothrombin time, partial prothrombin time, complete blood counts, and platelet counts performed every 4–6 hours. Urokinase was infused via the basilic vein in 1 patient and from the femoral vein in 2 patients. After urokinase therapy, percutaneous transluminal angioplasty (PTA) at the obstruction site was performed first with an 8-mm, 3-cm balloon dilatation catheter, and then with successive dilatations using a 10-mm, 4-cm balloon in 2 patients and successive 12-mm and 15-mm valvuloplasty balloon catheters in another patient. A stent measuring 3 cm in length and 3 mm in external collapsed diameter was preloaded on a 7 French, 8-mm, 3-cm balloon catheter and then placed across the entire lesion to ensure adequate flow dynamics.

Outcome.—Five patients had complete resolution of their symptoms, and 1 had partial resolution (table). Two patients who had initial complete resolution had recurrences. One recurrence involved rethrombosis of the superior vena cava, which occurred twice and required percutaneous thrombectomy; the other recurrence involved restenosis requiring PTA of the SVC just distal to the stent. Both patients again had complete resolution of their symptoms after these second procedures.

Conclusion.—Intravascular stents are a valuable additional palliative treatment for patients with SVC syndrome.

▶ Contrary to my comments in Abstract 2–5, I am convinced that the judicious use of stents has a definite role in the palliation of patients with advanced malignancy and associated major venous obstruction. At our own institution, we have had a favorable experience similar to that reported in this article.—J.M. Porter, M.D.

Venous Stenoses in Patiens Who Undergo Hemodialysis: Treatment With Self-Expandable Endovascular Stents

Quinn SF, Schuman ES, Hall L, Gross GF, Uchida BT, Standage BA, Rosch J, Ivancev K (Good Samaritan Hosp, Portland, Ore; Oregon Health Sciences Univ, Portland; Naval Hosp, San Diego; Univ of Lund, Sweden)

Radiology 183:499–504, 1992   2–7

Background.—Surgical extension of vascular grafts is limited, and the results of angioplasty for venous stenoses have been so poor that some centers have abandoned the procedure. An alternative is to use an endovascular stent in a difficult stenosis.

Methods.—During a 32-month period, 25 modified, self-expandable endovascular stents were placed in 20 hemodialysis access sites in 19 patients. Twenty-one stenoses and 4 occlusions were managed by endovascular stenting. The stenoses were initially dilated using a high-pressure balloon.

Results.—Successful results were initially achieved in 18 of the 20 access sites. The stents were patent after a mean follow-up of 309 days. At 2 years, the primary patency rate was 25%; the secondary rate was 34%; and the tertiary rate was 42%. Morbidity occurred in 15% of the patients and there was 1 death. All complications (including the death, which was secondary to sepsis) occurred before the use of antibiotic prophylaxis and before the technique was refined. The results were best when a large vein without an acute angle, located away from venous confluences, was involved.

Conclusion.—Endovascular stents may be useful for treating large-vessel stenoses and occlusions at some anatomical sites, but their use at more common sites of stenosis is less well established.

▶ Although venous stents are of clear value in the treatment of large vein stenosis, especially when short-term palliation is the goal, they appear to be of limited value in the treatment of venous stenosis associated with hemodialysis shunts.—J.M. Porter, M.D.

Surveillance for Recurrent Stenosis After Endovascular Procedures: A Prospective Study

Miller BV, Sharp WJ, Shamma AR, Kresowik TF, Petrone S, Corson JD (Univ of Iowa, Iowa City)

Arch Surg 126:867–872, 1991 2–8

Introduction.—A prospective series of 89 endovascular procedures, performed during a 1-year period for chronic lower extremity ischemia, included 50 balloon angioplasties, 32 laser-assisted balloon angioplasties, and 7 atherectomies. The indication was claudication in 65.2% of the cases, critical ischemia in 30.3%, and a failing bypass in 4.5%.

Methods.—The segmental limb pressures were recorded preoperatively, and color duplex ultrasonography was done. The ankle-arm index was estimated postoperatively, and color duplex examination was performed at 1-week, 1-month, and then 3-month intervals. All levels of aortoiliac and infrainguinal disease were treated in these patients.

Results.—Immediate technical success was achieved in 89.8% of the patients, and life-table analysis showed a 9-month patency rate of 45.4% (Fig 2–3).

Conclusion.—Endovascular procedures are followed by restenosis in a significant proportion of cases. Critical assessment of these procedures is appropriate. The trend of treating patients with angiographically detected lesions without regard to the patients' symptomatic status is condemned.

▶ After endovascular therapy, a large number of patients with lower extremity symptoms were followed carefully by a group of observant surgeons. Despite the fact that two thirds of these procedures are performed for claudica-

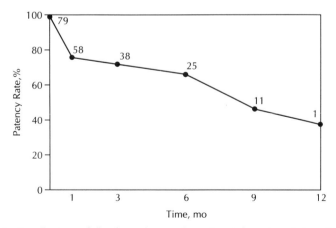

Fig 2–3.—Overall patency of all endovascular procedures attempted on primary lesions. (Courtesy of Miller BV, Sharp WJ, Shamma AR, et al: *Arch Surg* 126:867–872, 1991.)

tion only, a 9-month primary patency rate of only 45.4% was achieved. The authors appropriately advise restraint concerning the general acceptance of endovascular procedures. I agree. I continue to believe that there is far less to the entire field of endovascular intervention than what meets the eye.—J.M. Porter, M.D.

The Development of an Infected False Aneurysm Following Iliac Angioplasty
Cooper JC, Woods DA, Spencer P, Procter AE (Northern Gen Hosp, Sheffield, England)
Br J Radiol 64:759–760, 1991   2–9

Introduction.—Percutaneous transluminal angioplasty used for the treatment of peripheral vascular disease is relatively safe.

Case Report.—Man, 39, with a 4-year history of claudication in both legs underwent right transfemoral arteriography, which revealed 2 localized stenoses of the right external iliac artery and occlusion of the left superficial femoral artery. He underwent angioplasty to the 2 iliac stenoses and was discharged without complications. Two weeks later, he was readmitted with malaise, pyrexia, and increasingly severe pain in the right iliac fossa. Arteriography demonstrated a false aneurysm at the angioplasty site (Fig 2–4). Laparotomy revealed a 2-cm longitudinal split in the artery, with an associated infected false aneurysm. The arterial tear was repaired, and the aneurysm was ligated. After closure of the abdo-

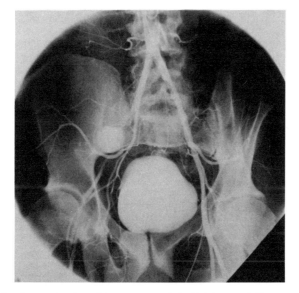

Fig 2–4.—Arteriogram showing a false aneurysm of the (right) external iliac artery. (Courtesy of Cooper JC, Woods DA, Spencer P, et al: *Br J Radiol* 64:759–760, 1991.)

men, a left-to-right femorofemoral crossover graft was performed. Recovery was uneventful.

Remark.—This apparently is the first reported case of an infected false aneurysm after angioplasty, and it is only the fifth report of a post-angioplasty false aneurysm.

▶ Isn't it remarkable that false aneurysms do not occur more frequently after balloon angioplasty?—J.M. Porter, M.D.

Septic Endarteritis of the Femoral Artery Following Angioplasty
Frazee BW, Flaherty JP (Univ of Chicago)
Rev Infect Dis 13:620–623, 1991   2–10

Introduction.—A patient who had septic endarteritis of the femoral artery after percutaneous transluminal coronary angioplasty was evaluated. Nine previously reported patients were reviewed.

Findings.—*Staphylococcus aureus* was the causative organism in all patients. Endarteritis developed in each case after repeat angioplasty or a repuncture (a second catheterization at the same site for diagnostic purposes). All patients were bacteremic, and most had formation of a pseudoaneurysm. Half the patients had distal embolism. Five of 6 evaluable patients had regional septic arthritis or osteomyelitis. The patients received antibiotics for 4–6 weeks and also had surgery—most often resection of the pseudoaneurysm and vascular bypass.

Recommendations.—Patients undergoing a percutaneous transluminal coronary angioplasty in the lower extremity should be watched for signs of septic endarteritis if repeated arterial catheterizations are performed. If a repeat arterial puncture is necessary, the other leg is preferable. Antibiotic prophylaxis should be used.

▶ These authors report on a worrisome group of 10 patients in whom septic endarteritis of the femoral artery developed after percutaneous transluminal coronary angioplasty. I wonder how many more of these patients have never been reported?—J.M. Porter, M.D.

Ultrasonic Energy: Effects on Vascular Function and Integrity
Fischell TA, Abbas MA, Grant GW, Siegel RJ (Stanford Univ Med Ctr, Stanford, Calif; Cedars-Sinai Med Ctr, Los Angeles)
Circulation 84:1783–1795, 1991   2–11

Background.—Delivery of ultrasonic energy by a flexible wire probe is a new approach to ablating atherosclerotic plaque. A perfused whole-vessel model, the rabbit thoracic aorta, was used to study the effects of ultrasonic energy at a level of 20 kHz.

Methods.—Energy was transmitted to vascular target sites using a ball-tipped titanium wire probe. The power output ranged from .7 to 5.5 W × 60 seconds, 42–230 joules. The effects of ultrasound energy on arterial vasomotor behavior were studied by long-axis ultrasonic imaging after precontraction with phenylephrine or KC1. In addition, plaque ablation was carried out in iliofemoral arteries obtained from human cadavers.

Results.—Ultrasonic energy produced dose-dependent relaxation in precontracted rabbit aortas, whether endothelium was present or not. The vessel wall warmed by less than 1°C with as much as 2 minutes of treatment at 5.5 W. No smooth muscle injury was found at power outputs that relaxed the vessels. Totally occluded iliofemoral vessel segments were recanalized by probe-tip power outputs of 2.9–5.5 W.

Implications.—Ultrasonic ablation of atherosclerotic disease is a relatively tissue-selective approach. The effects of mechanical ablation are much more marked in noncompliant arterial segments than in normal segments. The relaxing effect of ultrasonic energy may make this method especially safe when used in the coronary circulation.

▶ Transmission of ultrasound energy directly to a vascular target via a intraluminal wire probe is new to me. The authors' remarkable observation that such energy transfer at moderate power level results in vasodilatation, which apparently is unrelated to either muscle-cell injury or thermal effect, may have important therapeutic implications. Further information in this interesting area is awaited.—J.M. Porter, M.D.

Limitations of Balloon Angioplasty for Vein Graft Stenosis
Whittemore AD, Donaldson MC, Polak JF, Mannick JA (Brigham and Women's Hosp and Harvard Med School, Boston)
J Vasc Surg 14:340–345, 1991   2–12

Background.—A considerable number of autogenous infrainguinal reconstructions fail because of vein graft stenosis—most often developing near anastomoses. Fibrous intimal hyperplasia presumably is the cause. Percutaneous transluminal balloon angioplasty has been proposed as an alternative to surgical revision in the treatment of vein graft stenosis.

Series.—Balloon angioplasty was carried out in 30 patients with 54 stenotic lesions that had developed in autogenous vein grafts after infrainguinal arterial reconstruction.

Results.—The primary cumulative 5-year patency rate was 18% (Fig 2–5) and was not related to the length of the stenotic lesion or the need for initial thrombolytic treatment. When a single angioplasty sufficed,

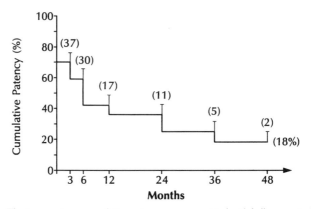

Fig 2–5.—The 4-year primary cumulative patency curve associated with balloon angioplasty for vein graft stenoses. (Courtesy of Whittemore AD, Donaldson MC, Polak JF, et al: *J Vasc Surg* 14:340–345, 1991.)

59% of the patients had a patent reconstruction at 3 years, compared with only 6% when repeated dilation was necessary.

Conclusion.—Balloon angioplasty is not a consistently effective means of providing long-term secondary patency when vein graft stenosis complicates infrainguinal arterial reconstruction.

▶ This study makes the point that angioplasty is not an effective means for correcting stenosis in vein grafts. The reason that this form of reconstruction performs less well than simple vein patch grafting is unclear (1). However, it should also be noted that angioplasty works less well in the superficial femoral arteries than it does in the higher flow vessels. The observation supports the conclusion that some form of pharmacologic, as opposed to surgical, therapy is needed for the correction of intimal hyperplasia and stenoses in blood vessels.—F.W. LoGerfo, M.D.

Reference

1. Whittemore AD, et al: *Ann Surg* 193:35, 1981.

3 Vascular Lab and Imaging

Effects of Ionic and Nonionic Radiographic Contrast Agents on Endothelial Cells In Vitro

Owens MR, Ribes JA, Marder VJ, Francis CW (Univ of Rochester School of Medicine and Dentistry, Rochester, NY)

J Lab Clin Med 119:315–319, 1992   3–1

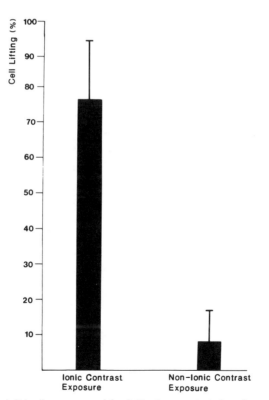

Fig 3–1.—Endothelial cells were exposed for 5-10 minutes to ionic (ioxaglate meglumine or diatrizoate meglumine) or nonionic (iohexol) contrast agents, then assessed for "cell lifting" by microscopic examination. Cell lifting after exposure to ionic contrast was significantly greater (P < .005). (Courtesy of Owens MR, Ribes JA, Marder VJ, et al: *J Lab Clin Med* 119:315-319, 1992.)

Background.—Adverse effects such as local pain and venous thrombosis reportedly are less frequent when newer, more expensive nonionic contrast agents are used in place of ionic materials.

Methods.—The effects of diatrizoate meglumine, iohexol, and ioxaglate meglumine or endothelial cells were examined in vitro by exposing cultured human umbilical vein cells to undiluted contrast media for 5–10 minutes. Exposed cells were examined microscopically for "cell lifting" (Fig 3–1).

Results.—Exposure of the cells to ionic contrast medium for 10 minutes led to lifting of 76% of the cells, compared with lifting of only 6% of those exposed to nonionic medium. In studying the adhesion of platelets in anticoagulated whole blood to everted segments of rabbit aorta, exposure of fresh vessels to ionic contrast medium increased platelet adhesion significantly (Fig 3–2). Greater adhesion was seen using stored vessels and, in this instance, contrast exposure did not increase adhesion further.

Conclusion.—These findings suggest that exposing endothelial cells to ionic contrast medium either alters their surface properties or exposes the intercellular matrix, which leads to platelet adhesion. These effects may contribute to the thrombotic potential of these agents.

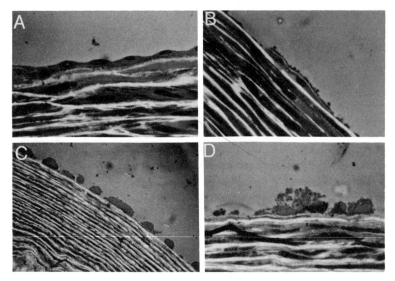

Fig 3–2.—The composite photomicrograph shows **A,** intact endothelial cells on the surface of a fresh, perfused aorta segment with no platelets attached. **B,** platelets attached to the endothelial cell surface and to the subendothelium of fresh vessel exposed to ionic contrast medium before perfusion. **C,** platelet clumps on the surface of a perfused, stored aortic segment. **D,** multiple platelet aggregates/thrombi covering the surface of a perfused, stored vessel. (Courtesy of Owens MR, Ribes JA, Marder VJ, et al: *J Lab Clin Med* 119:315–319, 1992.)

▶ These authors report that the old-fashioned ionic contrast agents have direct toxic effects on endothelial cells and increased platelet deposition compared with the newer, much more expensive nonionic contrast agents. Although these results are interesting, their clinical significance is uncertain, especially in light of the material presented in Abstract 3–2.—J.M. Porter, M.D.

Contrast Media-Related Thromboembolic Risks: Effects of Blood Mixed With Contrast Media in Contact With Angiographic Catheters
Corot C, Belleville J, Amiel M, Eloy R (Hôpital Pneumo-Cardiologique, Lyon, France)
Semin Hematol 28:54–59, 1991   3–2

Introduction.—Recent clinical studies have suggested that nonionic contrast media can produce an increased number of coronary occlusions during percutaneous transluminal coronary angioplasty.

Methods.—Generation of fibrinopeptide A (FpA) was examined in vitro with 5 different contrast media. In addition, 10 patients received injections of 50 mL of either ioxaglate (ionic) or iopamidol (nonionic) low-osmolality contrast media through a pigtail catheter in the pulmonary artery; after 10 minutes, the catheter was removed and examined.

Results.—The results of the FpA generation test are shown in Figure 3–3, which shows high FpA generation with the nonionic contrast media. Catheters exposed to ioxaglate had protein deposits and isolated platelets or small aggregates, but they had no formation of fibrin or

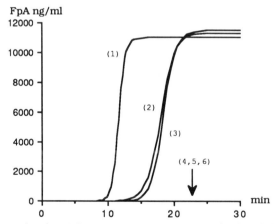

Fig 3–3.—The results of an FpA generation test on nonanticoagulated whole blood: theoretical sigmoid curves. The number *1*, indicates sodium chloride, .9%; *2*, iopamidol; *3*, Iohexol; *4*, Ioxaglate; *5*, Ioxitalamate; *6*, Diatrizoate. (Courtesy of Corot C, Belleville J, Amiel M, et al: *Semin Hematol* 28:54–59, 1991.)

thrombus. Those exposed to iopamidol exhibited platelet aggregates with intense fibrin formation and the presence of red cells.

Conclusion.—The use of nonionic low-osmolality contrast medium is a risk factor for thrombosis. A rigorous clinical trial comparing different contrast media used by the same radiologist (using identical catheters) is needed.

▶ These authors performed clinical studies examining FpA generation; they conclude that, compared with the old-fashioned ionic media, the nonionic contrast media present an increased risk for thrombosis in patients. A number of studies have now shown that the use of nonionic contrast media is associated with a clear increase in the incidence of coronary occlusion during percutaneous transluminal coronary angioplasty. The same must occur in peripheral arteriography (1).—J.M. Porter, M.D.

Reference

1. Eloy R, et al: *Clin Materials* 7:89, 1991.

A Modified Technique of Pre-Operative Aortography to Demonstrate the Complete Arterial Tree of the Lower Limb
Aston NO, Thomas ML, Burnand KG (St Thomas' Hosp, London)
J Cardiovasc Surg 32:360–365, 1991   3–3

Background.—The decision to reconstruct distal vessels cannot be made preoperatively without adequate arteriographic studies. Intraoperative arteriography increases operative time and, for technical reasons, may be of limited value. A modified technique of aortography that was designed to visualize the entire arterial tree was evaluated in 100 patients consecutively referred for aortography.

Methods.—The patients, who were being considered for their first arterial reconstruction, included 78 men and 22 women (mean age, 64 years and 63 years, respectively). The most frequent symptom was moderate claudication. Single-plane anteroposterior views were taken using translumbar aortography. Modifications to the standard technique included the use of a long injection time, 100 mL of iopamidol 370 at nearly 10 mL/sec; prolonged filming for approximately 30 sec; 3 films at 1 film/sec of ileofemoral, popliteal, and calf arteries; and multiple exposures of the feet, approximately 10 films at 1 film/sec. There were no complications or adverse reactions. Nearly 20% of the patients required a second injection identical to the first.

Results.—The aortograms were used to classify 18 limbs as having aortoiliac disease, 103 as having superficial femoral disease, 28 as having combined segment disease, and 51 as having generalized disease. The calf and ankle arteries were visualized in 98% of the limbs, and patency of the pedal arch was established in 92%. Most examination failures occurred in patients with combined segment disease, 14% of whom did not have visualization of the pedal arch.

Conclusion.—A modified aortographic technique is described, by which the entire arterial tree—from the aorta to the foot—can be demonstrated in most limbs with symptomatic chronic atherosclerotic disease. Using this technique, the surgeon can plan most peripheral vascular reconstructions without intraoperative arteriography. Successful bypass is not precluded by an incomplete pedal arch, but a patent complete arch does indicate the potential for long-term patency.

▶ High-quality arteriography with clear visualization of all arteries from the groin to the toe is mandatory for high-quality vascular surgery. Using a multitude of techniques (e.g., drugs, reactive hyperemia, hyperthermia, etc.), skilled angiographers should routinely obtain such studies in more than 95% of all patients. If you are continually faced with arteriograms with poor visualization below the knee and/or the need for intraoperative arteriography to define your operative target, then you do not have the right angiographers.—J.M. Porter, M.D.

Duplex Ultrasound Criteria for Diagnosis of Splanchnic Artery Stenosis or Occlusion

Moneta GL, Yeager RA, Dalman R, Antonovic R, Hall LD, Porter JM (Oregon Health Sciences Univ and VA Med Ctr, Portland)
J Vasc Surg 14:511–520, 1991   3–4

Background.—Duplex ultrasound scanning seems to be a promising means of detecting splanchnic artery stenosis and occlusion in patients with symptoms of chronic intestinal ischemia, but specific criteria are lacking.

Methods.—Mesenteric artery duplex scans and infradiaphragmatic lateral aortograms were acquired in 34 patients who had significant large artery atherosclerotic changes on angiography.

Results.—Ten superior mesenteric arteries and 16 celiac arteries exhibited at least 70% stenosis on angiography. Analysis of receiver-operator-characteristic (ROC) curves suggested that duplex-derived peak systolic velocity accurately predicted the presence of significant arterial stenosis. (Fig 3–4). Either a peak systolic velocity $\geq$ 275 cm/sec in the superior mesenteric artery or a lack of a flow signal predicted significant stenosis with a sensitivity of 89% and a specificity of 92%. A peak velocity of 200 cm/sec or more in the celiac artery was 75% sensitive and 89% specific for significant stenosis. The addition of end-diastolic velocity or calculated velocity ratio did not enhance predictions of splanchnic artery stenosis.

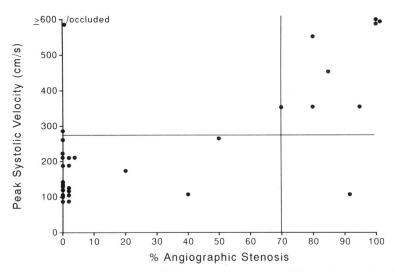

Fig 3–4.—Superior mesenteric artery (SMA) peak systolic velocities (PSV) as a function of angiographic stenosis in patients with visualization of their SMA by both angiography and duplex scanning, ($R = .68, P = .0001$ for angiographically patent SMAs). Note that the angiographic occlusions successfully identified by duplex scanning are positioned at the extreme upper right of the figure. The *horizontal line* indicates the proposed PSV (275 cm/sec) for detecting a $\geq$ 70% angiographic stenosis (*vertical line*) (Courtesy of Moneta GL, Yeager RA, Dalman R, et al: *J Vasc Surg* 14:511–520, 1991.)

Conclusion.—Patients whose peak systolic velocities are normal require no further assessment if the splanchnic vessels are well visualized. If duplex scanning identifies a high-grade lesion and appropriate symptoms are present, then angiography should be done. If the findings are equivocal and there is a normal to low-normal mesenteric peak systolic velocity, a postprandial study may be helpful.

▶ Visceral ischemia undoubtedly has been grossly underdiagnosed in the past. I believe the future of earlier diagnosis rests in the vascular laboratory; however, accurate testing requires experience and dedicated technologists. The development of precise criteria for duplex diagnosis is now occurring. A prospective validation of the criteria in this article was presented at the June, 1992 meeting of The Society for Vascular Surgery.—J.M. Porter, M.D.

A New Approach for Three-Dimensional Reconstruction of Arterial Ultrasonography
Franceschi D, Bondi JA, Rubin JR (University Hosps of Cleveland; Case Western Reserve Univ, Cleveland)
J Vasc Surg 15:800–805, 1992   3–5

Objective.—A computerized method was developed to create realistic 3-dimensional arterial images from 2-dimensional contiguous ultrasound

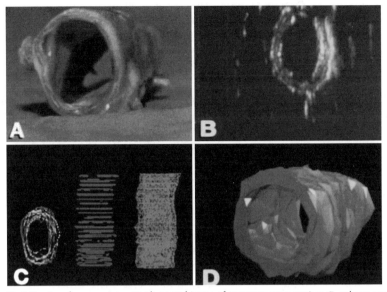

Fig 3–5.—**A,** cadaver specimen; **B,** ultrasound image of transverse cross section; **C,** polygon vectors "stacked" after edge tracing. Wireframe is produced by connecting contours with polygons. **D,** final 3-dimensional reconstruction. The model depicted consists of 1,796 polygons with 6,201 edges. (Courtesy of Franceschi D, Bondi JA, Rubin JR: *J Vasc Surg* 15:800–805, 1992.)

scan slices. The method was evaluated by performing 3-dimensional reconstructions of cadaver arteries.

Technique.—Images are digitized into a computer with a resolution of 512 × 480 pixels and a dynamic range of 8 bits/pixel (256 gray scale). After edge enhancement using convolution filters, the intraluminal and outer edges are traced and converted to a polygon vector within a defined 3-dimensional space. Serial cuts made 2 mm apart from each other are "stacked" into a 3-dimensional model, interpolating polyhedra between slices.

Results.—Three-dimensional reconstructions were made of 16 normal and arteriosclerotic distal aortas and common iliac arteries from fresh cadavers. The anatomically accurate reconstructions conveyed detailed surface information (Fig 3–5). Excellent correlation with gross observations was found when diameter, area, residual lumen, and percent stenosis were analyzed.

Conclusion.—This 3-dimensional reconstructive method is a reliable means of reproducing anatomical vascular findings.

▶ The near-term future of many imaging studies, including ultrasound, CT, and MRI, appears to be 3-dimensional image reconstruction. I am uncertain whether 3-dimensional image reconstruction is more of a novelty or a real assistance in vascular diagnosis.—J.M. Porter, M.D.

Comparison of Colour Doppler Ultrasound With Venography in the Diagnosis of Axillary and Subclavian Vein Thrombosis

Baxter GM, Kincaid W, Jeffrey RF, Millar GM, Porteous C, Morley P (Western Infirmary, Glasgow)

Br J Radiol 64:777–781, 1991   3–6

Background.—Encouraging results have been achieved using B-mode ultrasound with duplex ultrasonography to detect central venous occlusion. Color Doppler ultrasonography has proved advantageous in diagnosing venous thrombosis in the lower extremity. Therefore, this approach was compared with venography.

Patients and Methods.—Nineteen patients undergoing long-term renal dialysis were studied prospectively because of signs and symptoms, including intermittent edema, pain, and venous distension, in 30 upper extremities. In all but 5 patients, 2 or more central venous lines had been placed via the subclavian vein. The mean patient age was 52 years. Color Doppler ultrasonography and venography were done within 2 hours of each other.

Results.—Venography showed thrombosis in 8 extremities: subclavian vein thrombosis in 6 patients (combined with axillary vein thrombosis in 3) and isolated innominate venous thrombosis in 2. The superior vena cava was visible in only half the positive cases. The innominate vein was thrombosed in 2 of 4 patients in whom it was seen. Color Doppler ultrasonography missed one case of subclavian venous stenosis, but it made the primary diagnosis in all 8 patients with thrombosis. The innominate and internal jugular veins were consistently visualized. Ultrasonography was 89% sensitive and 100% specific for occlusion and stenosis combined.

Conclusion.—Color Doppler ultrasonography appears to be as accurate as venography in diagnosing axillary and subclavian thrombosis. It is noninvasive, involves no radiation exposure, and is less costly than venography.

▶ For several years, we have made our treatment decisions concerning lower extremity venous thrombosis entirely on the basis of duplex examinations, but we have been unwilling to do so in cases of upper extremity venous thrombosis, because reports have indicated that upper extremity duplex ultrasonography for venous thrombosis is relatively inaccurate. This careful study from Scotland shows very high accuracy with color duplex ultrasonography used in the diagnosis of axillary subclavian vein thrombosis. This has been our experience in the past year, and we are beginning to accept color duplex ultrasonography as a substitute for phlebography in the diagnosis of axillary subclavian venous thrombosis.—J.M. Porter, M.D.

Role of Transoesophageal Echocardiography in Evaluation of Cardiogenic Embolism
Black IW, Hopkins AP, Lee LCL, Jacobson BM, Walsh WF (Prince Henry/Prince of Wales Hosps, Sydney, Australia)
Br Heart J 66:302–307, 1991   3–7

Objective.—Whether transesophageal echocardiography can help in the assessment of some patients who either are at risk of cardiac embolism or have had embolism was examined in a prospective series of 100 patients who also underwent transthoracic echocardiography.

Methods.—The transesophageal study was carried out using a 5-MHz single-plane phased-array transducer. A total of 63% of the patients were seen after cerebral ischemia or peripheral arterial embolism, 23 before percutaneous balloon dilation of the mitral valve, and 14 before electrical cardioversion of atrial fibrillation.

Results.—The transthoracic study demonstrated possible sources of embolism in 4 patients. Transesophageal echocardiography demonstrated a total of 59 potential sources in 45 patients; left atrial spontaneous echo contrast was the most common finding. Sixty-eight percent of the patients in fibrillation showed a potential source of embolism on transesophageal study, as did 19% of the patients in sinus rhythm. Cardioversion was done without embolism occurring in patients without left atrial thrombus. Mitral valve dilatation was not performed in 3 patients who were found to have large thrombi in the left atrial appendage.

Conclusion.—Transesophageal echocardiography is more sensitive in detecting potential sources of cardiogenic embolism than is transthoracic examination; it also is a safe procedure.

▶ Few tests in vascular surgery have been more futile in the search for a cardiac source of peripheral embolization than transthoracic echocardiography. Without question, transesophagel echocardiography represents a dramatic improvement in the search for a source of embolism. I am certain this test will have widespread clinical usefulness.—J.M. Porter, M.D.

Detection of the Source of Arterial Emboli by Transesophageal Echocardiography: A Case Report
Rubin BG, Barzilai B, Allen BT, Anderson CB, Sicard GA (Washington Univ, St Louis)
J Vasc Surg 15:573–577, 1992   3–8

Background.—The combined percentage of emboli of noncardiac origin and those of unknown origin has remained constant at approximately 15%. Noncardiac causes are being recognized more frequently, but so-called cryptogenic emboli are becoming rare. In 1 case of acute lower extremity ischemia caused by embolism, initial studies failed to re-

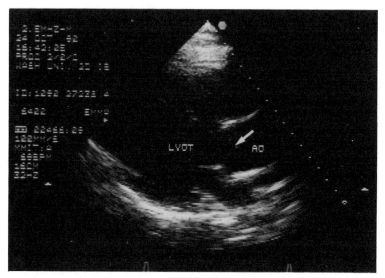

Fig 3–6.—A transthoracic echocardiographic (TTE) view of a region of aortic valve. The quality of the image is typical of resolution obtained on TTE. The left ventricular outflow tract (LVOT) and aorta (AO) are labeled, and the aortic valve leaflets are indicated (*arrow*). No valvular abnormalities were noted on this examination. (Courtesy of Rubin BG, Barzilai B, Allen BT, et al: *J Vasc Surg* 15:573–577, 1992.)

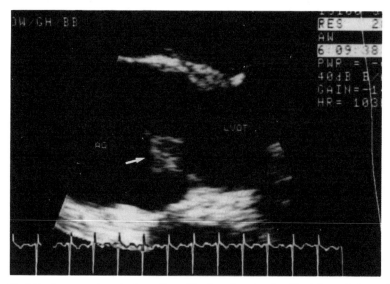

Fig 3–7.—A transesophageal echocardiographic view of aortic valve. The left ventricular outflow tract (LVOT) and aorta (AO) are indicated. The aortic valve is open, and a large echogenic mass (*arrow*) hanging off the inside of the valve cusp in the middle of the aortic flow lumen is easily seen. (Same area as depicted in Figure 3–6.) (Courtesy of Rubin BG, Barzilai B, Allen BT, et al: *J Vasc Surg* 15:573–577, 1992.)

veal the source, but subsequent transesophageal echocardiography demonstrated an aortic valve lesion.

Case Report.—Man, 49, had severe claudication in both calves and was found to have bilateral popliteal artery occlusions. Organized white material was removed from both vessels, and normal pulses returned. A standard transthoracic echocardiogram was interpreted as normal (Fig 3-6), but a transesophageal study demonstrated a mobile mass (size, 1 cm^2) on the right cusp of the aortic valve (Fig 3-7). Emergency valve replacement was carried out, and it yielded a friable mass that arose from an aortic valve leaflet and proved to be organized thrombus, as did the popliteal artery specimen.

Conclusion.—Transesophageal echocardiography is a sensitive measure that should be considered when a cardiac source of embolism is suspected, despite a normal transthoracic echocardiogram. It may be useful as the initial imaging study if embolism from the thoracic aorta is suspected.

▶ This case report clearly demonstrates the benefit of transesophageal echocardiography in the described patient.—J.M. Porter, M.D.

Effect of Temperature on Digital Systolic Pressures in Lower Limb in Arterial Disease

Sawka AM, Carter SA (Univ of Manitoba, Winnipeg; St Boniface Gen Hosp, Winnipeg, Man, Canada)
Circulation 85:1097–1101, 1992   3–9

Background.—The limitations of measuring ankle pressure have prompted interest in estimating systolic blood pressure in the toes, which reflect the overall obstruction of the extremity arteries down to the digits and are probably not affected by incompressibility of the tibial vessels. The digital pressures may, however, be influenced by temperature.

Methods.—A pneumatic cuff was used to measure systolic pressure in the great toe in 77 extremities with arteriosclerosis obliterans. Local temperature was altered by perfusing water through a cuff for 7 minutes. Flow was interrupted by a tourniquet to permit equilibration of the toe and water temperatures.

Results.—The mean toe pressure was significantly lower at a temperature of 10°C than it was during routine measurement or at 30°C (Fig 3-8). The pressure at 30°C was a mean of 10 mm Hg higher than during routine measurement, when the initial digital temperature was below 30°C, but not when it was higher.

Conclusion.—Falsely low systolic toe pressures may be recorded when toe temperature is low, probably because of delayed opening of the main digital arteries on deflation of the cuff. Measuring pressure at a

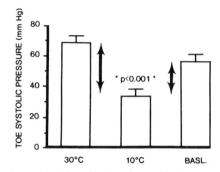

Fig 3–8.—Bar graphs showing the effect of local cooling and local warming on toe systolic pressure. *Abbreviation: BASL,* baseline. (Courtesy of Sawka AM, Carter SA: *Circulation* 85:1097–1101, 1992.)

warm local temperature will provide a more accurate assessment of the degree of arterial obstruction, and it possibly will provide a more accurate prediction of whether skin lesions will heal.

▶ This study indicates that an accurate measurement of great toe pressure can only be obtained when the toe temperature is at least 33°C. Before we use toe pressures in decision-making, such as prediction of wound healing, we must make certain that toe temperatures are in the required range when the toe pressure is measured.—J.M. Porter, M.D.

The Effect of Cooling on Toe Systolic Pressures in Subjects With and Without Raynaud's Syndrome in the Lower Extremities

Carter SA (Univ of Manitoba, Winnipeg, Man, Canada)
Clin Physiol 11:253–261, 1991   3–10

Introduction.—Previous studies have indicated that finger systolic pressures decrease precipitously during local and body cooling, especially in patients with vasospastic Raynaud's syndrome (RS). Such effects

Toe Systolic Pressures During Body Warming and Body Cooling

Group	Systolic pressure (mmHg)		
	Warming	Cooling	Difference
No Raynaud's syndrome	94 ± 4 (91)	71 ± 5 (67)	24 ± 4 (22)†
Raynaud's syndrome	79 ± 3 (78)*	21 ± 6 (8)*	58 ± 5 (62)*†

Note: The median values are shown in brackets.
* P <.01 from the group without Raynaud's syndrome.
† P <.01 from zero.
(Courtesy of Carter SA: *Clin Physiol* 11:253–261, 1991.)

of temperature on systolic pressures in the toes have not been reported previously. The effect of changes in local and body temperature on toe systolic pressures was examined in patients with RS and in normal controls.

Patients.—Toe systolic pressures were measured during local and body warming and cooling in 20 patients (age, 18–59 years) with RS of the toes and in 30 normal controls (age, 13–69 years). Half the patients with RS were women.

Results.—The systolic pressures were significantly lower in patients with RS under all experimental conditions (table). Pressures were significantly lower during body cooling than during body warming in both the patients and the controls. The mean decrease in pressure with body cooling was 58 mm Hg in patients with RS and 24 mm Hg in controls. During body cooling, toe pressures decreased to less than 30 mm Hg in 70% of the patients with RS, but in only 3% of the controls. Local cooling from 30°C to 10°C during body cooling resulted in a significant mean decrease in pressure of more than 40 mm Hg in both groups, with the toe pressure decreasing below 30 mm Hg in more than 90% of patients with RS and in 26% of normal controls.

Conclusion.—Body cooling and local temperature have an important role in the mechanism of vasospasm in the toes. This finding also has relevance to the diagnosis of RS in the lower extremities, in that erroneous low pressure values could be obtained in patients with arteriosclerotic occlusion whose feet are cold during the test.

▶ Not surprisingly, the toe pressure in patients with RS appears to decrease with cooling, just as finger pressure does. Patients with RS have a much greater decrease in toe pressure with cooling than do control patients. See also Abstract 3–9.—J.M. Porter, M.D.

Accuracy of Lower Extremity Arterial Duplex Mapping
Moneta GL, Yeager RA, Antonovic R, Hall LD, Caster JD, Cummings CA, Porter JM (Oregon Health Sciences Univ, Portland; Veterans Affairs Med Ctr, Portland, Ore)
J Vasc Surg 15:275–284, 1992   3–11

Objective.—A blinded, prospective study was undertaken in 150 patients referred for aortic and leg artery reconstruction to determine whether arterial duplex mapping of the lower extremity can supplement or possibly replace angiography.

Methods.—Starting at the aortic bifurcation, a 2- or 3-MHz probe was used to examine the common and external iliac vessels. The infrainguinal arteries were assessed using a 5-MHz transducer. Each lower extremity was classified on the basis of the history, physical findings, and 4-cuff segmental Doppler pressures.

TABLE 1.—Criteria for Clinical Classification of Lower
Extremity Arterial Occlusive Disease in Individual
Lower Extremities

Group	Clinical disease pattern	Criteria
A	No significant arterial occlusive disease	Palpable pedal pulse; ABI* ≥ 0.9
B	Aortoiliac (inflow) disease only	Diminished groin pulse; HTI † < 0.9; HTI ≤ ABI + 0.3
C	Infrainguinal (outflow) disease only ‡	Normal groin pulse; HTI ≥ 0.9 ABI < 0.9
D	Multilevel inflow and outflow disease ‡	Diminished groin pulse; HTI < 0.9 HTI ≥ ABI + 0.3

* ABI, ankle-brachial index (highest ankle Doppler-derived systolic pressure/highest brachial artery Doppler-derived systolic pressure).
† HTI, high thigh index (high-thigh Doppler-derived systolic pressure/highest brachial artery Doppler-derived systolic pressure).
‡ All patients with incompressible tibial arteries were classified as group C or D, depending on inflow status.
(Courtesy of Moneta GL, Yeager RA, Antonovic R, et al: *J Vasc Surg* 15:275–284, 1992.)

Results.—Eighty extremities lacked significant occlusive disease (group A, Table 1); 44 had aortoiliac disease; 117 had infrainguinal occlusive disease; and 45 had multilevel inflow and outfllow occlusive disease. All but 1% of the arterial segments that were seen angiographically proximal

TABLE 2.—Sensitivities, Specificities, Positive Predictive Values, and Negative Predictive Values for Duplex Scanning in Detecting a ≥ 50% Stenosis or Occlusion in Lower Extremity Arteries Proximal to the Tibial Vessels

Clinical group	Iliac	Common femoral	Deep femoral	Superficial femoral	Popliteal
A	100/100 *	− †	40/98	67/99	100/99
	100/100		67/95	80/98	80/100
B	94/100	82/100	100/97	77/99	− †
	100/92	100/94	83/100	91/96	
C	71/99	71/98	89/95	92/98	67/99
	83/98	71/98	80/97	99/91	96/92
D	92/98	80/100	83/97	78/97	69/96
	97/94	100/91	91/94	98/67	75/94
Total	89/99	76/99	83/97	87/98	67/99
	94/97	93/96	83/97	97/89	93/94

* Sensitivity/specificity positive predictive value/negative predictive value.
† Analysis not performed if fewer than 5 high-grade lesions are in a category.
(Courtesy of Moneta GL, Yeager RA, Antonovic R, et al: *J Vasc Surg* 15:275–284, 1992.)

to the tibial arteries were identified by duplex scanning, as were 91% of the angiographically visualized infrapopliteal artery segments. The pattern of clinical disease did not substantially influence the ability of duplex mapping to detect stenosis of 50% or greater in the iliofemoral-popliteal system (Table 2). The same was the case for more distal segments, except for the peroneal artery (Table 3).

Conclusion.—It soon will be appropriate to carry out prospective trials to determine when lower extremity arterial duplex mapping can substitute for angiography.

▶ I strongly suspect that, in the future, contrast arteriography and ionizing radiation will become almost a dinosaur in vascular imaging. This study shows that, even with today's technology, duplex mapping is sufficiently accurate to underlie decision-making in reference to lower extremity arterial occlusive disease. I suspect that the future will consist of MR for imaging and duplex mapping for flow data, and that the innovative combination of these 2 modalities will substantially replace contrast arteriography.—J.M. Porter, M.D.

TABLE 3.—Sensitivities, Specificities, Positive Predictive Values, and Negative Predictive Values of Duplex Scanning for Identifying Interruption of Tibial Artery Patency

Clinical group	Anterior tibial	Posterior tibial	Peroneal
A	80/85 *	− †	− †
	50/96		
B	100/100	100/100	100/72
	100/100	100/100	55/100
C	73/96	100/88	92/76
	92/85	76/100	73/94
D	73/89	63/92	60/61
	85/81	71/89	40/78
Total all groups	90/93	90/92	82/74
	84/88	77/97	62/90

* Sensitivity/specificity positive predictive value/negative predictive value.
† Analysis not performed for categories with fewer than 5 arteries with segmental or total occlusion.
(Courtesy of Moneta GL, Yeager RA, Antonovic R, et al: *J Vasc Surg* 15:275-284, 1992.)

Identifying Total Carotid Occlusion With Colour Flow Duplex Scanning

Mattos MA, Hodgson KJ, Ramsey DE, Barkmeier LD, Sumner DS (Southern Illinois Univ School of Medicine, Springfield)
Eur J Vasc Surg 6:204–210, 1992

3-12

Cumulative Data Comparing Conventional Duplex Scanning With
Arteriography for Detecting Total Internal Carotid Artery
Occlusion (8 Reports, 2,314 Arteries)

Duplex	Arteriography	
	Non-occlusion	Total occlusion
Non-occlusion	2076	23
Total occlusion	16	199

Notes: Sensitivity = 90%; specificity = 99%; positive predictive value = 93%; negative predictive value = 99%.
(Courtesy of Mattos MA, Hodgson KJ, Ramsey DE, et al: Eur J Vasc Surg 6:204-210, 1992.)

Background.—Conventional duplex scanning is unable to reliably distinguish between severe internal carotid stenosis and total occlusion. Color flow duplex scanning (CFS) helps in identifying internal and external carotid arteries, and it allows the simultaneous assessment of flow in multiple vessels in longitudinal and transverse views. Low Doppler-shift frquencies are accurately studied by using new "slow-flow" software technology.

Methods.—The internal carotid arteries were studied by CSF in 4,866 patients from July 1987 to January 1991. A total of 483 of these patients also underwent arteriography.

Results.—Color flow duplex scanning accurately differentiated total internal carotid occlusion from stenosis (table). All but 5 of 87 totally occluded vessels were detected by CFS, and the study was specific. The positive and negative predictive values were 93% and 99%, respectively. Most false positive results and all false negative results reflected interpreter error. In the last 2 years of the study, CFS was 100% accurate in distinguishing between carotid occlusion and stenosis.

Conclusion.—Color flow duplex scanning is a reliable noninvasive means of evaluating the internal carotid artery. It is the method of choice for studying the carotid bifurcation.

▶ This article raises a critically important point. A false positive duplex diagnosis of carotid occlusion, made when the patient actually has 99% stenosis, deprives the patient of the opportunity to have normal patency restored by an endarterectomy. We consider the potential consequence of an erroneous call in this area so significant that we routinely dictate such reports, including the statement: "The vascular laboratory cannot reliably differentiate between 99 percent stenosis and total occlusion. A contrast arteriogram is required for this differential and should be considered if warranted by clinical circumstances." We will continue to add this phrase until we establish a specificity in our laboratory of 100%, which is unlikely.—J.M. Porter, M.D.

Carotid Duplex Sonography: Bisferious Pulse Contour in Patients With Aortic Valvular Disease

Kallman CE, Gosink BB, Gardner DJ (VA Med Ctr, San Diego)
AJR 157:403–407, 1991   3–13

Introduction.—The bisferious waveform, defined as 2 distinct systolic peaks separated from a well-defined dicrotic notch, has been well described in direct pressure measurements from the brachiocephalic arteries of patients with significant aortic regurgitation; however, the presence of a bisferious pulse contour or retrograde diastolic flow has never been documented in the carotid duplex waveforms of patients with aortic valve disease. The presence of these carotid duplex waveform abnormalities in patients with known aortic valve disease was investigated, and the findings were correlated with the severity of valve regurgitation.

Patients.—The study population consisted of 25 men and 1 woman, aged 33–90 years, who had preoperative duplex carotid sonography and echocardiography before undergoing coronary artery bypass grafting or valve replacement. All patients had aortic regurgitation or combined aortic regurgitation and stenosis. The carotid duplex sonograms of 20 age-

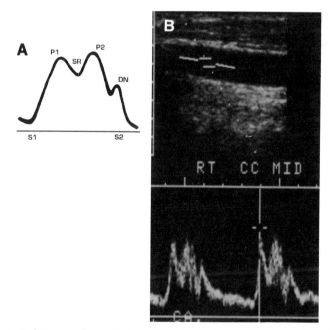

Fig 3–9.—Bisferious waveform with 2 systolic peaks. **A,** diagram shows 2 systolic peaks (P1, P2) separated by midsystolic retraction (SR). *Abbreviations:* DN, dicrotic notch; *S1,* first heart sound, caused by atrioventricular valves closing and pulmonic and aortic valves opening; *S2,* second heart sound, caused by aortic and pulmonic valves closing. **B,** duplex tracing of external carotid artery in man, 50, with moderate aortic regurgitation. (Courtesy of Kallman CE, Gosink BB, Gardner DJ: AJR 157:403–407, 1991.)

matched patients with a variety of cardiovascular diseases but no evidence of aortic valvular disease were also studied. The carotid duplex sonograms were examined by 2 radiologists for the presence of the bisferious waveform and diastolic flow reversal.

Results.—Thirteen patients (50%) with aortic regurgitation had bisferious waveforms on their carotid duplex sonograms (Fig 3–9), and 5 patients (19%) had significant retrograde diastolic flow. Three patients with retrograde diastolic flow also had bisferious waveforms. The other 2 patients had diastolic flow reversal without bisferious waveforms. In all, 15 patients (57%) had abnormal waveforms. Four patients with abnormal waveforms, who subsequently underwent aortic valve replacement, had normal waveforms after the operation. None of the 20 control patients had characteristic systolic or diastolic abnormalities.

Conclusion.—Because as many as one third of the patients with aortic regurgitation may not have a detectable murmur, carotid duplex sonography may be useful in identifying previously unsuspected aortic valvular disease.

▶ This is another important piece of information that may be detected by carotid duplex examination.—J.M. Porter, M.D.

Intravascular Ultrasound Assessment of the Renal Artery
Sheikh KH, Davidson CJ, Newman GE, Kisslo KB, Schwab SJ (Duke Univ, Durham, NC)
Ann Intern Med 115:22–25, 1991   3–14

Background.—Contrast angiography findings of atherosclerotic renal artery stenosis may overlap with those of fibromuscular dysplasia. Catheter-based intravascular ultrasound (US) imaging provides detailed real-time cross-sectional images of the arterial lumen and, unlike angiography, can image below the intimal surface. The results of intravascular US imaging in normal renal artery segments and in stenotic segments treated by percutaneous transluminal balloon angioplasty were studied.

Methods.—Renal artery segment images from 4 randomly selected normal subjects without known renal disease were compared with images from 4 patients with known renal artery stenosis before and after balloon angioplasty. Each patient was examined with digital angiography and with an intravascular ultrasound imaging system.

Results.—Digital angiography and ultrasonography were closely correlated in determining arterial lumen diameter and cross-sectional area (Fig 3–10). In normal segments, ultrasonography provided structural information on the normal arteries' intimal, medial, and adventitial wall layers that were not visualized by angiography (Fig 3–11). In 5 stenotic segments, ultrasonography and angiography attributed different numbers to atherosclerosis or fibromuscular dysplasia. After renal angioplasty, an-

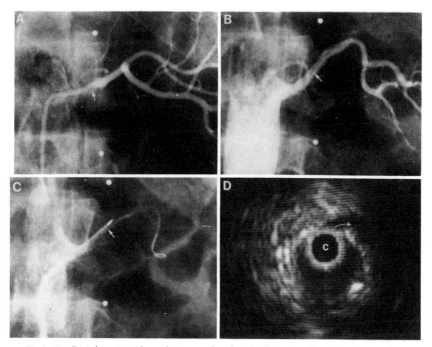

Fig 3–10.—Digital angiography and intravascular ultrasound imaging during renal angioplasty. **A,** angiogram before angiography showing atherosclerotic narrowing of the proximal left renal artery (*arrow*). **B,** angiogram after angiography indicating a dissection of the vessel wall (*arrow*) indicated by the radiolucent stripe in the vessel lumen. **C,** fluoroscopic image of the ultrasound catheter positioned within the arterial lumen. The ultrasound transducer (*arrow*) shows the point at which cross-sectional images are obtained. **D,** intravascular ultrasound image after angioplasty showing the dissection of the vessel wall (*arrow*) noted on the angiogram. (Courtesy of Sheikh KH, Davidson CJ, Newman GE, et al: *Ann Intern Med* 115:22–25, 1991.)

giography revealed 1 arterial dissection, but 3 were visualized with ultrasound.

Conclusion.—Catheter-based intravascular ultrasound imaging of the renal artery correlated well with renal angiography in assessing artery size. Ultrasonography provided structural information not obtainable by angiography alone, allowing better characterization of arterial pathology.

▶ Will intravascular ultrasound continue to be an interesting novelty, or will it become an important diagnostic tool?—J.M. Porter, M.D.

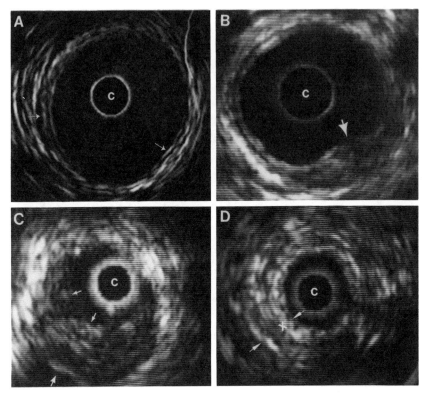

Fig 3–11.—Intravascular ultrasound images of renal arteries. **A,** normal renal artery with trilayered appearance. The ultrasound catheter is labeled C. The arterial lumen is echo-free and has a smooth interface with the arterial wall. The echogenic intimal layer, hypoechoic medial layer, and outer echogenic adventitial layers are indicated (*arrows*). **B,** renal artery with a minor degree of plaque (*arrow*). Intimal thickening in the region of plaque and in plaque-free areas is also present. The angiogram appeared normal. **C,** stenosis caused by atherosclerotic plaque. The predominantly hypoechoic plaque is demarcated by the 2 *inner arrows* that indicate the interface with the arterial lumen and the *outer arrow* that demarcates the arterial wall. **D,** stenosis caused by fibromuscular dysplasia. The interface of the intima with arterial lumen and the media with adventitia are indicated by arrows. *Abbreviation:* X indicates the intimal-medial interface. The intima and media are both echogenic, signifying elastin and collagen deposition in these arterial layers that is characteristic of fibromuscular dysplasia. (Courtesy of Sheikh KH, Davidson CJ, Newman GE, et al: *Ann Intern Med* 115:22–25, 1991.)

Sequential Intraluminal Ultrasound Evaluation of Balloon Angioplasty of an Iliac Artery Lesion

Tabbara MR, Mehringer CM, Cavaye DM, Schwartz M, Kopchok GE, Maselly M, White RA (Harbor-Univ of California Los Angeles Med Ctr, Torrance, Calif)
Ann Vasc Surg 6:179–184, 1992   3–15

Background.—Intravascular ultrasound imaging is emerging as an important method that can be used in conjunction with arteriography to assess arterial pathology. The method can accurately estimate the cross-

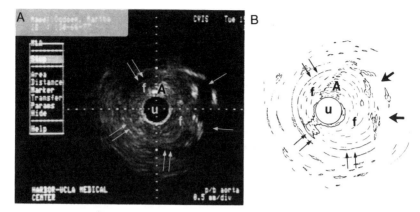

Fig 3–12.—**A,** intravascular ultrasound image and (**B**) artist's interpretation of the image of left iliac artery stenosis before dilation. The image is from the most narrow area of the angioplasty site, and it demonstrates calcification in the lesion (represented by bright echoes with shadowing beyond the site [*single arrows*]). *Double arrows* point to media of the artery wall. The vessel lumen is not easily visualized in this still photograph, because the intravascular ultrasound catheter occupies most of that space and is surrounded by soft echoes generated by a fibrous lesion (*f*). Structure identification was confirmed from dynamic images. A = images artifact produced by a wire on the side of the catheter for orienting images; *u* = ultrasound probe. The *dotted lines* at 90-degree intervals around the image enable calibration; *dots* are spaced .5 mm apart. (Courtesy of Tabbara MR, Mehringer CM, Cavaye DM, et al: *Ann Vasc Surg* 6:179–184, 1992.)

sectional area of the lumen and clearly define the morphology of the arterial plaque.

Case Report.—A 5F, 30-MHz intravascular ultrasound catheter used to image a localized 81% stenosis in the common iliac artery of a woman aged 52 years (Fig 3–12). The lesion was dilated using an 8-mm balloon, and it was imaged afterward by both arteriography (Fig 3–13) and ultrasonography (Fig 3–14). The same site was imaged again 2 months later, using an 8F, 20-MHz ultrasound catheter, when the patient underwent femoropopliteal bypass surgery. Sequential on-line calculations of the lesion's cross-sectional area and volume were acquired

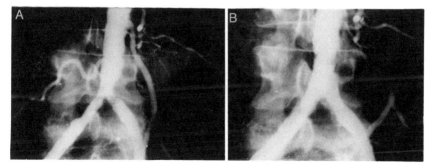

Fig 3–13.—Arteriograms of left iliac artery stenosis (**A**) before and (**B**) after balloon dilation. (Courtesy of Tabbara MR, Mehringer CM, Cavaye DM, et al: *Ann Vasc Surg* 6:179–184, 1992.)

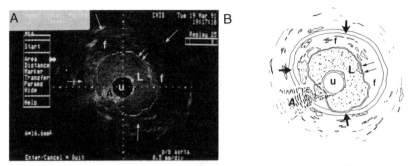

Fig 3–14.—**A,** an intravascular ultrasound image and (**B**) an artist's interpretation of the image of the most narrow part of stenosis after dilatation. The vessel wall is identified with *arrows*; fibrous plaque (*f*) is visible as soft echoes, and the vessel lumen is seen as a fine speckled pattern of echoes (L) generated by flowing blood. The lumen is outlined by a solid line (*double arrows*) produced on the image to enable calculation of the cross-sectional area. A = image artifact; *u* = ultrasound probe; *dots* are at .5-mm intervals. (Courtesy of Tabbara MR, Mehringer CM, Cavaye DM, et al: *Ann Vasc Surg* 6:179–184, 1992.)

by the ultrasound method. At the same time, the morphology of the fractured arterial plaque was clearly defined, and the distribution of calcification was visualized. Ultrasound imaging demonstrated intraluminal flaps that were not apparent on arteriography.

Conclusion.—Intraluminal ultrasonography can document the immediate and long-term effects of balloon angioplasty.

▶ Intravascular ultrasound confirms that the effects of balloon angioplasty appear to be similar to those of a bomb detonation within an artery. I am convinced that if vascular surgeons left an artery this mangled after arterial surgery, thrombosis would occur in 100% of patients. Undoubtedly the almighty, in her infinite wisdom, takes care of interventional radiologists.—J.M. Porter, M.D.

The Value of Duplex Scanning With Venous Occlusion in the Preoperative Prediction of Femoro-Distal Vein Bypass Graft Diameter
Davies AH, Magee TR, Jones DR, Hayward JK, Baird RN, Horrocks M (Bristol Royal Infirmary, Bristol, England)
Eur J Vasc Surg 5:633–636, 1991   3–16

Introduction.—The long saphenous vein is considered the best conduit for femorodistal vein bypass, but the minimum vein graft size that can safely be used and the effect of graft size on outcome are uncertain. A simple technique for predicting functional graft size was assessed in 35 patients who underwent femorodistal bypass, most of them for critical ischemia. Bypass extended to the distal popliteal artery in 14 patients and to the calf vessels in 21.

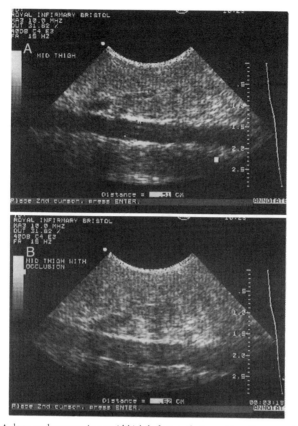

Fig 3–15.—**A,** long saphenous vein at midthigh before occlusion, with a diameter of 5.1 mm. **B,** a long saphenous vein occluded at 3 minutes, with a diameter of 6.2 mm. (Courtesy of Davies AH, Magee TR, Jones DR, et al: *Eur J Vasc Surg* 5:633–636, 1991.)

Methods.—The diameter of the long saphenous vein was determined preoperatively using a duplex scanner with a 10-MHz sector scanner head. The patients were examined lying on a couch at 15 degrees of reverse Trendelenberg tilt. Measurements were recorded at the groin, midthigh, and knee levels, and they were repeated with a cuff on the upper thigh inflated to 100 mm Hg for 3 minutes. The study was repeated at 1 week and at 2 months after surgery.

Results.—Scans demonstrating dilatation before and after vein occlusion are shown in Figure 3–15. Dilated vein diameter was a good predictor of functional graft size at both 1 week and 2 months after surgery (table). Dilatation occurred in all 5 patients whose measured vein diameter at the knee and mid-thigh was less than 3 mm.

Long Saphenous Vein Mean Diameter Measurements at the
Mid-Thigh and Knee

	Mean diameter (mm)			
	Non-dilated (mm)	Dilated (mm)	7 days (mm)	2 months (mm)
Mid-thigh	4.1 (2.5–8.0)	5.1 (3.2–8.4)	5.0 (3.0–9.1)	5.2* (3.4–8.9)
Knee	3.9 (1.2–7.2)	4.8 (3.1–8.0)	4.8 (3.3–7.9)	4.9** (3.3–8.0)

Note: Ranges in parentheses.
* Analysis of variance: P < .05.
† Analysis of variance P < .025.
(Courtesy of Davies AH, Magee TR, Jones DR, et al: Eur J Vasc Surg 5:633–636, 1991.)

Conclusion.—Hopefully, this simple method of predicting functional vein graft size will increase the rate of use of the long saphenous vein in reconstructive vascular surgery.

▶ We have found duplex scanning to be of value in directing vein harvest for bypass in selected patients, especially those with multiple redo procedures. Perhaps the technique described in this study will permit a more accurate preoperative assessment of vein size. Despite our ability to use veins less than 3 mm in diameter, I have found their use to be associated with a disturbingly high failure rate, and I have almost come to prefer prosthetics to veins of this size.—J.M. Porter, M.D.

Color-Flow Duplex Scanning for the Surveillance and Diagnosis of Acute Deep Venous Thrombosis

Mattos MA, Londrey GL, Leutz DW, Hodgson KJ, Ramsey DE, Barkmeier LD, Stauffer ES, Spadone DP, Sumner DS (Southern Illinois Univ, Springfield)
J Vasc Surg 15:366–376, 1992   3–17

Background.—Color-flow scanning more accurately identifies veins below the knee than conventional duplex imaging does, and it permits veins to be surveyed longitudinally. The accuracy of the technique for detecting acute deep venous thrombosis was examined.

Methods.—Both color-flow scanning and phlebography were performed prospectively in 77 extremities of 75 patients who were clinically suspected of having venous thrombosis. In addition, 190 limbs of 99 patients who were at high risk of having thrombosis postoperatively were assessed.

TABLE 1.—Incidence and Location of Deep Venous
Thrombosis by Patients According to Study Group

| | *No. (%) of patients with DVT in the specified segment* | | |
	Diagnostic (N = 75)	*Surveillance (N = 99)*	*p value*
Any segment	40 (53%)	42 (42%)	NS
AK	32 (43%)	3 (3%)	*p* < 0.001
BK	35 (47%)	41 (41%)	NS
CF	18 (24%)	1 (1%)	*p* < 0.001
SF	32 (43%)	3 (3%)	*p* < 0.001
POP	27 (36%)	9 (9%)	*p* < 0.001
TP	33 (44%)	39 (39%)	NS

Abbreviations: CF, common femoral; SF, superficial femoral; POP, popliteal; TP, tibioperoneal.
Percentages represent the number of patients with thrombi in the specified venous segment (or combination of segments) of either limb divided by the total number of patients in each study group.
(Courtesy of Mattos MA, Londrey GL, Leutz DW, et al: *J Vasc Surg* 15:366–376, 1992.)

Results.—Thrombi were about equally frequent above and below the knee in the diagnostic group, but they were far more frequent in below-knee veins in the surveillance group (Tables 1 and 2). The extent of thrombosis is shown in Table 3. Color-flow scanning was 100% sensitive and 98% specific above the knee in symptomatic patients, and it was

TABLE 2.—Incidence and Distribution of Deep Venous
Thrombosis by Limbs According to Study Group

| | *No. (%) of limbs with DVT in the specified segment* | | |
	Diagnostic (N = 77)	*Surveillance (N = 190)*	*p value*
Any segment	40 (52%)	44 (23%)	*p* < 0.001
AK	32 (42%)	3 (2%)	*p* < 0.001
BK	35 (47%)†	43 (23%)	*p* < 0.001
CF	18 (23%)	1 (0.5%)	*p* < 0.001
SF	32 (42%)	3 (2%)	*p* < 0.001
POP	27 (36%)†	9 (5%)	*p* < 0.001
TP	33 (44%)†	41 (22%)	*p* < 0.0003

Percentages represent the number of limbs with thrombi in the specified venous segment (or combination of segments) divided by the total number of limbs in each study group.
† Denominator N = 75, 2 limbs not studied below knee.
(Courtesy of Mattos MA, Londrey GL, Leutz DW, et al: *J Vasc Surg* 15:366–376, 1992.)

TABLE 3.—Extent of Thrombi in Limbs With Deep
Venous Thrombosis

	Diagnostic	Surveillance	p value
Occluding	58% (23/40)	11% (5/44)	p < 0.00002
Nonoccluding	42% (17/40)	89% (39/44)	p < 0.00002
Isolated			
AK	9% (3/32)	33% (1/3)	NS
BK	23% (8/35)	95% (41/43)	p < 0.001
TP	15% (5/33)	83% (34/41)	p < 0.001

(Courtesy of Mattos MA, Londrey GL, Leutz DW, et al: *J Vasc Surg* 15:366–376, 1992.)

94% sensitive and 75% specific below the knee. In the surveillance group, the study was only 55% sensitive in detecting thrombi—more than 90% of which were limited to the tibioperoneal veins. The study had negative predictive values of 100% for diagostic extremities and 88% for surveillance extremities. The positive predictive values were 80% for diagnostic extremities and 89% for surveillance extremities.

Conclusion.—Color-flow scanning is a highly accurate means of detecting thrombi above and below the knee in patients with symptomatic acute deep venous thrombosis. Below-knee thrombi are not as accurately identified in asymptomatic patients who are at risk of thrombosis, and the role of the study in this group of patients remains uncertain.

▶ Most of us have learned to pay careful attention to the comments of Dr. David Sumner, who is a very careful observer. I am convinced that most experienced vascular labs have achieved an accuracy in venous thrombosis diagnosis, both above and below the knee, that rivals contrast phlebography. However, Dr. Sumner and others point out that if we are doing population surveillance studies rather than deep venous thrombosis symptomatic diagnostic studies, below-knee accuracy decreases considerably. This is important information.—J.M. Porter, M.D.

Assessment of Normal and Abnormal Erectile Function: Color Doppler Flow Sonography Versus Conventional Techniques
Schwartz AN, Lowe M, Berger RE, Wang KY, Mack LA, Richardson ML (Univ of Washington, Seattle; Stevens Mem Hosp, Edmonds, Wash)
Radiology 180:105–109, 1991   3–18

Background.—The biophysical events that occur during erection were recently studied by duplex Doppler spectral waveform analysis. Color Doppler flow sonography was used to assess the cavernosal arteries and thus determine the systolic/diastolic velocities and spectral waveform changes before and during erection in men with normal and abnormal erectile function.

Methods.—The subjects were 10 healthy volunteers with normal erectile function and 39 patients with abnormal erectile function. Each subject underwent color Doppler flow imaging and spectral waveform analysis before and after intracorporal injection of papaverine and phentolamine mesylate.

Results.—The normal group showed a characteristic spectral waveform pattern corresponding to increased intracorporal pressure, with diastolic velocities being increased during early tumescence but later decreasing to 0. This pattern was not seen in patients who had abnormal arterial inflow, abnormal venous sinusoidal leakage, or both. The mean peak systolic velocity was lower in patients with abnormal arterial inflow. Waveforms progressed to—but not beyond—phase 1 or 2 in patients with severe venous sinusoidal incompetence; diastolic flow remained positive. In patients with both abnormal arterial inflow and abnormal venous sinusoidal outflow, the waveform changes reflected both processes.

Conclusion.—Color Doppler flow sonography can provide useful insights into normal and abnormal erectile function. Cavernosal arterial integrity and venous sinusoidal competence can be assessed noninvasively by analysis of peak diastolic/systolic velocities and waveforms, along with systolic occlusion pressures.

▶ Duplex sonography can provide important information concerning erectile function. I wonder, however, whether many vascular laboratories or vascular surgeons are engaged in the treatment of these patients.—J.M. Porter, M.D.

A Comparison of Transcranial Doppler and Cerebral Blood Flow Studies to Assess Cerebral Vasoreactivity

Dahl A, Lindegaard K-F, Russell D, Nyberg-Hansen R, Rootwelt K, Sorteberg W, Nornes H (Univ of Oslo)
Stroke 23:15–19, 1992   3–19

Introduction.—The value of transcranial Doppler ultrasonography for assessing cerebral vasoreactivity was examined in 43 patients whose symptoms suggested the presence of cerebrovascular disease.

Methods.—The findings on transcranial Doppler examination of the middle cerebral artery were compared with regional cerebral blood flow in the same territory. Flow was estimated by the radioxenon inhalation technique and by single-photon emission CT. Studies were repeated after intravenous injection of 1 g of acetazolamide.

Results.—The absolute increase in cerebral blood flow correlated significantly with the percent increase in velocity (Fig 3–16). Control limits were ascertained in healthy subjects (Tables 1 and 2). The 2 methods

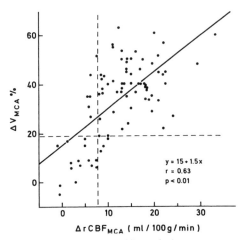

Fig 3–16.—Scatterplot of percent increase in middle cerebral artery time mean velocity (V_{MCA}) and absolute increase in regional cerebral blood flow in the corresponding perfusion territory ($rCBF_{MCA}$) after administration of acetazolamide in 43 patients (86 hemispheres). *Broken lines* show control limits (i.e., 5% fractile of controls). (Courtesy of Dahl A, Lindegaard K-F, Russell D, et al: *Stroke* 23:15–19, 1992.)

TABLE 1.—Regional Cerebral Blood Flow Values in 20 Controls

	Basal V_{MCA} (cm/sec)	Increase (%)	Range (%)	5% fractile (%)
Right V_{MCA}	63.6 (12.9)	33.4 (11.0)	18.3–53.0	19
Left V_{MCA}	63.7 (13.5)	34.6 (11.0)	18.6–53.3	19
Asymmetry in increase (right–left side)		−1.6 (7.6)	−14.5 to 12.5	−14, 12*

Note: Basal values, increase, and 5% fractile of increase in regional cerebral blood flow ($rCBF$) in the middle cerebral artery perfusion territory ($rCBF_{MCA}$) after administration of acetazolamide, 1 g. The values are mean, with SDs in *parentheses.*
* Represents the 95% fractile when subtracting increase on the left from the right side.
(Courtesy of Dahl A, Lindegaard K-F, Russell D, et al: *Stroke* 23:15–19, 1992.)

TABLE 2.—Transcranial Doppler Ultrasound Findings in 20 Controls

	Basal values (ml/100 g/min)	Increase (ml/100 g/min)	Range (ml/100 g/min)	5% fractile (ml/100 g/min)
Right $rCBF_{MCA}$	56.0 (7.8)	16.5 (4.7)	7.5–23.5	7.6
Left $rCBF_{MCA}$	55.2 (7.8)	16.4 (4.3)	7.5–25	7.6
Both sides	55.6 (7.8)	16.5 (4.5)	7.5–25	7.6
Asymmetry in increase (right–left side)		0.14 (1.9)	−3 to 4.5	−3, 4.4*

Note: Basal values, the increase, and 5% fractile of increase in time mean middle cerebral artery velocities (V_{MCA}) after injection of acetazolamide, 1 g. The values are mean with SDs in parentheses.
* Represents the 95% fractile when subtracting increase on the left from the right side.
(Courtesy of Dahl A, Lindegaard K-F, Russell D, et al: *Stroke* 23:15–19, 1992.)

yielded comparable assessments of vasoreactivity in 86% of the middle cerebral territories examined. The Doppler study detected all territories with markedly reduced blood flow. Only 1 hemisphere with a normal flow response to acetazolamide had reduced vasoreactivity on Doppler study.

Conclusion.—Transcranial Doppler ultrasonography with acetazolamide can be used to determine the clinical import of reduced cerebral perfusion reserve.

▶ The observation that cerebral blood flow correlates closely with transcranial Doppler measurement of cerebral blood flow velocity is, of course, of considerable potential importance. The ultimate usefulness of transcranial Doppler ultrasonography remains to be determined. I suspect that it will prove quite useful, but only in a small number of highly selected patients.—J.M. Porter, M.D.

Transcranial Doppler-Estimated Versus Thermodilution-Estimated Cerebral Blood Flow During Cardiac Operations: Influence of Temperature and Arterial Carbon Dioxide Tension
van der Linden J, Wesslén Ö, Ekroth R, Tydén H, von Ahn H (Univ Hosp, Uppsala, Sweden)
J Thorac Cardiovasc Surg 102:95–102, 1991   3–20

Background.—The transcranial Doppler technique is an effective, noninvasive method of monitoring cerebral perfusion with high temporal resolution. The ability of the transcranial Doppler technique to estimate cerebral blood flow changes during deep hypothermic cardiac operations was evaluated.

Methods.—In 7 patients, flow velocity changes in the middle cerebral artery (MCA) measured by the transcranial Doppler technique were compared with simultaneous measurements of venous blood flow in the ipsilateral internal jugular vein during 11 preset stages of the procedure. A thermodilution catheter was used to determine the jugular venous blood flow. Arterial carbon dioxide tension was varied during normothermia and during deep hypothermia. To facilitate comparisons, MCA flow velocity and jugular venous blood flow values were normalized by relating all values to the awake level (100%).

Results.—During the awake state, the mean jugular venous blood flow was 382 mL/min, and the mean MCA flow velocity was 45.1 cm/sec. The correlation of the combined data from all 7 patients was .77. At deep hypothermia, the mean MCA flow velocity was 49.9% of the awake levels; the mean jugular venous blood flow was 38.3% and the mean cerebral metabolic rates for oxygen were 20.6% (thermodilution-estimated rate) and 22% (Doppler-estimated rate) of the awake level (Fig 3–17). Variations in arterial carbon dioxide tension induced significant changes

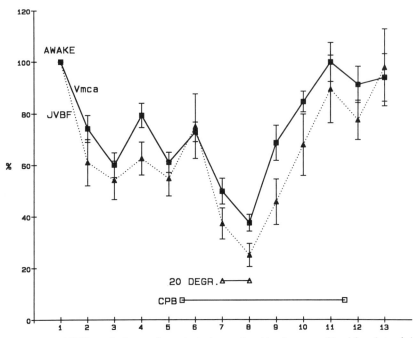

Fig 3–17.—Middle cerebral artery flow velocity (*squares*) and jugular venous blood flow (*triangles*) expressed in percent of individual awake values at 11 preset stages, from the awake state until after operation, including cardiopulmonary bypass (CPB) and deep hypothermia. Represents combined data from 7 patients. The values are mean ± standard error of mean. (Courtesy of van der Linden J, Wesslén Ö, Ekroth R, et al: *J Thorac Cardiovasc Surg* 102:95–102, 1991.)

in the 2 flow estimates both during normothermia before cardiopulmonary bypass and at deep hypothermia during bypass.

Conclusion.—The flow velocity of the MCA is a valid estimate of changes in volume flow through the brain. The noninvasive, continuous transcranial Doppler technique provided information similar to the invasive, noncontinuous thermodilution technique. The transcranial Doppler technique appears to be the preferred method for monitoring cerebral blood flow changes during cardiac surgery.

▶ These authors conclude that not only is transcranial Doppler an accurate method with which to assess brain blood flow, but it may also be the preferred method for monitoring cerebral blood flow during cardiac surgery. See Abstract 3–19.—J.M. Porter, M.D.

Transcranial Doppler for Detection of Cerebral Ischaemia During Carotid Endarterectomy
Jørgensen LG, Schroeder TV (Univ of Copenhagen)
Eur J Vasc Surg 6:142–147, 1992   3–21

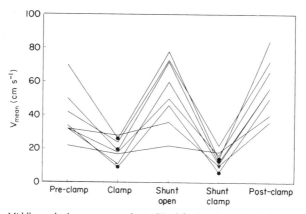

Fig 3–18.—Middle cerebral artery mean velocity (V_{mean}) for 8 patients who had temporary shunt during internal carotid artery endarterectomy. *Circles,* patients with electroencephalographic (EEG) flattening immediately after cross-clamping; *triangle,* patient who had EEG changes only at cross-clamping of the shunt. (Courtesy of Jørgensen LG, Schroeder TV: *Eur J Vasc Surg* 6:142–147, 1992.)

Background.—Cerebral ischemia can complicate carotid endarterectomy, and some patients require a temporary shunt to prevent such an event. Several methods of monitoring have been attempted to determine which patients require a shunt.

Methods.—Transcranial Doppler sonography was assessed in 44 patients with ipsilateral focal cerebrovascular symptoms who underwent carotid endarterectomy. Surgery was done under halothane-N_2O anesthesia with moderate hypocapnia. Eight patients received a temporary shunt because of contralateral carotid occlusion, a low stump pressure, or flattening on the electroencephalograph.

Results.—The mean middle cerebral arterial flow velocity decreased from 38 cm/sec^{-1} to 28 cm/sec^{-1} during cross-clamping and rose to 42 cm/sec^{-1} after removal of the clamp (Fig 3–18). A clamp value below 30 cm/sec^{-1} and a mean clamp/preclamp velocity ratio below .6 accurately reflected a cerebral blood flow of less than 20 mL/100 g^{-1}/min^{-1}. A ratio below .4 detected all 3 patients who exhibited EEG flattening. Stump pressures less accurately reflected the state of cerebral perfusion.

Conclusion.—Intraoperative transcranial Doppler sonography is a more accurate way of detecting patients with low cerebral blood flow than the estimation of carotid stump pressure.

▶ What is the role of transcranial Doppler monitoring during carotid surgery? For selective shunters, it may be the ultimate method to determine the need for shunting. More enlightened surgeons, such as your editor, shunt routinely and don't have to worry with this.—J.M. Porter, M.D.

Duplex Ultrasonographic Insonation and Visualization of Intracerebral Arteries

Montefusco-von Kleist CM, Rhodes BA (Merle West Med Ctr, Klamath Falls, Ore)
Angiology 42:812–818, 1991
3–22

Background.—The development of 2-MHz Doppler ultrasound has recently allowed direct, noninvasive interrogation of intracranial and intracerebral vessels. The inability of existing techniques to image the intracerebral artery walls clearly has limited the clinical application of transcranial Doppler ultrasonography, preventing identification and description of lesions. The instrumentation and examination methods for transcranial duplex ultrasonography of the intracerebral arteries were investigated.

Methods.—Ten healthy volunteers, aged 22–42 years, and 4 patients with neurologic symptoms were assessed. Optimal visualization was provided by a 2.25-MHz tightly curved phased-array probe with a 20-mm radius of curvature, and a 2-MHz pulsed Doppler. The initial step in examination was color-flow visualization of near- and far-field regions for both temporal and occipital sites. This maneuver enabled rapid identification and localization of the intracerebral arteries. Visualization of the

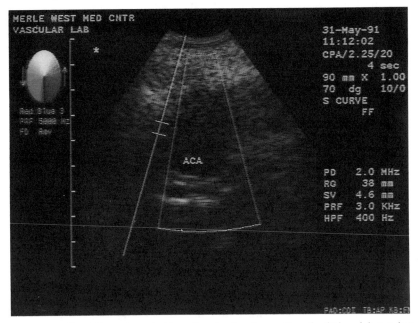

Fig 3–19.—This ACA was imaged without the color-flow feature. Note the thickened, hyperechoic vessel walls and roughened intima. These features are consistent with the presence of atherosclerotic disease. (Courtesy of Montefusco-von Kleist CM, Rhodes BA: *Angiology* 42:812–818, 1991.)

arteries in the longitudinal or transverse projections was achieved by rotation of the probe around its long axis. When needed, image magnification (2×) in real time was used to assist the operator in identifying arterial wall structural features.

Results.—A clear view of the middle cerebral (MCA) and anterior cerebral (ACA) arteries was obtained through temporal placement of the tightly curved phased-array probe. The 2.25-MHz curved phased-array probe was used for imaging the anterior cerebral artery (ACA) (Fig 3–19). Arterial wall features were enhanced by discontinuing the color-flow feature. The thickened, hyperechoic vessel walls and roughened intima indicate atherosclerotic changes. This patient, although free of neurologic symptoms, had a 22-year history of smoking cigarettes.

Conclusion.—These preliminary results are encouraging. The new ability to image the intracerebral vessels and insonate them at the same time should provide an unsurpassed advantage in diagnosing cerebrovascular disease.

▶ Equipment manufacturers are now making probes that are suitable for the imaging of intracranial vessels. This requires very low frequency for depth of penetration, with the attendant indistinct images. These authors suggest that the use of imaging and sequential Doppler interrogation of the intracranial vessels to detect areas of localized stenosis ultimately may be as useful as it is with other arteries in the body. I doubt it, but they may be right.—J.M. Porter, M.D.

The Correlation Between Three Methods of Skin Perfusion Pressure Measurement: Radionuclide Washout, Laser Doppler Flow, and Photoplethysmography
Malvezzi L, Castronuovo JJ Jr, Swayne LC, Cone D, Trivino JZ (Morristown Mem Hosp, Morristown, NJ; Columbia Univ College of Physicians and Surgeons, New York)
J Vasc Surg 15:823–830, 1992   3–23

Background.—Skin perfusion pressure (SPP) is an accurate gauge of tissue perfusion and, therefore, is of use in determining the proper amputation level and in assessing the prognosis of patients with ischemic foot ulcers. Skin perfusion pressure is the external pressure needed to stop the microcirculatory washout of intradermally deposited pertechnetate. However, washout measurements typically require 20 minutes each, necessitating both an immobile limb and frequent analgesia.

Methods.—Isotopic estimates of SPP were acquired simultaneously with measurements made by placing a laser Doppler probe or a photoplethysmographic probe with a transparent polyvinylchloride plastic blood pressure cuff (Fig 3–20). The pressure applied to the skin is transmitted by the bladder surface rather than by the surface of a rigid probe.

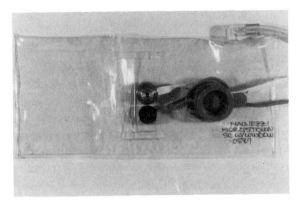

Fig 3–20.—Transparent polyvinylchloride plastic bladder with laser Doppler and PPG probes inserted. (Courtesy of Malvezzi L, Castronuovo JJ Jr, Swayne LC, et al: *J Vasc Surg* 15:823–830, 1992.)

The cuff is inflated to a suprasystolic pressure over the site of intradermally injected technetium 99m and then deflated in decrements of 10mm Hg at 3-minute intervals.

Results.—No reliable photoplethysmographic readings were available in 7 of the 13 extremities examined. The coefficient of correlation between SPP measurements when the isotopic and laser Doppler methods were compared was .991 (Fig 3–21).

Conclusion.—Estimating SPP using the laser Doppler technique is a simple means of noninvasively determining perfusion at the bedside. The results correlate closely with those of isotopic SPP measurements.

▶ In all likelihood, laser Doppler flowmetry is the best way to measure skin perfusion pressure. The obvious question, however, is whether the measurement of skin perfusion pressure has any particular value. Somehow I have never found the laboratory determination of optimal amputation healing site to be a burning clinical issue. The low specificity of all prior methods to

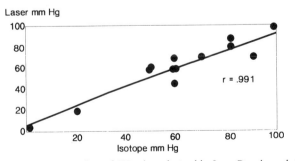

Fig 3–21.—Linear regression analysis of SPP values obtained by Laser Doppler and those obtained by ^{99m}Tc radionuclide washout ($r = .991$). (Courtesy of Malvezzi L, Castronuovo JJ Jr, Swayne LC, et al: *J Vasc Surg* 15:823–830, 1992.)

quantitatively determine amputation sites has been widely reported. This method, however, may be useful in other situations. See Abstract 3–24.—J.M. Porter, M.D.

Laser Doppler Flowmetry in Evaluation of Cutaneous Wound Blood Flow Using Various Suturing Techniques
Zografos GC, Martis K, Morris DL (Queen's Med Centre, Nottingham, England)
Ann Surg 215:266–268, 1992   3–24

Introduction.—It is important to be accurate in assessing blood flow to cutaneous wounds in abdominal surgery, because the blood supply to a wound is a major factor influencing wound healing.

Methods.—Blood flow was measured on either side of an abdominal incision and in uninjured control skin in 63 consecutive patients who had abdominal surgery. Clips, mattress sutures, and subcuticular sutures were used in 3 groups of 21 patients respectively. Studies were performed 1 and 5 days postoperatively using an infrared laser Doppler flowmeter.

Results.—Blood flow was significantly greater on postoperative day 1 than on postoperative day 5. The blood flow also was greater in wounds repaired with subcuticular sutures than in the other 2 groups.

Conclusion.—Wounds may begin to heal sooner after subcuticular suturing of an abdominal incision. The laser Doppler flowmeter is a useful means of estimating blood flow in surgical wounds.

▶ Few problems in lower-extremity revascularization surgery or abdominal vascular surgery are more maddening than recalcitrant incisional wound healing problems, which are frequently accompanied by the development of .5 cm to 1 cm of gangrenous necrosis along the incision. This usually delays the patient's hospitalization interminably. In recent years, we have moved exclusively to the subcuticular skin closure on all vascular incisions, and we have noted a remarkable decrease in our wound healing problems, which has more than compensated for the slight extra time required in the operating room. This important study provides objective support for this clinical decision.—J.M. Porter, M.D.

Magnetic Resonance Imaging of Renal Carcinoma With Extension Into the Vena Cava: Staging Accuracy and Recent Advances
Myneni L, Hricak H, Carroll PR (Univ of California, San Francisco)
Br J Urol 68:571–578, 1991   3–25

Objective.—The findings at MRI and CT examination were compared in 16 patients with surgically confirmed interior vena cava thrombi sec-

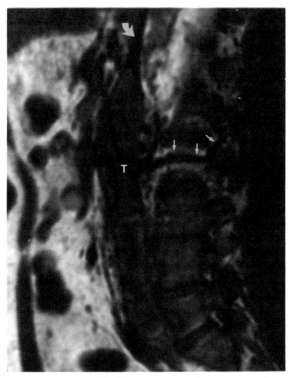

Fig 3–22.—Large tumor thrombus (T) of the extrahepatic inferior vena cava demonstrated on a sagittal T1-weighted 1.5-T image. Normal flow in the intrahepatic inferior vena cava is seen. The *white arrows* represent lumbar collateral vessels. (Courtesy of Myneni L, Hricak H, Carroll PR: *Br J Urol* 68:571–578, 1991.)

ondary to renal carcinoma. The 5 women and 11 men were aged 40–74 years.

Results.—Magnetic resonance imaging accurately detected tumor thrombus in the inferior vena cava in all 16 patients (Figs 3–22 and 3–23), and CT detected thrombus in 14. The cephalad extent of tumor thrombus was demonstrated in all cases but 1 on MRI, and in 11 cases by CT. Both the level of extension and the presence of thrombus in the hepatic veins were more easily seen on MRI studies. Invasion of the inferior vena caval wall was correctly identified by MRI in 7 cases and by CT in only 1. Gradient recall acquisition in steady state (GRASS) imaging, which was done in 8 patients, identified the thrombus as consisting of tumor or blood clot, or both.

Conclusion.—Magnetic resonance imaging is better than CT for demonstrating the extent of thrombosis in patients with renal carcinoma. The use of GRASS imaging allows differentiation of the tumor from blood thrombus.

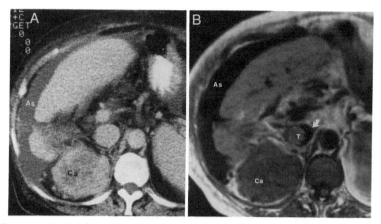

Fig 3–23.—A right-sided renal carcinoma (*Ca*) with tumor extension in the extrahepatic portion of inferior vena cava: **A,** CT, and **B,** corresponding T1-weighted .35-T MR image. On the CT scan, the inferior vena cava is prominent, but there is no difference in density to indicate the presence of tumor thrombus. On MRI, tumor thrombus (*T*) is seen in the inferior vena cava, with residual flow seen along its right lateral margin (*arrow*). Ascites (*As*) is also noted. (Courtesy of Myneni L, Hricak H, Carroll PR: *Br J Urol* 68:571–578, 1991.)

▶ Without question, both MRI and CT provide excellent visualization of the unusual patient with renal cell carcinoma extension into the vena cava. Preoperative knowledge of this problem is essential for optimal operative planning.—J.M. Porter, M.D.

Impact of Magnetic Resonance Imaging on the Management of Diabetic Foot Infections

Durham JR, Lukens ML, Campanini DS, Wright JG, Smead WL (Ohio State Univ, Columbus)
Am J Surg 162:150–154, 1991   3–26

Background.—Optimal treatment of the infected diabetic foot requires a quick and reliable method of defining the presence of abscess cavities, cellulitis, and osteomyelitis. Magnetic resonance imaging (MRI) may provide such a method. The usefulness of MRI in directing surgery for preservation of the infected diabetic foot was investigated in a retrospective/prospective study.

Methods.—Eighteen patients (12 men and 6 women; mean age, 54 years) with diabetes and apparent foot infection were studied. The mean duration of foot symptoms was 7 days. Half had palpable pedal pulses, and 67% had erythema. Magnetic resonance imaging was done as part of the initial assessment in 12 patients and as part of a postoperative evaluation for persistent fever in 6 patients. The decision to operate was made by the attending surgeon using the results of the MRI examination. The mean follow-up was 12 months. Patients were assigned to groups based on clinical presentation without initial MRI.

Results.—Ten patients (group I) had definite cellulitis without suspected abscess; 2 patients, (group II) were thought to have a deep-seated abscess; and 6 patients (group III) had persistent fever and leukocytosis after apparently adequate drainage and débridement of an abscess. In group I, MRI showed cellulitis only in 5 patients and osteomyelitis in addition to cellulitis in 3; all of these patients responded to bed rest and intravenously administered antibiotics. In the other 2 patients in group I, MRI revealed an unexpected deep-seated abscess, which was locally drained. Magnetic resonance imaging allowed precise definition of abscesses in group II. In group III, MRI found undrained pockets of purulence in 2 patients.

Conclusion.—Magnetic resonance imaging appears to offer several advantages in evaluation of the diabetic foot, including increased soft tissue contrast and muliplanar imaging capability. It allows the most accurate drainage of abscesses and prevents unnecessary surgical exploration.

▶ We have all been impressed by the occasional diabetic foot abscess that burrows into unusual anatomical sites and is usually accompanied by few, if any, clinical symptoms. Traditionally, we have had to widely dissect abscesses to find their various pockets, a method which sometimes creates considerable tissue damage. Precise localization of diabetic foot infection with MRI may be a real advance.—J.M. Porter, M.D.

The Comparative Evaluation of Three-Dimensional Magnetic Resonance for Carotid Artery Disease

Wilkerson DK, Keller I, Mezrich R, Schroder WB, Sebok D, Gronlund-Jacobs J, Conway R, Zatina MA (Univ of Medicine and Dentistry of New Jersey–Robert Wood Johnson Med School; Laurie Imaging Ctr, New Brunswick, NJ)
J Vasc Surg 14:803–811, 1991
3–27

Background.—Three-dimensional (3-D) MR angiography offers an alternative to conventional contrast angiographic assessment of the carotid bifurcation. It is noninvasive, avoids ionizing radiation, and is less expensive than contrast angiography.

Methods.—Thirteen patients with extracranial carotid artery disease underwent bilateral 3-D MR angiographic studies. Three of them had a permanent stroke. Bilateral contrast studies and duplex imaging also were done. After acquiring a sagittal localization MR image for centering, the cervical artery anatomy was assessed using a gradient-echo pulse sequence. The reformatted tissue volume was subjected to computer-ray tracing to produce multiple projection images (Fig 3–24).

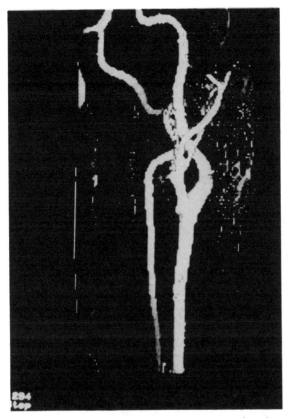

Fig 3–24.—A 3-D MR angiogram in a normal volunteer. Note the ease of visualization of the carotid bifurcation and vertebral artery. (Courtesy of Wilkerson DK, Keller I, Mezrich R, et al: *J Vasc Surg* 14:803–811, 1991.)

Results.—Adequate MR studies were achieved in all patients. The common, external, and internal carotid vessels and the distal vertebral arteries generally were readily identified as patent, stenotic (Fig 3–25), or occluded. The basilar artery was visualized in 4 of the 13 patients. Disease of the carotid siphon could not be evaluated by 3-D MR angiography. A few MR studies suggested complete short-segment internal carotid occlusion when the artery was clearly patent (although severely narrowed) on contrast angiography. The MR study was 92% sensitive in detecting 50% to 99% stenoses (table).

Conclusion.—It may be difficult to interpret high-grade stenoses by 3-D MR angiography, and ulcerations are not demonstrated accurately. At present, this study is most useful when the duplex examination is not

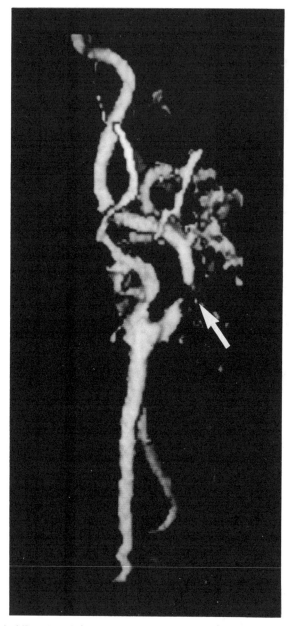

Fig 3–25.—An MR angiogram demonstrates a critical stenosis in the internal carotid artery (*arrow*). Note loss of the MR signal at the site of stenosis with immediate vessel reconstruction. We interpret this finding as a 99% stenosis. (Courtesy of Wilkerson DK, Keller I, Mezrich R, et al: *J Vasc Surg* 14:803–811, 1991.)

Comparison of 3-D Angiography and Conventional Angiography
(% Stenosis)

Conventional angiography

3-D MR	0	0-15	16-49	50-79	80-99	100
0	1	—	—	—	—	—
0-15	—	1	—	—	—	—
16-49	—	1	7	1	—	—
50-79	—	—	1	4	—	—
80-99	—	—	—	3	5	—
100	—	—	—	—	—	2
Uninterpretable	—	—	—	—	—	—

(Courtesy of Wilkerson DK, Keller I, Mezrich R, et al: *J Vasc Surg* 14:803–811, 1991.)

interpretable, when severe contrast allergy is present, or when the patient refuses invasive testing.

▶ As noted in Abstract 3–5, modern imaging is moving increasingly toward 3-D display. I am certain that, in the near future, MRI is going to include improvement in the performance of MR angiography. Perhaps 3-D MR angiography will be an important portion of this improvement.—J.M. Porter, M.D.

Detection of Internal Carotid Artery Stenosis: Comparison of MR Angiography, Color Doppler, Sonography, and Arteriography
Polak JF, Bajakian RL, O'Leary DH, Anderson MR, Donaldson MC, Jolesz FA
(Brigham and Women's Hosp, Boston; Harvard Med School, Boston)
Radiology 182:35–30, 1992   3–28

MRI Findings of Internal Carotid Artery Stenosis Severity as a Function of Angiographic Findings

Stenosis Severity with MR Angiography	Stenosis Severity with Angiography*			Total
	<50%	≥50%	100%	
<50%	9	1	0	10
≥50%	5	22	0	27
100%	0	0	4	4
Total	14	23	4	41

*Excludes 1 case of subtotal occlusion.
(Courtesy of Polak JF, Bajakian RL, O'Leary DH, et al: *Radiology* 182:35–40, 1992.)

Introduction.—Two-dimensional time-of-flight MR angiography can detect bifurcations of the carotid artery as well as blood flow and stenoses. The results obtained using this technique were compared with the outcome of Doppler sonography and angiography in patients with possible stenoses of the carotid artery.

Methods.—Twenty-three consecutive patients with a suspected diagnosis of carotid artery stenosis underwent 2-dimensional time-of-flight MR angiography, Doppler sonography, and contrast angiography of the carotid artery. The angiographic procedure served as the standard for comparison of the detection methods. The 10 women and 13 men had an average age of 65.4 years. The stenosis was diagnosed by blind review, with a 50% or greater narrowing of the width of the carotid's lumen or the occurrence of a signal gap serving as a sign of stenosis.

Results.—Among the 23 internal carotid arteries examined, 14 showed less than 50% narrowing of the width of the lumen in the enhanced angiogram. In the 13 symptomatic patients, a stenosis of at least 50% width reduction was demonstrated on the symptomatic side. Occlusion of 50% or more, or stenosis at the carotid bifurcation was found in 67%. The diagnostic sensitivity of the MR angiography procedure in the detection of carotid stenosis was .96. Five of 22 cases had a positive diagnosis of a large stenosis on visualization of the MR angiogram (table). The diagnostic specificity of the MR angiogram in 14 normal arteries was .64, with 5 false positive results. The sonography procedure detected 22 of the 23 stenoses, for a sensitivity of .96. A statistical correlation occurred between the narrowing viewed by MR angiography and the peak systolic velocity based on the color Doppler sonogram.

Conclusion.—Two-dimensional time-of-flight MR angiography can aid in the detection of stenoses of the carotid artery when combined with sonographic examination of the vessel.

▶ As I stated earlier, I believe that the combination of MR angiography and duplex Doppler sonography will greatly diminish the future need for contrast arteriography.—J.M. Porter, M.D.

Biological Classification of Soft-Tissue Vascular Anomalies: MR Correlation

Meyer JS, Hoffer FA, Barnes PD, Mulliken JB (Harvard Med School, Boston)
AJR 157:559–564, 1991   3–29

Background.—Magnetic resonance imaging is helpful in showing the extent of arteriovenous and lymphatic malformations, but the term "hemangioma" is often used generically. The term has been applied to combinations of infantile hemangiomata and venous malformations with confusing radiologic findings.

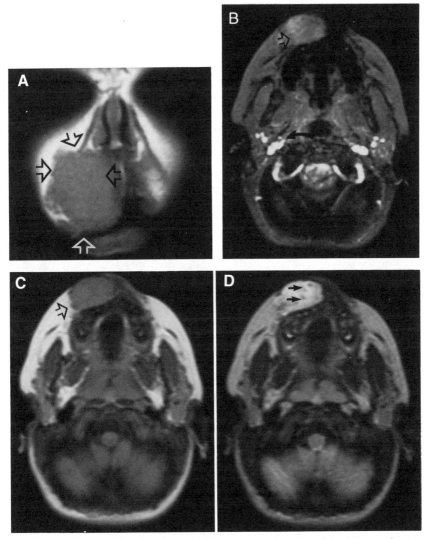

Fig 3–26.—Boy, 4 years, with a compressible blue venous malformation of the right upper lip. **A,** a coronal T1-weighted SE presaturation MR image show an intermediate-intensity lesion (*arrows*) with no flow voids. **B,** an axial GRASS image with gradient-moment nulling shows an intermediate-intensity lesion (*open arrow*) and a high-intensity flow in the normal vessels outside malformation (*solid arrow*). **C,** an axial proton-density SE presaturation image shows an intermediate-intensity homogeneous lesion (*arrow*). **D,** an axial T2-weighted SE presaturation image shows a high-intensity mass containing low-intensity punctate areas (*arrows*) suggesting early calcification or hemosiderin deposition. Note displacement of the teeth posterior to mass. This venous malformation was later sclerosed, then resected. (Courtesy of Meyer JS, Hoffer FA, Barnes PD, et al: *AJR* 157:559–64, 1991.)

Methods.—Magnetic resonance imaging was performed in 23 patients with vascular anomalies, including 5 with hemangiomas, 3 with arteriovenous malformations, 3 with venous malformations, 6 with lymphatic malformations, and 6 with lymphaticovenous malformations. Imaging used T1-weighted longitudinal spin-echo and T2-weighted axial spin-echo sequences with presaturation superiorly and inferiorly.

Results.—The hemangiomas were high-flow lesions containing solid tissue that appeared to be intermediate in intensity on T1-weighted SE presaturation images and bright on T2-weighted SE presaturation images. The arteriovenous malformations also exhibited high flow and flow voids on SE presaturation images. No solid tissue abnormality was evident. The venous malformations were slow-flow lesions (Fig 3–26), which typically had a less intense signal from the venous space on gradient-recalled echo images with gradient-moment nulling than on T2-weighted SE presaturation images. All lymphatic malformations exhibited slow flow. Two of them were cystic. The lymphaticovenous malformations also had slow-flow characteristics.

Conclusion.—Consistent MRI findings are obtained when vascular anomalies are classified as infantile hemangiomas and vascular malformations.

▶ Magnetic resonance imaging should be considered in the evaluation of all patients with significant soft tissue vascular developmental anomalies. This study presents helpful classification information.—J.M. Porter, M.D.

Diagnosis of Abdominal Venous Thrombosis by Means of Spin-Echo and Gradient-Echo MR Imaging: Analysis With Receiver Operating Characteristic Curves

Arrivé L, Menu Y, Dessarts I, Dubray B, Vullierme M-P, Vilgrain V, Najmark D, Nahum H (Hôpital Beaujon, Clichy; Hôpital Saint-Louis, Paris)
Radiology 181:661–668, 1991   3–30

Objective.—The accuracy of spin-echo (SE) and gradient-echo (GRE) MRI for diagnosing abdominal venous thrombosis was studied in 72 patients who were clinically suspected of having thrombosis.

Methods.—Images of 292 abdominal veins were reviewed in a blinded manner by 3 radiologists using 7 levels of diagnostic confidence. Corroborative studies demonstrated thrombosis in 95 instances. Both SE and GRE images were acquired in all patients.

Results.—Blood clot thrombus was present in 86 vessels and tumor thrombus was seen in 9 others (Fig 3–27). Analysis of receiver-operating-characteristic (ROC) curves showed that SE images alone were 76% sensitive at a specificity of 90%, and 63% sensitive at a specificity of 95%. With GRE images alone, sensitivities were 74% and 58%, respectively.

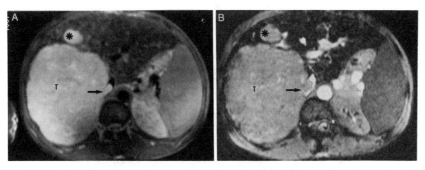

Fig 3–27.—Magnetic resonance images of tumor thrombus of the inferior vena cava in a patient with a large heptocellular carcinoma of the right lobe of the liver. **A,** SE (1,800/30) image shows a partially obstructing caval thrombus (*arrow*) with a signal intensity similar to that of the main tumor mass (*T*). Another lesion (*asterisk* in **A** and **B**) is well depicted. **B,** GRE (60/19) image shows tumor thrombus (*arrow*) with imtermediate signal intensity similar to that of the tumor (*T*). (Courtesy of Arrivé L, Menu Y, Dessarts I, et al: *Radiology* 181:661–668, 1991.)

Combining the 2 types of images yielded sensitivities of 88% and 82%, respectively.

Conclusion.—Combining SE and GRE imaging can help determine whether confusing patterns of intravascular signal intensity represent a patent or thrombosed vessel. The MRI approach remains limited in assessing small vascular structures because of suboptimal spatial resolution.

▶ These authors present convincing evidence that MRI can reliably detect a number of visceral venous thromboses that are difficult to detect with conventional angiography.—J.M. Porter, M.D.

Magnetic Resonance Angiography of Abdominal Vessels: Early Experience Using the Three-Dimensional Phase-Contrast Technique
Vock P, Terrier F, Wegmüller H, Mahler F, Gertsch Ph, Souza SP, Dumoulin CL (Univ of Berne, Switzerland; General Electric Co, Schenectady, NY)
Br J Radiol 64:10–16, 1991   3–31

Introduction.—Magnetic resonance phase-contrast angiography (MRA) is an alternative to radiologic methods of angiography that entail exposure to ionizing radiation and a risk of side effects from contrast medium. Duplex sonography may fail to depict deeper abdominal vessels clearly.

Methods.—Abdominal MRA is based on the 3-dimensional acquisition of 3 sequences sensitive to a single flow direction. The 20 patients and 13 controls examined received no antiperistaltic medication and were allowed to breathe normally during the 3 11-minute acquisition periods.

Results.—The normal aorta, superior mesenteric artery, renal arteries, inferior cava, and portal vein were demonstrated most consistently (Fig 3–28). Of 9 stenosed or occluded renal arteries, 8 were demonstrated by

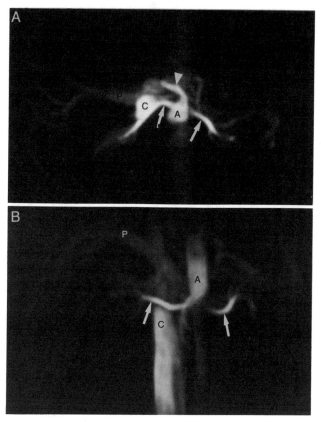

Fig 3-28.—Normal 3-dimensional phase-contrast MRA of the abdomen. **A**, axial view of 128 slices collapsed using the maximum intensity method. **B**, anteroposterior projection of the same data shown in **A**. A indicates aorta; C, inferior vena cava; *short arrows*, renal arteries; *arrowhead*, superior mesenteric artery; P, portal vein. Note the decrease of flow signal in the infrarenal aorta and, less obviously, in the suprarenal inferior vena cava. (Courtesy of Vock P, Terrier F, Wegmüller H, et al: *Br J Radiol* 64:10-16, 1991.)

MRA (Fig 3-29), which missed only a single minimal stenosis. No false positive studies were obtained. In several patients with portal hypertension, MRA depicted more venous collaterals than conventional angiography, especially in the paravertebral region.

Conclusion.—If further studies confirm MRA as an accurate procedure, it could become an important means of evaluating abdominal vascular disorders such as renal artery stenosis and portal hypertension.

▶ This study presents more information on the usefulness of MRA in the evaluation of abdominal vascular structures.—J.M. Porter, M.D.

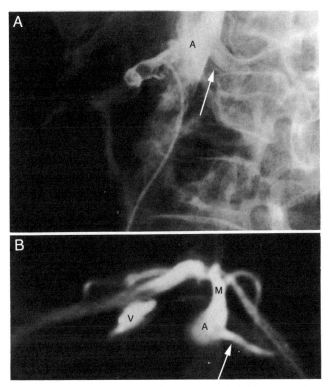

Fig 3–29.—Embolic occlusion of the right renal artery documented by conventional angiography (**A**) and by MRA (**B**); the axial view demonstrates normal flow in the left renal (*arrow*) and superior mesenteric artery (M), but no flow signal in the right renal artery. *Abbreviations:* A indicates aorta; V, inferior vena cava. (Courtesy of Vock P, Terrier F, Wegmüller H, et al: *Br J Radiol* 64:10–16, 1991.)

Muscle Perfusion With Technetium-MIBI in Lower Extremity Peripheral Arterial Diseases

Sayman HB, Urgancioglu I (Istanbul Univ, Turkey)
J Nucl Med 32:1700–1703, 1991
3–32

Background.—Contrast angiography does not adequately image the small vessels of an extremity. Radionuclide studies do demonstrate tissue perfusion. A new tracer, ^{99m}Tc-methoxy-isobutyl-isonitrile (^{99m}Tc-MIBI), which was developed chiefly to image myocardial perfusion, has proved helpful for skeletal muscle perfusion studies.

Methods.—Muscle perfusion in the lower extremities was assessed in 18 symptomatic patients with claudication and 6 control patients referred for myocardial perfusion studies. The new tracer was also used in treadmill exercise testing.

Results.—Radionuclide activity normally is symmetrically distributed both at rest and after exercise (Fig 3–30). Some patients with claudica-

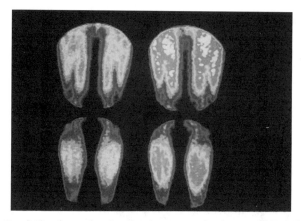

Fig 3–30.—Rest (left) and stress (right) studies showing even distribution of ^{99m}Tc-MIBI in the lower extremity muscles of a normal case. (Courtesy of Sayman HB, Urgancioglu I: *J Nucl Med* 32:1700–1703, 1991.)

tion had increased activity on the side of occlusion at rest, which on exercise increased on the other side only, presumably reflecting resting compensatory hyperemia (Fig 3–31). Other patients with proved collateral vessels had low counts that were ipsilateral to the occlusion at rest and an increase on exercise. Patients who lacked collateral vessels exhibited a perfusion difference between the legs at rest, which increased after exercise.

Conclusion.—Muscle perfusion studies with ^{99m}Tc-MIBI are a simple and accurate means of evaluating patients with arterial disease in the lower extremity. The myocardium is imaged at the same time without further preparation.

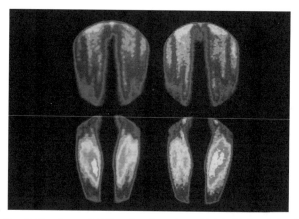

Fig 3–31.—Rest (left) and stress (right) studies of a patient with left-sided occlusive disease showing resting compensatory hyperemia on left calf. (Courtesy of Sayman HB, Urgancioglu I: *J Nucl Med* 32:1700–1703, 1991.)

▶ Without question, radionuclide studies can detect diminished muscle perfusion in ischemic extremities. The real question, however, is whether this has any particular clinical usefulness. I suspect it does not.—J.M. Porter, M.D.

Radionuclide Limb Blood Flow in Peripheral Vascular Disease: A Review of 1100 Measurements
Parkin A, Robinson PJ, Martinez D, Wilkinson D, Kester RC (St James's Univ Hosp, Leeds, England)
Nucl Med Commun 12:835–851, 1991   3–33

Background.—Doppler estimates of the ankle/brachial systolic pressure ratio are useful in screening for occlusive arterial disease, but the

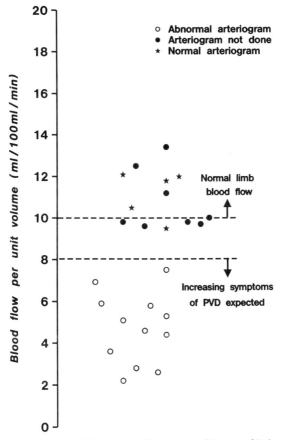

Fig 3–32.—Limb blood flow in 25 diagnostic problem patients. (Courtesy of Parkin A, Robinson PJ, Martinez D, et al: *Nucl Med Commun* 12:835-851, 1991.)

findings are poorly reproducible. Radionuclide studies based on the intramuscular injection of radioxenon or pertechnetate are a sensitive means of detecting peripheral vascular disease, as is first-pass radionuclide arteriography.

Methods.—A simple method of measuring total below-knee extremity blood flow is based on the use of technetium-99m-labeled red blood cells and a gamma camera. This method was used to evaluate 72 patients, 39 of whom successfully completed 4 treadmill tests.

Results.—The normal range of blood flow was 10–22.3 mL/100 mL of tissue/min. The flow rates in the symptomatic extremities of patients with arterial disease ranged from 9 mL/100 mL tissue/min in mild claudication to less than 1 mL/100 mL of tissue/min in those with rest pain (Fig 3–32).

Applications.—Radionuclide measurements of extremity blood flow, apart from helping to solve diagnostic problems, proved useful in defining the severity of peripheral vascular disease, and also in ascertaining the response to treatment after angioplasty or bypass surgery.

▶ These authors are quite enthusiastic about the usefulness of determinations of radionuclide limb blood flow in patients with peripheral vascular disease. I am unconvinced, but remain reasonably open-minded. See my comments for Abstract 3–32.—J.M. Porter, M.D.

Imaging of the Renal Arteries: Value of MR Angiography
Debatin JF, Spritzer CE, Grist TM, Beam C, Svetkey LP, Newman GE, Sostman HD (Duke Univ Durham, NC)
AJR 157:981–990, 1991   3–34

Introduction.—The value of MR angiography for visualizing the renal arteries and detecting renovascular disease was compared with that of conventional angiography. Twenty-five patients were studied for possible renovascular hypertension, and 8 potential kidney donors were assessed.

Methods.—Each of 33 MR studies consisted of axial 2-dimensional (2-D) phase-contrast, coronal 2-D phase-contrast, and coronal 2-D time-of-flight acquisitions. All were completed within 48 hours of conventional angiography. The 3 MR image sets were interpreted both independently and together. Only the proximal 35 mm of each renal artery was assessed.

Results.—Renal artery disease was best evaluated with coronal phase-contrast images (Fig 3–33). Combined axial and coronal phase-contrast imaging demonstrated all dominant renal arteries and detected 13 of 15 stenoses, with a sensitivity of 87% and a specificity of 97%.

Conclusion.—Biplanar MR angiography has considerable potential as a noninvasive screening measure for evaluating renovascular disease. Modifications such as the use of a surface coil and gradient reordering

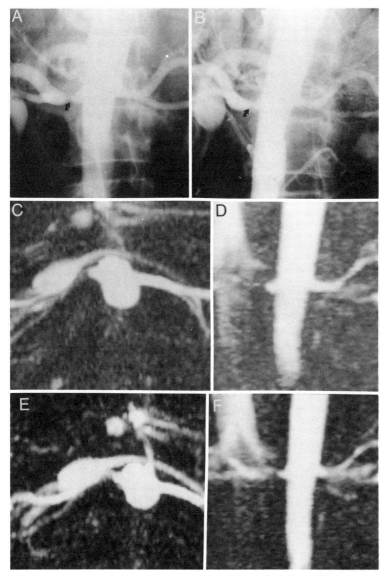

Fig 3–33.—**A**, conventional arteriogram shows high-grade stenosis (75% to 99%) in the proximal right renal artery (*arrow*) of a man, 35. **B**, arteriogram shows reduction to a moderate lesion (*arrow*) after percutaneous transluminal angioplasty. Axial (**C**) and coronal (**D**) preangioplasty maximum-pixel-intensity projection (MIP) phase-contrast images show extended area of signal void (more than 5 mm) in the proximal right renal artery with reconstitution of signal distally. Axial (**E**) and coronal (**F**) postangioplasty MIP phase-contrast images show a reduced area of signal void (less than 5 mm) corresponding to moderate lesion (50% to 75%). Stenosis was correctly detected and graded on phase-contrast MR angiography both before and after angioplasty. (Courtesy of Debatin JF, Spritzer CE, Grist TM, et al: *AJR* 157:981-990, 1991.)

may help in assessing distal renal artery disease, especially in patients with fibromuscular dysplasia.

▶ Magnetic resonance angiography has the potential not only to image the renal arteries to detect stenosis, but also to quantitatively assess blood flow. This can be achieved without the use of contrast agents or radiation. These are major and significant clinical advances, and with improved instrumentation and technology, reliable noninvasive renal artery imaging should be possible in the near future.—C. Zarins, M.D.

4 Nonatherosclerotic Conditions

Takayasu's Arteritis in Children
Morales E, Pineda C, Martínez-Lavín M (Instituto Nacional de Cardiologia Ignacio Chávez, México City)
J Rheumatol 18:1081–1084, 1991   4–1

Introduction.—Takayasu's arteritis, which is rarely recognized in children, was studied in 26 children (20 girls and 6 boys; mean age, 11.7 years) seen in a 20-year period.

Clinical Features.—Most children were seen with signs of generalized inflammation (Table 1). Pulse abnormalities were a constant feature, and

TABLE 1.—Outstanding Clinical Features of 26 Children
With Takayasu's Arteritis

	Number	(%)
General Symptoms		
Asthenia, weight loss, fever	17	(65)
Cardiovascular		
Alteration of pulses	26	(100)
Arterial hypertension	22	(85)
Heart failure	17	(65)
Epistaxis	7	(27)
Claudication of the limbs	8	(31)
Rheumatologic		
Arthritis	17	(65)
Neurologic		
Headache	13	(50)
Convulsions	3	(12)
Hemiplegia	2	(8)
Dermatologic		
Nodular skin eruptions	5	(19)
Gastrointestinal		
Abdominal pain, vomiting	13	(50)
Lymphatic		
Lymphadenopathy	10	(38)

(Courtesy of Morales E, Pineda C, Martínez-Lavín M: *J Rheumatol* 18:1081–1084, 1991.)

TABLE 2.—Outstanding Laboratory Abnormalities in
Children With Takayasu's Arteritis

	Number/ Number Tested	(%)
Positive PPD	11/15	(73)
Hemoglobin < 12 g	17/26	(65)
Leukocytosis	10/26	(38)
C-reactive protein > 3+	18/22	(81)
Increased immunoglobulins	12/20	(60)
Antistreptolysin 0 > 250 U	11/23	(48)
CH50 < 80 U	7/16	(44)
Antinuclear antibodies	7/17	(42)
Rheumatoid factor	3/16	(19)
Proteinuria > 0.5 g/l	12/26	(46)
Hematuria	7/26	(27)
Creatinine > 1.5 g/l	5/26	(19)
Increased sedimentation rate > 50 mm/h (Westergren)	19/26	(85)

(Courtesy of Morales E, Pineda C, Martínez-Lavín M: *J Rheumatol* 18:1081–1084, 1991.)

all but 4 patients had arterial hypertension. The most common neurologic abnormality was severe headache. Half the patients had gastrointestinal symptoms, and 10 had lymphadenopathy. A positive purified protein derivative test and low hemoglobin were each found in more than half the patients tested (Table 2).

Management and Outcome.—Apart from treatment to control hypertension and heart failure, 7 patients received steroids. Some systemic manifestations responded, but the pulse abnormalities persisted. An-

TABLE 3.—Causes of Death in 9 Children With
Takayasu's Arteritis

Cause	Number
Cardiorenal failure	2
Purulent peritonitis	1
Sudden death*	1
Aortic rupture during surgery	1
Ruptured aneurysm of subclavian artery	1
Ischemic cerebrovascular event	1
Hemorrhagic cerebrovascular event	1
Ventricular fibrillation	1

* Autopsy was not performed.
(Courtesy of Morales E, Pineda C, Martínez-Lavín M: *J Rheumatol* 18:1081–1084, 1991.)

tituberculosis treatment, which was given to 6 children, was ineffective. Bypass surgery succeeded in 1 of 3 attempts. There were 9 deaths during a mean follow-up of 5 years (Table 3). Half the surviving patients require constant treatment for hypertension and/or heart failure.

Conclusion.—The association between Takayasu's arteritis and tuberculosis remains uncertain, but there are suggestions that mycobacterial infection may have a pathogenetic role. Steroid therapy has not lessened arterial obstruction. This is an aggressive illness, carrying a 5-year mortality of 35% in this series.

▶ The most important message to be taken away from this paper is that Takayasu's arteritis in the pediatric age group is frequently an aggressive—even lethal—disease, with a mortality of 35% at 5 years. These children occasionally require vascular surgery for aneurysm or stenosis, but the vascular repairs are unsuccessful with distressing frequency.—J.M. Porter, M.D.

Non-Specific Aorto-Arteritis (Takayasu's Disease) in Children
Sharma S, Rajani M, Shrivastava S, Kaul U, Kamalakar T, Talwar KK, Saxena A (All India Inst of Med Sciences, New Delhi)
Br J Radiol 64:690–698, 1991   4–2

Objective.—Nonspecific aorto-arteritis, or Takayasu's disease, has been documented infrequently in children. Panaorto-arteriography using digital-subtraction angiography was performed in 32 children (16 years of age and younger) who had a clinical diagnosis of nonspecific aorto-arteritis. The findings were assessed.

Data Analysis.—There were 21 female and 11 male patients (mean age, 10.8 years; age range, 18 months–16 years). The most common clinical features were hypertension, diminished arterial pulses, and bruits; congestive cardiac failure occurred in 12 patients. All patients had more than 1 obstructive lesion (table), which usually involved the abdominal aorta (75%) and the renal arteries (62.5%) (Fig 4–1). In contrast, aneurysms were uncommon (15.6%) and predominantly involved the descending thoracic aorta. Percutaneous transluminal angioplasty was performed in 8 patients with uncontrollable hypertension. The initial success rate was 80%, and the mean follow-up period was 9 months. Restenosis occurred in 1 patient 5.5 months after initial success; the lesion was successfully redilated.

Conclusion.—Takayasu's arteritis in children is not uncommon. Obstructive lesions are frequent, usually involving the abdominal aorta and renal arteries. Digital subtraction angiography is usually adequate for establishing the diagnosis. The preliminary results of percutaneous transluminal angioplasty in the management of these children are en-

Sites of Arterial Involvement ($n = 32$)

Vessels involved	Number of patients	%
Aortic arch	3	9.4
Thoracic aorta	13	40.6
Abdominal aorta	24	75.0
Renal arteries	20	62.5
Renal arteries, unilateral	10	31.25
Renal arteries, bilateral	10	31.25
Subclavian artery	13	40.6
Subclavian artery, left	10	31.25
Subclavian artery, right	1	3.1
Subclavian artery, both	2	6.2
Left carotid artery	5	15.6
Superior mesenteric artery	6	18.7
Innominate artery	2	6.2
Femoral artery	4	12.4
Aneurysm formation	5*	15.6
Descending thoracic aorta	4	—
Abdominal aorta	1	—
Left common iliac artery	1	—
Right renal artery	1	—
Pulmonary artery ($n = 20$)	5	25.0
Obstruction of lobar branch	3	—
Peripheral pruning of both pulmonary arteries	2	—

* Two patients had multiple aneurysms.
(Courtesy of Sharma S, Rajani M, Shrivastava S, et al: *Br J Radiol* 64:690–698, 1991.)

couraging, but further long-term follow-up is necessary to establish its efficacy.

▶ Patterns of arteriographic disease were assessed in 32 consecutive children with Takayasu's disease. Obstructive arterial lesions were seen in all patients and commonly involved the abdominal aorta and renal arteries. Thoracic aortic aneurysm occurred in approximately 15% of the patients. The extensive and serious arterial involvement occurring in this condition accounts for the extreme mortality. See Abstract 4–1.—J.M. Porter, M.D.

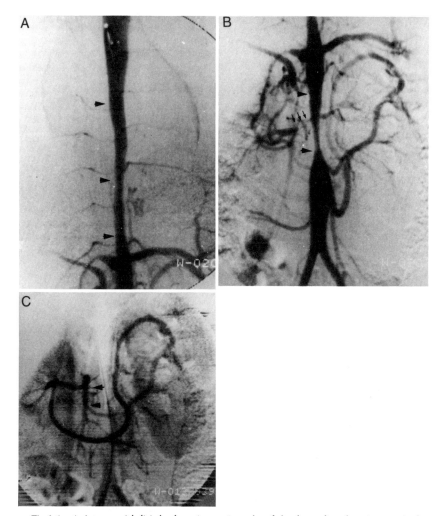

Fig 4–1.—A, intra-arterial digital subtraction angiography of the descending thoracic aorta in the anteroposterior view, showing a long segment narrowing of the descending aorta (*arrowheads*). **B,** intra-arterial digital subtraction angiography of the abdominal aorta in the same patient, showing a long segment narrowing of the perirenal segment (*open arrowhead*) with right renal artery stenosis, occlusion of the superior mesenteric artery (*small arrowheads*) and a large meandering collateral. **C,** late frame of the same study showing retrograde filling of the occluded superior mesenteric artery (*arrowheads*) by the meandering collateral. (Courtesy of Sharma S, Rajani M, Shrivastava S, et al: *Br J Radiol* 64:690–698, 1991.)

Carotid Lesions Detected by B-Mode Ultrasonography in Takayasu's Arteritis: "Macaroni Sign" as an Indicator of the Disease

Maeda H, Handa N, Matsumoto M, Hougaku H, Ogawa S, Oku N, Itoh T, Moriwaki H, Yoneda S, Kimura K, Kamada T (Osaka Univ Med School, Japan; Yao Municipal Hosp, Osaka, Japan)
Ultrasound Med Biol 17:695–701, 1991   4–3

Introduction.—Takayasu's arteritis, a nonspecific inflammatory disease, usually localizes in the elastic arteries of the aorta and its chief branches. When this condition occurs in the carotid artery, the patient may experience disturbances of vision and neurologic symptoms. With the advent of the B-mode high-resolution ultrasound technique, alterations of the carotid's lumen and arterial wall (which are responsible for these symptoms) can be seen noninvasively.

Methods.—All 23 patients with Takayasu's arteritis who were being studied were women (mean patient age, 38 years). The diagnosis of Takayasu's arteritis resulted from clinical examinations, the presence of symptoms, a physical examination, serologic assays, and aortography. All patients underwent contrast angiography of the ascending aorta.

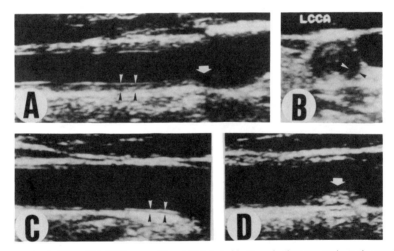

Fig 4–2.—A diffuse thick IMC pattern (**A** and **B**) detected by B-mode ultrasonography in the carotid artery of the patients with Takayasu's arteritis compared with the normal pattern (**C**) and atheromatous plaque (**D**) detected in the carotid arteries of a normal subject and a patient who had a stroke, respectively. In the lateral view (**A**), as denoted by *arrowheads*, diffuse circumferential thickening of IMC can clearly be seen throughout the common carotid artery (CCA). However, this pattern appears to break off at the upper extent (*an arrow*) of the CCA, and in the transverse view (**B**), a characteristic doughnut-like circumferential thick IMC is clearly demonstrated. In a usual case, however, the thick IMC could be detected only at the near- and far-wall interfaces in a projection when examinations in the different projections could reveal diffuse circumferential thickening of the IMC. In a normal carotid artery (**C**), the normal IMC pattern (*arrowheads*) was observed; in the carotid artery with atheromatous lesions (**D**) (*arrow*), only a localized thickening of the IMC (3.2 mm in thickness) could be detected. (Courtesy of Maeda H, Handa N, Matsumoto M, et al: *Ultrasound Med Biol* 17:695–701, 1991.)

Results.—The ultrasonograms of the carotid artery obtained from all patients demonstrated B-mode images of 2 parallel echogenic lines bisected by a hypoechoic or anechoic space. The inner echogenic line and the anechoic space corresponded to the intima-media complex (IMC). The IMC in 45 normal subjects demonstrated a maximal thickness of .3–.9 mm and, in 12 age-matched healthy women, it was .5–.8 mm. In the patients with Takayasu's arteritis, the ultrasound technique using the B-mode image of the carotid artery distinguished between the normal IMC pattern with a thickness of less than 1 mm (Fig 4–2C), and the diffuse thick IMC areas where the thickness was greater than 1 mm (Fig 4–2A and B). The carotid artery's B-mode image could also be classified according to patterns representing occlusion, dilatation, and no dilatation. Among the 46 carotid arteries studied, 34 demonstrated a diffuse thick IMC pattern. The presence of a neck bruit correlated with the ultrasonic finding of the carotid artery.

Conclusion.—The B-mode ultrasound technique can aid in the diagnosis and assessment of pathologic changes in patients with Takayasu's arteritis in the carotid artery. The detection of a diffuse thick IMC pattern characterizes the presence of this disorder.

▶ Characteristic circumferential arterial wall thickening of 1 or both common carotid arteries was routinely seen in young female adults with Takayasu's disease who were studied by B-mode ultrasound. This once more attests to the generalized arterial disease present in these patients. I suspect we will see more of this condition in the future. See also Abstracts 4–1 and 4–2.—J.M. Porter, M.D.

Urokinase Treatment of Neonatal Aortoiliac Thrombosis Caused by Umbilical Artery Catheterization: A Case Report
Smith PK, Miller DA, Lail S, Mehta AV (East Tennessee State Univ, Johnson City)
J Vasc Surg 14:684–687, 1991
4–4

Introduction.—Umbilical artery catheterization is complicated by aortoiliac thrombosis in approximately 1% of catheterized neonates. An infant who was effectively treated by urokinase infusion was evaluated.

Case Report.—Term infant, with meconium staining after cesarean section delivery, was in severe respiratory distress. Ventilation began shortly after birth, and a 5F umbilical artery catheter was placed for the delivery of hypertonic solutions, nutritional materials, and a number of drugs that can irritate the vascular endothelium. Sepsis was clinically evident on day 8, and blood cultures later yielded *Staphylococcus epidermidis*. On day 13, the infant had mottled, pulseless lower extremities and congestive heart failure. An ultrasound study revealed a thrombus that totally occluded the aorta and extended into both iliac arteries. A real-time study showed thrombus in the celiac and superior mesenteric arteries and in both renal arteries. A femoral pulse reappeared within 12 hours of urokinase infusion (4,400 units/kg bolus followed by 4,400 units/kg/hour). Fresh frozen plasma was given to produce a fibrinolytic state. Thrombus blocking the left renal artery was dissolved by local urokinase infusion. Subsequently aggressive heparin and warfarin therapy was required to achieve anticoagulation. At age 1 year, the child had good pulses and was developing normally, but she had a small left kidney.

Recommendation.—A study of similar cases of aortoiliac thrombosis in neonatal life suggested that medical and operative treatment are almost equally effective. It seems reasonable to try urokinase therapy first.

▶ The authors of this informative article make the observation that their review of the literature indicates that the reported medical and surgical treatment of neonatal catheter-associated thrombosis seems to produce equal results; this leads them to conclude that urokinase therapy is preferable to surgery as the initial treatment for these frequently critically ill infants. I believe the authors' recommendations are reasonable.—J.M. Porter, M.D.

Aortic Thrombosis After Umbilical Artery Catheterization in Neonates: Prevalence of Complications on Long-Term Follow-Up
Seibert JJ, Northington FJ, Miers JF, Taylor BJ (Univ of Arkansas for Med Sciences; Arkansas Children's Hosp, Little Rock)
AJR 156:567–569, 1991   4–5

Introduction.—A previously reported study showed that of 81 neonates who were studied for aortic thrombosis by abdominal sonography after umbilical artery catheterization, 21 were found to have aortic clots. All but 4 of the infants had extensive thrombi producing at least 40% stenosis of the aortic area.

Methods.—Data on 10 of the affected infants who were followed up at ages 36–42 months were compared with the data on 7 age-matched controls.

Results.—Of the 10 infants with a history of aortic thrombosis, 3 had blood pressures greater than the 95th percentile, and 6 had blood pressures between the 50th and 95th percentiles. Four children were below the fifth percentile for height. Of 9 study infants, 7 had a discrepancy of .5–2 cm in thigh or calf circumference, and 1 had a significant leg length discrepancy. Sonography showed no residual clot in the aorta or renal vessels, and Doppler flow studies were consistently normal. Of 7 control infants, 1 was hypertensive 1 had leg-length discrepancies.

Conclusion.—The long-term effects of thrombi secondary to umbilical artery catheterization remain uncertain. None of these infants were treated, but these findings suggest that the need for treatment should be reevaluated. These infants should have careful long-term follow-up, with special attention to hypertension and leg length discrepancy.

▶ The incidence of hypertension and leg growth abnormalities occurring years after untreated umbilical artery catheter-induced aortic thrombosis in children is disturbing. The obvious question is whether children with either thrombolytic or surgical treatment fare any better than this control group without specific treatment. At present, we do not know.—J.M. Porter, M.D.

Microvascular Reconstruction of Major Arteries in Neonates and Small Children
LaQuaglia MP, Upton J, May JW Jr (Children's Hosp Med Ctr; Massachusetts Gen Hosp, Boston)
J Pediatr Surg 26:1136–1140, 1991   4–6

Background.—Arterial injuries are uncommon in small children. When they occur, they are usually iatrogenic and have a catastrophic result. Nine cases of successful major arterial reconstruction performed during the first 2 years of life (using microvascular methods) were discussed.

Cases.—The median age at repair was 28 days. Half the children were revascularized in the first month of life. All were at risk for tissue necrosis. Eight children had had iatrogenic injuries, which were related to invasive catheter manipulation in 6 cases and operative technique in 2. In the ninth patient, the subclavian artery had been sacrificed during excision of a malignant tumor. Femoral repairs were done in 5 cases, subclavian in 1, brachial in 1, posterior tibial in 1, and radial artery in 1. In 1 case, direct arterial repair of a brachial artery was done; in another, it was done with a transected superficial femoral artery. Reversed saphenous vein grafts were used in the rest of the children. Iatrogenic dissection of the ipsilateral iliac artery required the use of a femofemoral bypass graft to attain adequate inflow in 1 patient. No operative deaths

Types of Repair, Vessel Diameters, and Outcomes

Case No.	Follow-Up (d)	Type of Graft	Artery Repaired	Proximal Diameter (mm)	Distal Diameter (mm)	Patency	Survival
1	10	None	Brachial	0.7	0.7	Patent	Died
2	1	Vein	Femoral	2.0	2.0	Patent	Died
3	21	Vein	Femoral	2.0	2.0	Patent	Alive
4	542	Vein	Femoral	2.0	2.0	Patent	Alive
5	4,052	Vein	Femoral	2.0	2.0	Stenosis*	Alive
6	516	Vein	Subclavian	1.8	1.8	Patent	Died
7	1,826	Vein	Posterior tibial	1.0	0.8	Patent	Alive
8	1,449	None	Femoral	2.2	2.2	Patent	Alive
9	1,085	Vein	Radial	1.2	0.5	Patent	Alive

* Pulse volume recordings showed severe stenosis, but the limb was viable.
(Courtesy of LaQuaglia MP, Upton J, May JW Jr: *J Pediatr Surg* 26:1136–1140, 1991.)

occurred. There were no reexplorations, and normal perfusion was restored to all involved extremities (table).

Conclusion.—Microvascular technique permits early, successful arterial reconstruction and limb salvage in neonates and small children. Continuous follow-up of patients undergoing vascular procedures in infancy is needed.

▶ The remarkable achievement of 100% actuarial arterial repair patency at a mean follow-up of 18 months is noted. These authors believe that an 8-20 power magnification operating microscope and 9-0 to 11-0 sutures are important in achieving these dramatic results.—J.M. Porter, M.D.

Peripheral Vascular Disease in Patients With Systemic Lupus Erythematosus
McDonald J, Stewart J, Urowitz MB, Gladman DD (Wellesley Hosp, Univ of Toronto, Ont, Canada)
Ann Rheum Dis 51:56–60, 1992   4–7

Background.—Atherosclerotic disease, especially that involving the coronary arteries, can develop prematurely in patients with systemic lupus erythematosus. Ten patients with lupus who were seen with intermittent claudication or gangrene were studied. They were among 563 patients included in a prospective follow-up series, and they were matched with other patients with lupus for age, gender, demographic characteristics, and risk factors.

Results.—The activity of lupus was similar in the study patients and controls, as were the values for partial thromboplastin time and the prevalence of cardiolipin antibody. A similar number of patients received steroids and had a family history of atherosclerosis. The groups did not differ with respect to hyperlipidema, smoking status, hypertension, or the use of oral contraceptives. A longer duration of lupus and longer steroid use were both risk factors for peripheral vascular disease. Eight of the 10 patients had co-existing coronary artery disease or transient ischemic attacks.

Conclusion.—Peripheral vascular disease develops earlier in patients with systemic lupus than in the general population. At particular risk are those patients with a longer duration of lupus and those using steroids for some time. Most of these patients also had coronary artery disease as well as peripheral vascular disease.

▶ I have always wondered—but have been unable to determine—whether long-term steroid use is, in itself, a risk factor for atherosclerosis progression. These authors suggest that it may be.—J.M. Porter, M.D.

Peripheral Gangrene Associated With Kawasaki Disease

Tomita S, Chung K, Mas M, Gidding S, Shulman ST (Northwestern Univ, Chicago; Univ of California, San Diego; Univ of Miami, Fla; Kurume Univ, Japan)
Clin Infect Dis 14:121–126, 1992　　　　　　　　　　　　　　　4–8

Background.—Kawasaki disease (KD), which was first described in 1967, was initially thought to be a benign disease without sequelae; however, the complications of coronary artery aneurysms and the occasional involvement of other medium-sized arteries are now well known. A rare but serious complication of severe peripheral ischemia with resultant gangrene was described in 3 American infants and reviewed in 8 patients, including only 1 in Japan, whose case reports were previously reported.

Patients.—Japan has the greatest incidence of KD, but this complication has been reported only once in that country. Among the reported cases, the ethnic distribution is 6 whites, 2 blacks, 2 Asians, and 1 American Indian. In these 11 infants, at least 9 had associated giant coronary aneurysms and 8 had associated peripheral arterial aneurysms. In 8 infants, the subtle manifestations of KD delayed the diagnosis and initiation of therapy until ≥ 14 days after onset. Peripheral ischemia was noted 15–31 days after onset.

Findings.—The pathogenesis of KD probably includes a combination of local peripheral arteritis, arteriospasm, thrombosis peripherally and/or more proximally, and cardiogenic shock. Anti-inflammatory therapy affects the active arteritis and is central to the control of the peripheral arterial disease in KD. Recommended treatment to prevent the potentially devastating consequences of progressive gangrene includes the combination of anti-inflammatory (salicylates and intravenous gamma globulin), vasodilator (prostaglandin E_1 or sympathetic block), and thrombolytic and anticoagulant therapies. Corticosteroids should be avoided because of an increased risk of coronary abnormalities, although there is some evidence that they may be helpful in cases of cardiogenic shock.

Conclusion.—The 3 American infants with KD complicated by peripheral extremity gangrene bring the total of reported cases to 11. Recommended therapy includes anti-inflammatory agents, vasodilative agents or methods, and thrombolytic and/or anticoagulant agents to attempt to prevent progressive gangrene.

▶ To date, most of the children reported in whom peripheral gangrene has developed in association with KD have had associated coronary and peripheral arterial aneurysms. The precise vascular cause of the gangrene is unclear, but it may involve vasculitis, thrombosis, or arterial embolism.—J.M. Porter, M.D.

Vascular Involvement in Behçet's Disease

Koç Y, Güllü I, Akpek G, Akpolat T, Kansu E, Kiraz S, Batman F, Kansu T, Balkanci F, Akkaya S, Zilei T (Hacettepe Univ, Ankara, Turkey)
J Rheumatol 19:402–410, 1992   4–9

Background.—Behçet's disease (BD) is a multisystemic disorder characterized by vasculitis, recurrent oral and genital ulcerations, and uveitis. At its onset, there may be manifestations of vascular involvement alone.

Patients.—Of 137 patients with BD who were seen in Turkey in 1986-1990, 38 (27.7%) had vascular involvement, which included subcutaneous thrombophlebitis or major vascular lesions (table).

Findings.—The ratio of males to females was greater in the patients with vascular involvement. The most frequent vascular abnormality is venous thrombosis. Arterial aneurysms and/or thrombosis occurred in only 4 of 137 patients. Subcutaneous thrombophlebitis was the most prevalent vascular manifestation, and these patients were more likely to have major venous occlusions in the lower extremities and inferior vena cava. Arterial lesions made up only 12% of the vascular complications.

Conclusion.—Vascular involvement is a prominent component of BD.

▶ Behçet's disease is being recognized with greater frequency, and it is certainly being reported in the literature with greater frequency than it was previously. In a remarkable clinical series, 38 of 137 patients had significant vascular involvement which, in the overwhelming majority of patients, was

Frequency and Types of Involvement in 38 Patients With Vascular BD		
Involvement Site	No.	Percent
1. Venous		
Subcutaneous thrombophlebitis	18	47.3
Vena cava superior	6	15.8
Vena cava inferior	6	15.8
Femoral	4	10.5
Cerebral sinus	3	7.9
Subclavian	2	5.2
Hepatic	1	5.2
Brachial	1	2.6
Axillary	1	2.6
2. Arterial		
Pulmonary	3	7.9
Carotid	1	2.6
Popliteal	1	2.6
Radial	1	2.6

venous thrombosis of both superficial deep and visceral veins. The distinct possibility of venous or arterial thrombotic disease in patients with BD must be considered.—J.M. Porter, M.D.

Neurologic Involvement in Behçet Disease: Imaging Findings in 16 Patients
Banna M, El-Ramahi K (King Faisal Specialist Hosp, Riyadh, Saudi Arabia)
AJR 157:867–872, 1991   4–10

Background.—As many as 25% of patients with Behçet disease (BD) have neurologic manifestations. Computed tomography is of little diagnostic value in these cases. The MRI findings in 16 patients with CNS involvement by BD were reviewed. They represent 44% of all such patients seen in a 10-year period (Fig 4-3).

Findings.—Only 2 of 21 CT studies showed equivocal findings of brain-stem atrophy. Two of 4 angiograms gave conclusive evidence of dural venous sinus thrombosis. Nine patients had MRI abnormalities consisting of high signal intensity foci on T2-weighted images. The lesions decreased in size after treatment with steroids—either alone or combined with immunosuppressive agents. In some instances, they disappeared.

Conclusion.—A wide range of systems may be involved by BD. Japanese researchers believe that the basic brain lesion is a chronic relapsing inflammatory-cell infiltration around venules and capillaries, and occasionally around arteries. The finding of small high-signal foci on T2-

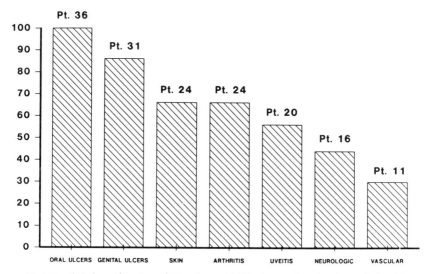

Fig 4–3.—Clinical manifestations of 36 patients with BD who constituted study population. (Courtesy of Banna M, El-Ramahi K: *AJR* 157:867–872, 1991.)

weighted MRI can help diagnose cerebral BD. The primary differential diagnoses include multiple slcerosis, brain-stem infarction, and rhombo-encephalitis.

▶ Neurologic manifestations accompany BD in 10% to 25% of patients. Although CT evaluation of the CNS has been relatively unrewarding, this study indicates remarkable findings from MRI evaluation of the CNS in a number of these patients. The primary abnormalities consist of abnormally high signal intensity foci on T2-weighted images. These lesions diminished or disappeared with corticosteroid or immunosuppressive drugs in a number of patients.—J.M. Porter, M.D.

False Aneurysm of the Abdominal Aorta in Behçet's Disease
Smith EJ, Abulafi M, McPherson GA, Allison DJ, Mansfield AO (Royal Postgraduate Med School, London)
Eur J Vasc Surg 5:481–484, 1991   4–11

Background.—Large arteries are not commonly involved in Behçet's disease (BD), but lesions in such arteries tend to be more severe and progressive. In a patient with BD, a false aneurysm of the abdominal aorta developed.

Case Report.—Man, 28, with BD had abdominal and back pain. Ultrasound examination showed an aortic dissection below the level of the renal arteries and an associated thrombus on the posterior wall. The patient was managed nonoperatively. On a subsequent readmission for persistent back pain, digital subtraction angiography showed a false aneurysm arising from the posterior wall of the lumbar aorta. In view of the active BD, surgery was not performed, but the false aneurysm was embolized. A second embolization was performed 1 month later for a newly formed extension of the sac. Subsequent definitive surgery was performed when the patient had signs of a leaking aneurysm, and when his BD was considered less active. The infrarenal aorta was replaced with a Dacron graft, and a Dacron cuff was sutured over the proximal and distal anastomoses to prevent further aneurysm formation. Follow-up at more than 3 years showed no recurrence of false aneurysm or further complications.

Conclusion.—In the presence of active BD, reconstructive surgery for false aneurysm of the aorta is associated with a high incidence of complications. A nonoperative interventional approach by embolization of the false aneurysm can control aneurysmal progression until the underlying disease is less active. Definitive surgery can then be performed with less likelihood of postoperative complications.

▶ Large artery involvement, although uncommon, may be seen in patients with BD. This interesting patient had a false aneurysm of the abdominal aorta that initially was treated nonoperatively because of the risk of surgical complications during active Behçet's vasculitis.—J.M. Porter, M.D.

Efficacy of Ketanserin in the Therapy of Raynaud's Phenomenon: Thermometric Data
Arosio E, Montesi G, Zannoni M, Perbellini L, Paluani F, Lechi A (Istituto di Clinica Medica e Medicina del Lavoro, Verona, Italy; Univ of Verona, Italy)
Angiology 42:408–413, 1991   4–12

Introduction.—Ketanserin has been proposed as a treatment for Raynaud's phenomenon because it inhibits the vasospasm-potentiating effect of serotonin.

Methods.—After a 2-week washout period during which placebo was administered, ketanserin, 40 mg, was given twice daily for 15 days to 12 patients with stable Raynaud's phenomenon. Computerized thermometry was used to assess circulation in the fingers at 23°C, after cold testing at 10°C, and after thermal recovery.

Results.—There was no marked symptomatic change, but administration of ketanserin did reduce the number of daily attacks and reduce their duration. Finger temperatures, especially those at baseline and after recovery, increased during treatment.

Conclusion.—Ketanserin appears to promote circulation in the fingers and reduce vasospasm in patients with Raynaud's phenomenon.

▶ Our experience indicates that only approximately 10% of patients with Raynaud's syndrome have sufficiently severe symptoms to warrant drug therapy. Objective assessment of response to drug treatment is almost impossible, because there is no generally agreed on method by which objective reponse can be detected. The interesting antiseratonin drug, ketanserin, may be of limited value in vasospastic Raynaud's phenomenon.—J.M. Porter, M.D.

Retrospective Comparison of Iloprost With Other Treatments for Secondary Raynaud's Phenomenon
Watson HR, Belcher G (Burgess Hill, West Sussex, England)
Ann Rheum Dis 50:359–361, 1991   4–13

Background.—Patients with secondary Raynaud's phenomenon generally have not been adequately managed by any single method. Iloprost is a chemically stable prostacyclin analogue that is more effective than placebo in treating Raynaud's phenomenon secondary to connective tissue disease.

Methods.—Infusions of iloprost were given to 127 patients with Raynaud's episodes secondary to connective tissue disease. In 84 patients, the results of other treatments were available. More than 85% of the patients had systemic sclerosis. Iloprost was infused at a rate of as much as 2 ng/kg/min for 6–8 hours.

Results.—Patients found infusion of iloprost to be helpful in 58% of the 84 cases in which previous treatments had been tried. Only 43% of these patients had found other treatment to be helpful. Half the 48 patients who had not previously responded to any treatment did respond to iloprost.

Conclusion.—Intravenously administered iloprost is a useful treatment for patients with severe secondary Raynaud's phenomenon, even those who have failed to respond to other measures.

▶ I do not believe long-term intravenous therapy with iloprost is appropriate treatment for Raynaud's attacks. We and others, however, have found it useful for symptomatic treatment of patients who have extremely painful ischemic digital ulcerations associated with autoimmune disease, especially scleroderma. I continue to be unclear as to the mechanism of benefit that some claim persists long after the cessation of drug administration. This has not been our experience. On balance, I think this drug is modestly useful for the symptomatic treatment of painful digital ulceration.—J.M. Porter, M.D.

Encephalo-Omental Synangiosis in the Management of Moyamoya Disease
Havlik RJ, Fried I, Chyatte D, Modlin IM (Yale Univ, New Haven, Conn)
Surgery 111:156–162, 1992   4–14

Introduction.—Moyamoya disease is a chronic occlusive cerebrovascular disorder characterized by a stenosed distal internal carotid artery and by the development of a fine vascular network at the base of the brain. Often, the anterior and/or middle cerebral arteries also are involved. Cerebral ischemia is manifested as repeated episodes of hemiplegia, dysarthria, and involuntary movements.

Case Report.—Man, 43, had a right periventricular infarct and, subsequently, episodes of left arm weakness and numbness that lasted up to several hours. He had several episodes of slurred speech. Angiography showed bilateral internal carotid and middle cerebral stenoses with multiple collateral vessels at the base of the brain. A right temporal artery–middle cerebral bypass relieved symptoms for 2 years, when angiography showed moyamoya vessels, multiple anterior and middle cerebral stenoses, and a patent bypass. A scan demonstrated reduced perfusion in the area of the right basal ganglia and parietal cortex. Perfusion improved after an omental pedicle graft was placed through a subcutaneous tunnel on the right cerebral cortex. The symptoms resolved dramatically in the 2.5 years since the procedure was performed, and left-sided function improved considerably.

Conclusion.—These data suggest that omental transposition may be used either as an adjunct to or in place of superficial temporal artery–middle cerebral artery bypass to treat moyamoya disease.

▶ This disease appears to be distinctly uncommon in America; however, vascular surgeons who treat carotid disease should be familiar with its existence. Therefore, I have included this discussion. One simply cannot evaluate the efficacy of omental transplantation from a single case.—J.M. Porter, M.D.

Temporal Arteritis With Low Erythrocyte Sedimentation Rate: A Review of Five Cases
Wise CM, Agudelo CA, Chmelewski WL, McKnight KM (Wake Forest Univ, Winston-Salem, NC)
Arthritis Rheum 34:1571–1574, 1991   4–15

Background.—Temporal (giant cell) arteritis is a systemic vasculitis chiefly involving the cranial arteries. It is primarily seen in individuals older than 50 years of age. Most of the patients have an increased erythrocyte sedimentation rate (ESR).

Methods.—Five patients with biopsy-proved temporal arteritis and an ESR below 50 mm/hr were compared with 25 other patients with a high ESR, and with 10 patients with negative temporal artery biopsy specimen results and a low ESR.

Findings.—The patients with low-ESR temporal arteritis resembled the other groups, except for a higher mean hemoglobin level than the high-ESR group. There also was a history of polymyalgia rheumatica or steroid therapy in 4 of 5 patients. Apparently, even low-dose steroid therapy is able to reduce the ESR in patients with temporal arteritis.

Conclusion.—Comparatively few patients with temporal arteritis have a low ESR, and steroid therapy probably has a role in many of these patients.

▶ Giant cell arteritis usually is encountered in vascular surgical practice because of axillary-brachial arterial involvement, but it occasionally is encountered because of carotid involvement. A high sedimentation rate is regarded by many as a requirement for the diagnosis of this disease, but it seems clear that a small number of patients who have giant cell arteritis do, in fact, have a low ESR. These authors note that many patients with low ESR with giant cell arteritis have a prior history of steroid therapy which may have affected the ESR.—J.M. Porter, M.D.

Temporal Artery Biopsy Technique: A Clinico-Anatomical Approach

Scott KR, Tse DT, Kronish JW (Univ of Miami School of Medicine)
Ophthalmic Surg 22:519–525, 1991   4–16

Introduction.—Temporal artery biopsy is required to establish a diagnosis of temporal arteritis. A technique based on the branching patterns of the superficial temporal artery, the fascial layers, and the site of the temporal branches of the facial nerve was described.

Technique.—The frontal branch of the artery is usually selected for biopsy. However, if only the parietal branch is clinically involved, then it, rather than the frontal branch, should be selected for surgery. The "danger zone" (Fig 4-4) outlines the area in which an incision may cause significant facial nerve injury. If the arterial biopsy in the danger zone is required, the surgeon must take care to remain external to the superficial temporal fascia to avoid injury to the facial nerve branches that run just deep to the fascia. The artery is superficial. When local signs are absent, a distal segment of the frontal branch should biopsied. Wound closure is best done in 2 separate layers.

▶ There may be more here than many people want to know about temporal artery biopsy. Nonetheless, it seems obvious that careful incision placement is critical, both in avoiding nerve injury and in assuring adequate arterial biopsy.—J.M. Porter, M.D.

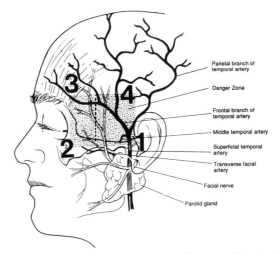

Fig 4–4.—Anatomy of the superficial temporal artery. The "danger zone" for the facial nerve is outlined by the following reference points: (*1*) the tragus of the ear; (*2*) the junction of the zygomatic arch and the lateral orbital rim; (*3*) 2 cm above the level of the superior orbital rim and in a line directly superior to 2; and (*4*) superior to the tragus and in horizontal alignment with 3. The *vertical dotted line* defines the site of the cross-sectional diagram and is not an incision line. (Courtesy of Scott KR, Tse DT, Kronish JW: *Ophthalmic Surg* 22:519–525, 1991.)

**Visual Recovery in Two Patients After Intravenous Methylpredniso-
lone Treatment of Central Retinal Artery Occlusion Secondary to Gi-
ant-Cell Arteritis**
Matzkin DC, Slamovits TL, Sachs R, Burde RM (Montefiore Med Ctr/Albert
Einstein College of Medicine, New York)
Ophthalmology 99:68–71, 1992   4–17

Background.—Giant cell arteritis may present with marked loss of vision in 1 eye. Without treatment, there is significant risk that vision will
be lost in the fellow eye within 1–10 days. The usual cause is anterior
ischemic optic neuropathy, but central retinal artery occlusion or retinal
ischemia also may be responsible.

Cases.—Two patients with biopsy-proved giant cell arteritis had central retinal artery occlusion and lost acuity to the point of no light perception. Methylprednisolone, 15–30 mg/kg/day, was given intravenously, and both patients regained baseline visual acuity. The patients
received prednisone after discharge from the hospital. Both were followed up for at least a year after the event.

Discussion.—Past reports have suggested that useful vision does not
often return in giant cell arteritis, especially when light perception is lost.
Why these patients, both of whom had arteritic central retinal artery occlusion, regained excellent vision is uncertain, but early, aggressive steroid treatment may well prove helpful in these cases.

▶ I was unaware that there was any prospect for vision recovery in patients
with central retinal artery occlusion associated with giant cell arteritis. The
remarkable vision recovery that occurred in these 2 patients after administration of intravenous methylprednisolone suggests that this therapy should at
least be considered in such patients.—J.M. Porter, M.D.

Surgical Management of the Thoracic Outlet Compression Syndrome
Davies AH, Walton J, Stuart E, Morris PJ (Univ of Oxford, Oxford, England)
Br J Surg 78:1193–1195, 1991   4–18

Background.—There is continuing disagreement as to whether the
first rib should be removed in the presence of a cervical rib to relieve
thoracic outlet compression syndrome (TOCS).

Patients and Management.—Fifty-eight patients had surgery during
1975–1988 for TOCS; 22 of these patients had a cervical rib. Three
fourths of the patients had vascular symptoms (many of them with a neurologic component), whereas 19% of the patients had neurologic symptoms only (Table 1). Thirty-six patients had the first rib excised, 19 had a
cervical rib removed, 2 patients had fibrous bands divided, and 1 had resection of a large transverse process.

TABLE 1.—Nature of the Presenting Symptoms in 58 Patients With and Without a Cervical Rib

Symptoms	No. of patients
Presence of a cervical rib	
Arterial	5
Raynaud's	1
Arterial/neurological	8
Neurological	6
Venous	2
Total	22
Absence of a cervical rib	
Arterial	7
Raynaud's	2
Arterial/neurological	9
Neurological	5
Venous	10
Other	3
Total	36

(Courtesy of Davies AH, Walton J, Stuart E, et al: Br J Surg 78:1193–1195, 1991.)

TABLE 2.—Symptomatic Outcome of Surgery in 21 Patients With a Cervical Rib and in 32 Without

	Total no. of patients	Cure	Improvement	No improvement
Presence of a cervical rib				
Arterial	5*	4	1	
Raynaud's	1		1	
Arterial/ neurological	8	8		
Neurological	5	5†		
Venous	2	2		
Total	21	19	2	0
Absence of a cervical rib				
Arterial	6	3	2‡	1
Raynaud's	2		2	
Arterial/ neurological	7	6		1
Neurological	5	3		2
Venous	9	5	4	
Other	3	2	1	
Total	32	19	9	4

* One patient had fibrous bands divided.
† Two patients had first rib excision.
‡ One patient had fibrous bands divided, and the other had a transverse process removed.
(Courtesy of Davies AH, Walton J, Stuart E, et al: Br J Surg 78:1193–1195, 1991.)

Results.—Thirty-eight patients (72%) were cured of their symptoms, and another 11 improved significantly. Comparable results were achieved by excising a cervical rib or the first rib (Table 2).

Conclusion.—Patients with TOCS who have a cervical rib are adequately treated by excision of the cervical rib alone.

▶ A remarkable 38% of the patients in this thoracic outlet series had cervical ribs. The authors conclude that, in symptomatic patients, excision of the cervical rib alone is adequate and concomitant excision of the first rib is not required. I note with interest, however, that 62% of the patients did not have a cervical rib. Thus, it appears that thoracic outlet surgery in the absence of bony abnormality has reared its ugly head in Great Britain.—J.M. Porter, M.D.

Endoscopic Transthoracic Sympathectomy in the Treatment of Hyperhidrosis
Edmondson RA, Banerjee AK, Rennie JA (King's College Hosp, London)
Ann Surg 215:289–293, 1992   4–19

Introduction.—Axillary hyperhidrosis may be managed by excising the eccrine glands; however, if there is palmar involvement, sympathectomy is the only satisfactory option that yields lasting results. The results of 50 endoscopic transaxillary dorsal sympathectomies performed during a 5-year period were reviewed.

Technique.—An incision is made in the anterior axillary line over the third rib space, avoiding the long thoracic nerve. A Verres needle is inserted after clamping the side of the endotracheal tube, and the lung is slowly deflated by instilling carbon dioxide interpleurally. A laparoscope is inserted to visualize the upper sympathetic chain. A second small incision is made over the fourth interspace to insert a diathermy probe, and the second through fourth ganglia (with their interconnecting fibers) are treated.

Results.—The procedure improved or eliminated symptoms of hyperhidrosis in most patients. All but 8% of the patients were satisfied with the outcome. Three fourths of the patients had compensatory sweating, and half had gustatory sweating; however, these effects were widely accepted by the patients. No patient had permanent Horner's syndrome.

Conclusion.—Endoscopic transaxillary dorsal sympathectomy is a simple, effective, and inexpensive surgical treatment for hyperhidrosis of the upper extremity. Only an overnight hospital stay is required.

▶ Hyperhidrosis, although uncommon, is encountered with sufficient frequency that vascular surgeons should have a plan of action for the condition. Topical application of various aluminum chloride-based compounds may be tried first; partial axillary skin excision is another option. Thoracic sympathec-tomy traditionally gives good results; Performing the procedure through an endoscope may be an improvement, although a short axillary third interspace thoracotomy seems to work perfectly well.—J.M. Porter, M.D.

Arterial Thromboembolic Complications of Inflammatory Bowel Disease: Report of Three Cases

Novotny DA, Rubin RJ, Slezak FA, Porter JA (Akron City Hosp, Akron, Ohio; Northeastern Ohio Universities College of Medicine, Rootstown, Ohio; Muehlenberg Hosp, Plainfield, NJ)

Dis Colon Rectum 35:193–196, 1992   4–20

Introduction.—Thrombembolism involving both the arterial and venous systems is a recognized problem in patients with inflammatory bowel disease. As many as one third of all patients have extra-intestinal manifestations.

Patients.—In 3 patients with active pancolonic ulcerative colitis, arterial thromboembolic complications developed before operative treatment. A woman, 34, who had colitis for 11 years and had a history of migratory phlebitis and axillary venous thrombosis, also had leg ischemia secondary to clot in the distal aorta and extending to the common iliac artery. A man, 38, who had bloody diarrhea for 18 months had several extra-intestinal manifestations, including superficial phlebitis and popliteal artery embolism. An elderly woman with a long history of ulcerative colitis had small bowel ischemia resulting from superior mesenteric artery embolism. Ischemic necrosis of the ileostomy developed after surgery, necessitating revision. The patient died postoperatively of massive stroke.

A Survey.—Reports from 262 members of the American Society of Colon and Rectal Surgeons yielded data on 57 patients, including these patients, who had a total of 68 thromboembolic events (table). Approximately two thirds of these events were deep venous thromboses and/or pulmonary emboli. These complications resulted in 4 deaths.

Thromboembolic Complications	
Deep venous thromboses and/or pulmonary emboli	40
Cerebrovascular accidents	10
Venous occlusions (not deep venous thromboses)	8
Arterial occlusions	8
Other	2
Total number of events	68

(Courtesy of Novotny DA, Rubin RJ, Slezak FA, et al: *Dis Colon Rectum* 35:193-196, 1992.)

Conclusion.—Arterial thromboembolic complications of inflammatory bowel disease can produce significant morbidity. Colectomy may be necessary, because long-term anticoagulation is limited by the risk of gastrointestinal tract bleeding.

▶ Extra-intestinal manifestations of inflammatory bowel disease occur in almost one third of patients. Arterial and venous thromboembolic complications are well-recognized accompaniments of inflammatory bowel disease in a number of patients, although the pathophysiologic mechanisms are unknown.—J.M. Porter, M.D.

What Happens to Patients With Non-Vascular Leg Pain?
Varty K, van Dorpe J, Johnston JAS, Campbell WB (Royal Devon and Exeter Hosp, Exeter, England)
BMJ 303:1516, 1991   4–21

Background.—Nonvascular leg pain refers to pain in the leg or foot that suggests arterial occlusive disease despite the absence of such disease.

Methods.—A total of 525 patients with pain in the leg or foot were referred to a vascular surgery clinic during a 3-year period; 55 of these had nonvascular pain diagnosed when arterial disease was excluded by clinical observation, stress testing, and Doppler ultrasonography. The median follow-up was 27 months.

Course.—Thirteen patients were referred to other specialists who made a diagnosis—most often of lumbar spinal disease (table). Eleven of

Conditions Causing Nonvascular Leg
Pain in 13 Patients Who Received
Diagnosis After Referral to
Other Specialists

Diagnosis	No*
Spinal stenosis	3
Sciatica	3
Lumbar spondylosis	2
Peripheral neuropathy	2
Multiple sclerosis	2
Osteoarthritis of hip	1
Morton's neuroma	1

* One patient had both spinal stenosis and peripheral neuropathy.
(Courtesy of Varty K, van Dorpe J, Johnston JAS, et al: *BMJ* 303:1516, 1991.)

the 36 patients who had no diagnosis improved clinically, whereas 17 remained unchanged and 8 became worse. Six patients had evidence of mild arterial disease at follow-up, but the symptoms were consistent with arterial insufficiency in none of these patients.

Conclusion.—After significant arterial disease is ruled out by Doppler study, most patients with nonvascular leg pain can be reassured. Less than one fourth of the patients had symptomatic deterioration.

▶ This is a curious paper. What happens to patients with leg pain who are referred to vascular surgeons but turn out not to have a vascular cause of their leg pain? This study indicates that almost one third of the patients eventually will have another diagnosis established; of the remaining patients, nearly one half persist with unchanged symptoms, one fourth improve, and one fourth deteriorate. Interestingly, no patients had evidence of significant arterial disease during follow-up.—J.M. Porter, M.D.

Femoral Pseudoaneurysm From Drugs of Abuse: Ligation or Reconstruction?

Padberg F Jr, Hobson R II, Lee B, Anderson R, Manno J, Breitbart G, Swan K (Univ Hosp and St Michael's Med Ctr, Newark, NJ; VA Med Ctr, East Orange, NJ)
J Vasc Surg 15:642–648, 1992   4–22

Background.—Arterial pseudoaneurysms may form when drugs are self-injected in the groin, and an infected pseudoaneurysm that goes untreated may cause serious complications or death. How best to manage these lesions is not clear. Eighteen patients with femoral artery aneurysms treated in 1981–1989 were reviewed.

Methods.—Concern about the risk of amputation if the femoral artery was acutely interrupted prompted a reluctance to limit initial management to ligation and débridement. Six patients had femoral artery ligation primarily, whereas 12 underwent arterial reconstruction by vein patch angioplasty or by an autogenous or prosthetic bypass graft. The

	No. patients	Total No. reoperations for arterial complications	No. amputations	Mortality (%)
Comparative Outcome of Ligation and Revascularization				
Ligation	6	2	0	0
Reconstruction	12	13	3	0

(Courtesy of Padberg F Jr, Hobson R II, Lee B, et al: *J Vasc Surg* 15:642–648, 1992.)

most common site of treatment was the femoral bifurcation. Limb viability was estimated intraoperatively from the presence of an audible Doppler signal at the ankle.

Results.—Three of the 12 patients having revascularization required amputation, and 13 required secondary arterial surgery in addition to débridement and skin grafting. None of the patients having primary ligation and débridement required amputation (table).

Conclusion.—Primary ligation is indicated to control the septic focus and to eliminate the risk of hemorrhage in these cases. Revascularization is considered only when the absence of a Doppler signal at the ankle indicates acute limb ischemia.

▶ Direct vascular repair of infected arterial pseudoaneurysms at sites of illicit drug injection are associated with an inordinate incidence of graft infection, thrombosis, and hemorrhage. These authors convincingly demonstrate that, if there is a persistence of an audible Doppler signal at the ankle after temporary arterial occlusion, simple arterial ligation is the preferable means of treatment. I certainly agree that revascularization should be considered only in those patients with limb-threatening ischemia associated with simple ligation.—J.M. Porter, M.D.

Adventitial Cystic Disease of the Popliteal Artery: Early Recurrence After CT Guided Percutaneous Aspiration

Sieunarine K, Lawrence-Brown MMD, Kelsey P (Royal Perth Hosp, Perth, Australia)
J Cardiovasc Surg 32:702–704, 1991   4–23

Introduction.—Adventitial cystic disease of the popliteal artery is a rare cause of peripheral vascular insufficiency. Percutaneous aspiration has been proposed if the cyst is found before the artery is totally occluded.

Case Report.—Man, 55, had intermittent claudication for 2 months, with absent left popliteal and posterior tibial pulses and a weak dorsalis pedis pulse. A smooth spiral defect was found in the popliteal artery (Fig 4–5). Knee flexion to 90 degrees occluded the vessel (Fig 4–6). A large cyst indenting the anteromedial arterial wall was seen on CT. Attempted aspiration failed, but the patient's walking improved. The symptoms recurred after a few weeks. Thick fluid was aspirated under CT guidance, improving the lumen (Figs 4–7 and 4–8). Claudication returned within 6 months, when angiography confirmed incomplete compression of the popliteal artery. A 5- × 2-cm fusiform cyst was deroofed, and pulses were present 2 months later; the ankle/brachial pressure ratio exceeded unity in both lower extremities.

Conclusion.—If the artery is patent, percutaneous aspiration offers treatment with minimal trauma. Complete decompression may be diffi-

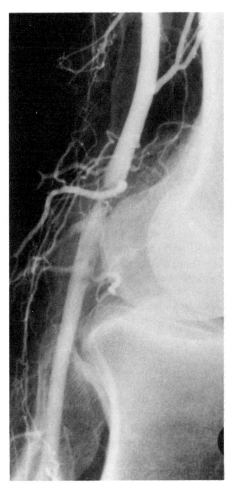

Fig 4–5.—Photograph illustrating compression of the artery. (Courtesy of Sieunarine K, Lawrence-Brown MMD, Kelsey P: *J Cardiovasc Surg* 32:702–704, 1991.)

cult to achieve, and later recurrence is a possibility that mandates long-term follow-up.

▶ I am not surprised that percutaneous cyst aspiration resulted in a recurrence. I am hard pressed to understand why the cyst would not recur. I believe surgery is the treatment of choice, and that lesion excision with segmental interposition vein grafting is the general procedure of choice.—J.M. Porter, M.D.

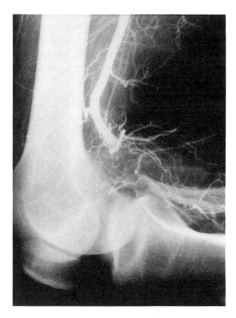

Fig 4–6.—Photograph illustrating the complete occlusion of the artery with 90-degree flexion of the knee. (Courtesy of Sieunarine K, Lawrence-Brown MMD, Kelsey P: *J Cardiovasc Surg* 32:702–704, 1991.)

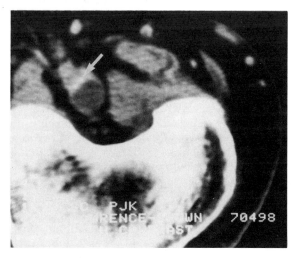

Fig 4–7.—A CT scan of the popliteal fossa showing dye (*arrow*) in the compressed lumen of the artery. (Courtesy of Sieunarine K, Lawrence-Brown MMD, Kelsey P: *J Cardiovasc Surg* 32:702–704, 1991.)

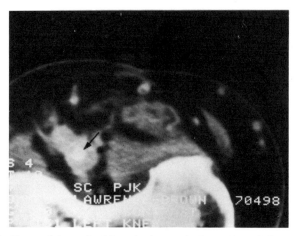

Fig 4–8.—A CT scan of the popliteal fossa (at the same level as in Fig 4–7) showing an improved lumen (*arrow*) after aspiration. (Courtesy of Sieunarine K, Lawrence-Brown MMD, Kelsey P: *J Cardiovasc Surg* 32:702–704, 1991.)

Treatment of Painful Diabetic Neuropathy With Topical Capsaicin: A Multicenter, Double-Blind, Vehicle-Controlled Study

Donofrio PD, for the Capsaicin Study Group (Wake Forest Univ, Winston-Salem, NC)
Arch Intern Med 151:2225–2229, 1991   4–24

Objective.—The pain of diabetic neuropathy is often refractory to simple analgesic treatment. Other treatments have been tried, but in many patients, their usefulness has been limited by side effects. Topically administered capsaicin has been useful in relieving the pain of postherpetic neuralgia and postmastectomy pain syndrome. A controlled, multicenter trial was conducted to ascertain the efficacy of .75% capsaicin cream in relieving the pain of diabetic neuropathy or radiculopathy.

Methods.—The analysis included 252 patients at 12 centers. The patients were randomly assigned to receive capsaicin or vehicle cream, which was applied to painful areas 4 times a day for 8 weeks. The mean patient age was 60 years, with nearly equal sex distribution; most patients had peripheral polyneuropathy. The physician's global evaluation and visual analogue scales were used to record intensity and relief of pain at 2-week intervals.

Results.—At the final visit, 69.5% of the capsaicin group had improvement on the physician's global evaluation scale vs. 53.4% of the vehicle group. Pain intensity decreased in 38.1% of the capsaicin group vs. 27.4% of the vehicle group, and pain relief improved in 58.4% of the capsaicin group vs. 45.3% of the vehicle group. Capsaicin results were statistically superior to vehicle cream alone. Capsaicin caused transient burning, sneezing, and coughing, but it was otherwise well tolerated.

Conclusion.—In patients with painful diabetic neuropathy, topically administered capsaicin cream appears to be a safe and effective treatment, given either alone or as an adjunct. It does cause an initial, transient burning, but it offers the advantages of safety, easy reversal of toxic reactions, and absence of systemic side effects and drug interaction.

▶ Our patients continue to explore unconventional herbal remedies for a variety of ailments. This paper suggests that the active ingredient in red pepper may be of some benefit in relieving the pain of diabetic neuropathy. What's next, garlic?—J.M. Porter, M.D.

Arteriopathy and Coarctation of the Abdominal Aorta in Children With Mucopolysaccharidosis: Imaging Findings
Taylor DB, Blaser SI, Burrows PE, Stringer DA, Clarke JTR, Thorner P (Univ of Toronto; Royal Perth Hosp, Pert, West Australia; British Columbia Children's Hosp, Vancouver, Canada)
AJR 157:819–823, 1991   4–25

Introduction.—In children with mucopolysaccharidosis I (MPS I), significant vascular disease can develop at an early age. Lesions are most prevalent in the coronary arteries, heart valves, endocardium and myocardium, and aorta. The lower aorta and the visceral and renal arteries tend not to be involved.

Methods.—In 1972–1990, 24 infants and children with MPS I were examined; in 8, arterial hypertension developed. In 5 of the hypertensive children, there was clinical evidence of aortic coarctation. Aortic imaging was performed in 4 hypertensive children, 3 of whom had clinical coarctation; 3 had Hurler's syndrome (MPS I H) and 1 had Scheie's syndrome.

Results.—Only 1 of the 4 patients had an abnormal ascending aorta, but all 4 had involvement of the abdominal aorta by multiple asymmetrical lesions of the aortic wall and/or abrupt, concentric aortic narrowing (Fig 4–9). The lumbar arteries were occluded in 2 patients, and major visceral arteries were abnormal in 3. Both wall lesions and stenoses at arterial origins were observed. Autopsy in one patient revealed aortic irregularity caused by deposition of mucopolysaccharide within the intima.

Conclusion.—As many as a third of patients with MPS I are hypertensive. Cardiovascular disease is found in all forms of MPS. Symptomatic children with a relatively favorable outlook may be candidates for surgical or transcatheter treatment of vascular disease. Aortic narrowing may contribute to both hypertension and claudication in these patients. Ob-

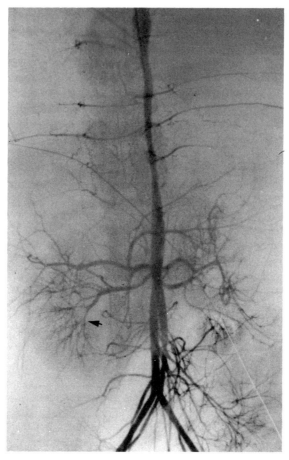

Fig 4–9.—Aortography in a boy, 4 years, with MPS I H. Aortography performed through an axillary artery shows severe, irregular, and diffuse narrowing of the suprarenal thoracoabdominal aorta, with occlusion of the multiple intercostal arteries and focal stenosis of the proximal superior mesenteric artery. Note also the caliber changes involving branches of renal arteries (*arrow*). (Courtesy of Taylor DB, Blaser SI Burrows PE, et al: AJR 157:819–823, 1991.)

structive aortic lesions may be detected sonographically or by MRI, reserving angiography for children who may be treatable.

▶ The mucopolysaccharidoses comprise a complex group of inherited disorders that are characterized by a deficiency of lysosomal enzymes. Widespread coronary, cardiac, and aortic lesions have been described in these patients. In this report, 33% of all children with MPS who were encountered at one institution were found to have significant narrowing of the abdominal aorta. Hypertension is frequent in these patients.—J.M. Porter, M.D.

Cerebral Vasculitis Associated With Cocaine Abuse

Fredericks RK, Lefkowitz DS, Challa VR, Troost BT (Wake Forest Univ, Winston-Salem, NC)
Stroke 22:1437–1439, 1991   4–26

Introduction.—Both angiographic and pathologic studies have suggested a relationship between cocaine abuse and cerebral vasculitis. In 1 patient, confirmed cerebral vasculitis occurred in temporal relation to the use of cocaine alone.

Case Report.—Woman, 24, was found acting very inappropriately after using cocaine both intravenously and intranasally. She also had used ethanol on a daily basis. The bizarre behavior was accompanied by dysphasia, ataxia, and hypertonic extremities. The patient was globally confused and exhibited right-left dissociation. A right frontal brain biopsy specimen, which was taken from an area of white matter change on MRI, revealed foci of interstitial edema near the small arteries and enlarged perivascular spaces containing proteinaceous material. Some small arterioles exhibited endothelial swelling and white cell infiltrates. The patient improved somewhat while undergoing high-dose intravenous steroid therapy.

Conclusion.—This patient suggests the existence of a non-necrotizing form of small vessel arteritis associated with cocaine abuse. These findings resemble those reported previously in connection with the abuse of amphetamines and of multiple drugs. The vascular changes may result from either hypersensitivity angiitis or angiospasm. The findings support the existence of a non-necrotizing cerebral arteritis in cocaine abusers.

▶ This case and others indicate that a non-necrotizing small vessel arteritis may be associated with cocaine use. This may occur in the brain (as shown in this paper), and it also occurs in other sites, especially the intestine.—J.M. Porter, M.D.

Genetic Linkage of the Marfan Syndrome, Ectopia Lentis, and Congenital Contractural Arachnodactyly to the Fibrillin Genes on Chromosomes 15 and 5

Tsipouras P, for the International Marfan Syndrome Collaborative Study (Univ of Connecticut Health Ctr, Farmington)
N Engl J Med 326:905–909, 1992   4–27

Background.—The Marfan syndrome is a common genetic disorder of the connective tissue that affects the musculoskeletal, cardiovascular, and ocular systems. The syndrome has been linked to the fibrillin gene on chromosome 15, fibrillin being a large glycoprotein constituent of elastin-containing microfibrils in many tissues. Congenital contractural arachnodactyly, which shares some features of Marfan syndrome, has been linked with the fibrillin gene on chromosome 5.

Objective and Methods.—Specific markers for the fibrillin genes were used for genetic linkage analysis in 28 families with Marfan syndrome and in 8 other families with various phenotypically related disorders, including congenital contractural arachnodactyly, ectopic lentis, mitral valve prolapse syndrome, and annuloaortic ectasia. Two informative markers are available, a (TAAAA)n for the fibrillin gene on chromosome 15 and a (GT)n for the fibrillin gene on chromosome 5.

Findings.—Genetic linkage was confirmed between the Marfan syndrome and fibrillin 15, with a maximum lod score of 25.6. Ectopia lentis also was linked with this gene, whereas congenital contractural arachnodactyly was linked with fibrillin 5. Neither mitral valve prolapse syndrome nor annuloaortic ectasia was linked to either fibrillin gene, although studies of fibrillin 15 for MVP syndrome were uninformative.

Conclusion.—Marfan syndrome is genetically linked with the fibrillin gene on chromosome 15, and it appears to be caused by mutations in this gene. Genes coding for other structural proteins of microfibrils may be involved in some forms of mitral valve prolapse and annuloaortic ectasia.

▶ Marfan syndrome has long been recognized as a condition with important cardiovascular abnormalities. The molecular biologic linkage of this condition to a mutation in a single fibrillin gene on chromosome 15 is another indication of the importance that molecular biology may have in defining a variety of vascular conditions. Fibrillin is an important structural unit of the elastin-associated microfibrils, important structural components of many tissues throughout the body.—J.M. Porter, M.D.

Erythromelalgia: Review of Clinical Characteristics and Pathophysiology
Kurzrock R, Cohen PR (Univ of Texas MD Anderson Cancer Ctr, Houston; Univ of Texas, Houston)
Am J Med 91:416–422, 1991   4–28

Background.—Erythromelalgia was first described by Mitchell in the 1870s. Later, a distinction was made between the idiopathic and secondary types. Some have suggested that the disorder be called erythromelalgia to emphasize the increase in skin temperature.

Clinical Aspects.—Erythromelalgia is characterized by a burning sensation, warmth, and dermal erythema involving the feet or the hands, or both. Symptoms become worse by lowering the affected part or by exposure to heat, and they are relieved by cooling or elevation. An adult-onset form may be secondary to myeloproliferative syndrome and associated thrombocytosis, or it may be idiopathic. An early-onset form begins in childhood or adolescence and is idiopathic.

Diagnosis.—Erythromelalgia associated with thrombocythemia involves disordered platelet function that affects the microvasculature. It may precede the onset of myeloproliferative disease by several years; thus, blood cell counts should be monitored in all affected adults.

Management.—Effective treatment is not available for children who have isolated erythromelalgia. Adults, however, may be markedly helped by a single daily dose of acetylsalicylic acid.

▶ The important message is that erythromelalgia is frequently a devastating condition. It appears to occur in both a childhood and an adult form, and it may or may not be associated with myeloproliferative disease. The only variety that appears to be amenable to therapy is the adult type associated with myeloproliferation. The childhood type, for which there is no effective treatment, can be utterly devastating.—J.M. Porter, M.D.

MR Angiography of Takayasu Arteritis

Oneson SR, Lewin JS, Smith AS (Case Western Reserve Univ, Cleveland; Cleveland Clinic Found)
J Comput Assist Tomogr 16:478–480, 1992   4–29

Introduction.—Takayasu's arteritis is a chronic inflammatory disorder that involves the aorta, the arteries arising from it, and the pulmonary arteries. One patient with arteritis involving vessels to the neck and upper extremities was evaluated by both angiography and MR angiography in which a 3-dimensional time-of-flight technique was used.

Case Report.—Woman, 25, who previously was in good general health, suddenly had right-sided headache, slurred speech, and left-sided weakness. Dense left hemiparesis ensued with a depressed level of consciousness, and loud supraclavicular bruits were noted on both sides, radiating to the neck. The left radial pulse was much reduced and there was a 30 mm Hg difference in systolic pressures in the 2 arms. Intra-arterial contrast angiography showed complete occlusion of the right and left common carotid arteries at their origins and moderate narrowing of the right brachiocephalic artery. The left subclavian artery was markedly narrowed beginning just distal to its origin. Magnetic resource imaging of the head showed infarction of the right lentiform and caudate nuclei. Findings at MR angiography were similar to those at conventional angiography. Steroid and heparin were given; the patient had mild left arm weakness when discharged.

▶ The MR angiogram shows impressive results in this patient with presumed Takayasu's arteritis. The future of MR arteriography appears bright.—J.M. Porter, M.D.

Transesophageal Echocardiography in the Detection of Potential Cardiac Source of Embolism in Stroke Patients

Cujec B, Polasek P, Voll C, Shuaib A (University Hosp, Saskatoon, Saskatchewan, Canada)
Stroke 22:727–733, 1991 4–30

Objective.—The diagnostic yields of echocardiography by the transesophageal and transthoracic routes were compared in the detection of a potential cardiac source of embolism. A group of 63 patients with transient ischemic attacks or stroke was evaluated between 1989 and 1990.

Results.—Transthoracic echocardiography demonstrated a potential cardiac source of embolism in 9 patients, all of whom had heart disease. Transesophageal studies revealed a potential cardiac source of embolism in 26 patients, 7 of whom lacked clinical cardiovascular abnormalities. Abnormalities detected in this group of patients included an atrial septal aneurysm in 2; a patent foramen ovale in 2; a myxomatous mitral valve in 2; and thrombus of the left atrial appendage in 1. The 26 patients with an identified cardiac source of embolism were older, had atrial fibrillation more often, and had a larger left atrium than the others. In addition, they had left ventricular hypertrophy more frequently.

Conclusion.—Transesophageal echocardiography is more sensitive than the transthoracic technique in detecting a potential cardiac source of embolism in patients with cerebral ischemia.

▶ It is now very clear that transesophageal echocardiography (TEEC) is far more sensitive than transthoracic echocardiography (TTEC) in detecting a cardiac source of arterial embolism. Although the clinical implications of many abnormalities detected by TEEC are not yet established, it does appear that, in those patients without clinically evident cardiac disease, the likelihood of detecting a cardiac source of embolism with TTEC is so low that TTEC is not indicated. Under these circumstances, TEEC is clearly the preferred diagnostic test.—G.L. Moneta, M.D.

5 Perioperative Considerations

Mortality Over a Period of 10 Years in Patients With Peripheral Arterial Disease
Criqui MH, Langer RD, Fronek A, Feigelson HS, Klauber MR, McCann TJ, Browner D (Univ of California, San Diego School of Medicine, La Jolla)
N Engl J Med 326:381–386, 1992   5–1

Background.—Patients with intermittent claudication reportedly die at twice the usual rate, and overall mortality has been found to be substantially increased among those with large vessel peripheral arterial disease (LV-PAD).

Methods.—Segmental blood pressures were measured in 565 men and women (average age, 66 years) to detect LV-PAD. In addition, flow velocity was estimated by the Doppler ultrasound method. Sixty-seven subjects (12%) were found to have LV-PAD, and they were followed up for 10 years.

Results.—Nearly 62% of men with LV-PAD and 17% of those without the disease died during follow-up. The respective figures for women were 33% and 12%. After adjusting for age, gender, and other cardiovascular risk factors, subjects with LV-PAD had a relative risk of dying of 3.1. The risk ratio for cardiovascular death was 5.9, and that for death from coronary heart disease was 6.6. Increased risk remained after excluding subjects who had a history of cardiovascular disease at the outset. Subjects with severe, symptomatic LV-PAD had a 15-fold increase in mortality from coronary heart disease.

Recommendations.—Patients documented as having LV-PAD should be carefully evaluated for cardiovascular disease, and they should be treated for known cardiovascular risk factors—particularly smoking, hyperlipidemia, and hypertension.

▶ An alternate title for this paper may be: "Wheel, Rediscovery of The." Isn't it remarkable that the leading internal medicine journal in the world found it necessary to publish the observation that patients with large artery peripheral vascular disease have a considerably increased risk of death from cardiovascular causes?—J.M. Porter, M.D.

Transesophageal Doppler Cardiac Output Monitoring: Performance During Aortic Reconstructive Surgery

Perrino AC Jr, Fleming J, LaMantia KR (Yale Univ, New Haven, Conn)
Anesth Analg 73:705–710, 1991   5–2

Introduction.—Transesophageal Doppler (TED) monitoring can provide a continuous noninvasive record of cardiac output by estimating aortic flow velocity. A prospective study of TED monitoring was conducted in 42 patients undergoing aortic reconstructive study. Nearly 500 simultaneous measurements of TED cardiac output and thermodilution cardiac output were acquired.

Methods.—The aortic cross-sectional area is determined using a nomogram. A 20F esophageal stethoscope is inserted, and Doppler signals are calibrated with the ascending aortic flow signal obtained using a transcutaneous Doppler probe. Thermodilution cardiac output is measured at end-expiration as a reference standard. Data are acquired before, during, and after placement of an aortic cross-clamp.

Results.—Correlation between the Doppler and thermodilution estimates of cardiac output deteriorated when the aorta was clamped, but it improved after removal of the clamp (Fig 5–1). Changes in Doppler and thermodilution measurements also correlated closely in the pre- and postclamp phases. The TED measurements trended accurately during large changes in thermodilution cardiac output.

Conclusion.—Transesophageal Doppler monitoring of cardiac output is an accurate means of evaluating patients with severe aortoiliac disease who undergo reconstructive surgery. Limitations of the present TED method include difficult calibration, a need to reposition the probe, and poor performance when the aorta is clamped. Manipulating the aorta impairs the accuracy of TED cardiac output monitoring.

▶ I wonder whether intraoperative transesophageal cardiac output monitoring will ultimately prove to be useful. Deterioration of the correlation of thermodilution cardiac output with esophageal Doppler during aortic clamping is especially worrisome, and it indicates that this technique may be of limited usefulness.—J.M. Porter, M.D.

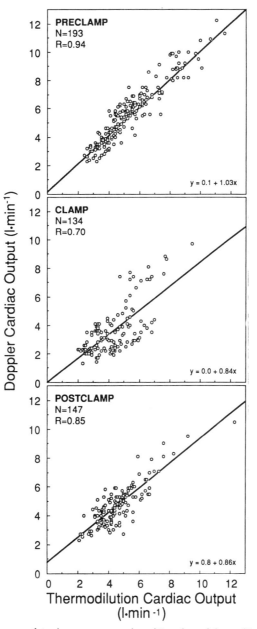

Fig 5–1.—Scattergrams of simultaneous transesophageal Doppler and thermodilution cardiac output measurements. Excellent correlation is seen in the preclamp and postclamp groups. (Courtesy of Perrino AC Jr, Fleming J, LaMantia KR: *Anesth Analg* 73:705–710, 1991.)

Dipyridamole Thallium-201 Scintigraphy as a Preoperative Screening Test: A Reexamination of Its Predictive Potential

Mangano DT, London MJ, Tubau JF, Browner WS, Hollenberg M, Krupski W, Layug EL, Massie B, the Study of Perioperative Ischemia Research Group (Univ of California, San Francisco; VA Med Ctr, San Francisco)

Circulation 84:493–502, 1991   5–3

Background.—Recent myocardial infarction and current congestive heart failure are uniformly recognized as predictors of perioperative cardiac morbidity, but the importance of other predictors remains controversial. Whether dipyridamole thallium-201 (^{201}T1 scintigraphy is useful in preoperative screening for perioperative myocardial ischemia and infarction was determined.

Methods.—One woman and 59 men who were undergoing elective vascular surgery had ^{201}T1 scintigraphy before their operation. The surgeon was blinded to the scintigraphy results. Myocardial ischemia was monitored intraoperatively by continuous 12-lead ECG and transesophogeal echocardiography (TEE); it was monitored postoperatively by continuous 2-lead ECG. Adverse perioperative outcomes included cardiac death, myocardial infarction, unstable angina, severe ischemia, or congestive heart failure.

Results.—Redistribution defects (defects that improved or reversed on delayed scintigrams) were seen in 37% of patients, persistent defects in 30%, and no defects in 33%. Fifty-four percent of adverse outcomes occurred in patients who did not have redistribution defects. Patients with such defects had no significant increase in the risk of an adverse outcome. Fifty-four percent of perioperative ECG and TEE episodes of ischemia and 58% of severe ischemic episodes developed in patients who did not have redistribution defects. The ^{201}T1 scintigraphy had a sensitivity of 40% to 54%, a specificity of 65% to 71%, a positive predictive value of 27% to 47%, and a negative predictive value of 61% to 82%.

Conclusion.—In this study of vascular surgery patients, routine screening use of ^{201}T1 scintigraphy does not appear to be warranted. The procedure has limited sensitivity in detecting perioperative ischemia or adverse cardiac outcome, and its negative predictive value appears to be lower than was previously thought. The primary difference in methodology between this study and multiple previous studies is that the treating physicians were blinded to the scintigraphy results.

▶ As may have been predicted, this paper has created a furor among cardiologists. These investigators have concluded that ^{201}T1 scintigraphy has limited sensitivity for the detection for perioperative ischemia and adverse cardiac outcomes. An important difference between this and previous studies is that in this study, the investigators taking care of the patients were unaware of the scan result; thus an unintentional source of bias may have been eliminated. This important article requires careful study.—J.M. Porter, M.D.

The Incidence of Perioperative Myocardial Infarction in General Vascular Surgery

Taylor LM Jr, Yeager RA, Moneta G, McConnell DB, Porter JM (Oregon Health Sciences Univ, Portland)
J Vasc Surg 15:52–61, 1991   5–4

Introduction.—A total of 491 patients having 534 general vascular operations in a 1-year period were monitored for perioperative myocardial infarction by ECG recording and determination of creatine phosphokinase isoenzymes. More extensive testing for coronary disease was limited to 31 patients (6%) who had unstable angina, uncontrolled arrhythmia, or severe congestive heart failure.

Results.—Three patients underwent coronary bypass surgery before the general vascular procedure. A total of 21 perioperative myocardial infarcts occurred, including 5 that were asymptomatic and detected by enzyme estimation only, and 16 that were symptomatic. Four of the latter infarcts were fatal. The relation of infarction to various types of vascular surgery is shown in the table. All 12 operative deaths were associated with urgent or emergent surgery, resulting in an urgent/emergent operative mortality rate of 4.8%. No deaths occurred in the 285 elective cases. The rate of perioperative infarction after elective surgery was 2.8%.

Conclusion.—Invasive coronary screening measures before vascular operation can be limited to carefully selected patients with severely

Incidence of Myocardial Infarction for Different Types of Operation

Operation Type (n)	Asymptomatic MI detected by CPK	Symptomatic MI (%)	Fatal MI (%)	Total MI(%)
Aortic (105)	1 (1.0%)3	3 (2.9%)	1(1.0%)	5(4.8%)
Carotid (87)	1 (1.1%)	4 (4.6%)	0	5(5.7%)
Infraing (207)	2 (1.0%)	3 (1.4%)	2 (1.0%)	7(3.4%)
Amputation (44)	0	0	0	0
Ax-femoral, Fem-fem (51)	1 (2.0%)	2 (3.9%)	0	3(5.9%)
Other* (40)	0	0	1 (2.5%)	1(2.5%)
Total (534)	5 (1.0%)	12 (2.2%)	4 (0.7%)	21 (3.9%)

*Includes visceral/renal, multilevel lower extremity, and brachiocephalic.
(Courtesy of Taylor LM Jr, Yeager RA, Moneta GL, et al: *J Vasc Surg* 15:52–61, 1991.)

symptomatic coronary artery disease. Widespread preoperative coronary screening appears unwarranted.

▶ Performance of detailed preoperative cardiac studies in peripheral vascular patients is clearly predicated on the assumption that severe reconstructible coronary arterial disease should be dealt with before vascular surgery. The only 2 reasons for dealing with the coronary disease first are to either (1) decrease vascular surgery perioperative mortality, or (2) increase longevity. This study indicates that the modern incidence of perioperative myocardial infarction in a center that does not practice extensive cardiac evaluation is already about as low as it is likely to become in this patient population. Thus, the only remaining issue is prolongation of life. To date, there has been no proof that this goal has been accomplished in a significant number of patients. Thus, I continue to believe that there is little justification for routine extensive coronary screening before elective vascular surgery.—J.M. Porter, M.D.

The Impact of Selective Use of Dipyridamole-Thallium Scans and Surgical Factors on the Current Morbidity of Aortic Surgery

Cambria RP, Brewster DC, Abbott WM, L'Italien GJ, Megerman JJ, LaMuraglia GM, Moncure AC, Zelt DT, Eagle K (Massachusetts General Hosp; Harvard Med School, Boston)
J Vasc Surg 15:43–51, 1992   5–5

Background.—Cardiac evaluation before vascular surgery remains a controversial issue. It is suggested that dipyridamole-thallium scanning be carried out selectively before surgery on the aorta, on the basis of clinical markers of coronary artery disease.

Methods.—The use of thallium scanning was reviewed in 202 patients having elective aortic reconstruction (151 for abdominal aortic aneurysm and 51 for aortoiliac occlusive disease).

Results.—Preoperative dipyridamole-thallium scanning was done in 29% of the patients. As a result, 11% of the patients had coronary angiography and 9% underwent coronary bypass grafting/percutaneous coronary angioplasty before aortic surgery. There was 1 cardiac death, 4% of patients had nonfatal myocardial infarction or unstable angina, and 6% experienced pulmonary complications. The factors associated with postoperative death or cardiopulmonary problems included an operating time longer than 5 hours, the presence of aortoiliac occlusive disease, and a history of ventricular ectopy. Both prolonged surgery and intraoperative myocardial ischemia predicted major cardiac complications.

Conclusion.—Thallium scanning guided by clinical markers of coronary artery disease will identify those patients requiring aortic reconstruction in whom invasive management of coronary disease before reconstruction is appropriate.

▶ These authors advocate selective use of dipyridamole-thallium cardiac scanning in preoperative vascular patients. They performed the test in 29% of their patients and found a 9% incidence of preoperative coronary grafting. Interestingly, their perioperative clinical outcome was virtually identical to that reported in Abstract 5–4. It appears that the Oregon group and the Massachusetts General group are reaching substantially different conclusions based on the same data.—J.M. Porter, M.D.

Comparison of Cardiac Morbidity Between Aortic and Infrainguinal Operations
Krupski WC, Layug EL, Reilly LM, Rapp JH, Mangano DT, Study of Perioperative Ischemia Research Group (Dept of Veterans Affairs Med Ctr; Univ of California, San Francisco)
J Vasc Surg 15:354–365, 1992   5–6

Objective.—Perioperative cardiac ischemic events were compared in a series of 53 patients having major abdominal vascular operations and in a group of 87 patients having infrainguinal vascular surgery. The respective average operating times were 421 and 459 minutes.

Methods.—Thirty-eight patients had dipyridamole-thallium cardiac scintigraphy preoperatively. The electrocardiogram and transesophageal echocardiogram were used to detect myocardial ischemia during surgery, and Holter monitoring was repeated 4 days postoperatively. The outcome events included cardiac death, nonfatal myocardial infarction, unstable angina, ventricular tachycardia, and congestive heart failure.

Results.—More patients in the infrainguinal group had diabetes, angina, and heart failure, but preoperative ECG and thallium scan abnormalities were similarly frequent in the 2 surgical groups. Echocardiography demonstrated intraoperative ischemia in 26% of the patients having aortic surgery and in 10% of those having infrainguinal procedures (Table 1). Outcome events were similarly frequent in the 2 groups (Table 2). Holter monitoring more often demonstrated postoperative ischemia in patients having infrainguinal operations.

Conclusion.—Patients requiring infrainguinal vascular reconstruction have cardiac disease more often than those who require aortic surgery, and they have a risk of cardiac events that is at least as great.

▶ The widespread perception is that major aortic surgery has a high likelihood of perioperative cardiac complications which, based on the magnitude of surgery, should certainly be greater than that expected after lower extremity vascular repair. It seems clear, however, that by the time significant lower extremity arterial ischemic symptoms develop, they almost invariably have severe associated coronary disease. This study documents (by a variety of methods) that adverse cardiac outcomes are at least as likely to occur after lower extremity arterial repair as after aortic operations.—J.M. Porter, M.D.

TABLE 1.—Perioperative Ischemia

| Study | No. of patients studied | No. of patients with abnormalities (% studies performed) | | p value* |
		Infrainguinal n = 87	Aortic n = 53	
Preoperative				
Standard 12-lead ECG†	140	60 (69)	28 (53)	0.08
Continuous 2-Lead ECG (Holter Monitor)‡	93	22 (37)	8 (24)	0.3
Dipyridamole-thallium scan§	38	7 (33)	6 (35)	0.8
Intraoperative				
Continuous 12-lead ECG‖	133	22 (26)	12 (23)	0.8
Continuous 2-lead ECG (Holter monitor)	139	32 (40)	16 (31)	0.4
Transesophageal echocardiography	133	8 (10)	13 (26)	0.02
Postoperative				
Continuous 2-lead ECG (Holter monitor)¶	133	46 (57)	16 (31)	0.005

* Infrainguinal vs. aortic.
† Indicates any abnormality, (e.g., myocardial infarction, arrhythmias, bundle branch block, and the like).
‡ Indicates ST segment changes suggestive of ischemia.
§ Reversible defect observed.
‖ Indicates ST segment changes suggestive of ischemia.
¶ Severe ischemia as defined by a 2-mm deviation of the ST segment from the baseline for ≥ 30 min.
(Courtesy of Krupski WC, Layug EL, Reilly LM, et al: *J Vasc Surg* 15:354–365, 1992.)

TABLE 2.—Postoperative Adverse Cardiac Outcomes

	Infrainguinal	*Aortic*	*p value**
Unstable angina†	1 (1%)	0 (0%)	0.7*
Myocardial infarction†	3 (3.5%)	0 (0%)	0.6*
Cardiac death†	3 (3.5%)	1 (2%)	0.9*
Ventricular tachycardia	7 (8%)	6 (11%)	0.7
Heart failure	9 (10%)	8 (15%)	0.6
Total outcome events	23 (26%)	15 (28%)	1.0

* Fisher's exact test.
† Total grave cardiac outcomes 8% vs. 2%, P = .3.
‡ Infrainguinal vs. aortic.
(Courtesy of Krupski WC, Layug EL, Reilly LM, et al: *J Vasc Surg* 15:354–365, 1992.)

Influence of Age on Results of Coronary Artery Surgery

Weintraub WS, Craver JM, Cohen CL, Jones EL, Guyton RA (Emory Univ, Atlanta

Circulation 84:226III–235III, 1991   5–7

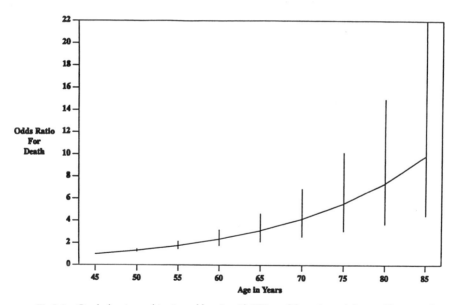

Fig 5–2.—Graph showing multivariate odds ratio with 95% confidence intervals by age. (Courtesy of Weintraub WS, Craver JM, Cohen CL, et al: *Circulation* 84:226III–235III, 1991.)

Background.—Coronary bypass surgery (CABG) is being performed increasingly in older and more seriously ill patients, and these patients have been consistently shown to be at higher risk for postoperative complications and in-hospital death. The importance of age in predicting complications and in-hospital mortality after CABG was evaluated.

Patients.—The study population consisted of 13,625 patients who underwent isolated first CABG between 1981 and 1989. There were 321 patients younger than 40 years of age, 1,758 aged 40–49 years, 4,167 aged 50–59, 5,049 aged 60–69, 2,184 aged 70–79, and 146 aged 80–89. Cardiac catheterization was performed in 8,767 patients, and the ejection fraction (EF) was available for 8,282 patients.

Results.—As patients aged, the proportion of women increased, the prevalence of severe angina and congestive heart failure (CHF) increased, and the severity of the distributions of the coronary stenoses increased. The incidence of complications resulting from neurologic events, wound infections, and mortality rates increased with each decade after age 40 years, particularly at ages 70–79 and 80–89. The mortality rates were .6% for patients aged 40–49 years, 1% for those aged 50–59, 1.9% for those aged 60–69, 5% for those aged 70–79, and 8.3% for those aged 80–89. Advanced age was the most significant independent correlate of neurologic events, wound infections, and in-hospital death (Fig 5-2). The other multivariate correlates of neurologic events were diabetes, hypertension, and angina severity. Angina class was the only other multivariate correlate of wound infections. Other correlates of in-hospital death were emergent operation, female gender, EF, coronary disease severity, diabetes, and a history of CHF. Periprocedural Q wave myocardial infarction (MI) was independent of age. Emergent operation was the most predictive and significant correlate of periprocedural MI, whereas hypertension, absence of a previous MI, and a normal EF were weaker correlates. The ability to predict any complication was relatively weak compared with the ability to predict in-hospital death.

Conclusion.—The relative infrequency of CABG performed in patients older than 80 years of age suggests that there already is strong selection against surgery in octogenarians. Furthermore, the risk of death and, to some extent, the risk of other complications may be predicted in advance on the basis of extensive clinical experience.

▶ As a group, vascular surgery patients are elderly. If one does extensive preoperative cardiac screening of vascular patients, a significant number of these patients may be referred for elective coronary bypass. This sobering report documents a striking relationship between coronary bypass mortality and age, with a mortality rate of 5% for the patients between 70 and 79 years of age and 8.3% for patients older than 80 years. This information must be seriously considered by the vascular surgeon before selecting extensive cardiac evaluation and possible coronary intervention in elderly patients before elective vascular surgery.—J.M. Porter, M.D.

Coronary Bypass Surgery Improves Survival in High-Risk Unstable Angina: Results of a Veterans Administration Cooperative Study With an 8-Year Follow-Up

Sharma GVRK, for the VA Unstable Angina Cooperative Study Group (VA Med Ctr, Roxbury, Mass)
Circulation 84:260III–267III, 1991   5–8

Introduction.—Earlier reports on unstable angina generally indicate no advantage of surgical over medical treatment, apart from better relief of symptoms. Because unstable angina includes a wide clinical spectrum, it seemed reasonable to randomize patients prospectively to medical or operative treatment based on their clinical evaluation.

Methods.—Of 468 patients with unstable angina, 374 were classified as type I, with progressive effort angina or recent rest angina; 94 had type II, with severe rest angina and ST-T changes on the ECG. Left ventricular function was abnormal in 27 of the type II patients.

Results.—During the 8-year follow-up, 45% of the patients assigned to medical treatment underwent surgery. However, intention-to-treat analysis indicated that crossover did not affect the conclusions of this study. Among the 27 type II patients with left ventricular dysfunction, those operated on did significantly better than those treated medically, with respective cumulative mortality rates of 13% and 46%. The cumulative mortality rates did not differ significantly in the other subgroups.

Conclusion.—Long-term follow-up of patients with unstable angina led to the identification of high-risk clinical subgroups whose mortality and morbidity could be improved by operative treatment. However, only 27 of 468 entering patients (6%) were in the group benefitting from surgery.

▶ This is an extremely important study. A total of 468 patients with unstable angina were randomized to conventional medical therapy or coronary bypass. Follow-up to 8 years revealed a significant survival benefit in favor of surgery only in those patients with severe rest angina with ST-T changes on the EKG *and* evidence of abnormal left ventricular function. Remarkably, only 27 of 468, or 6% of the total randomized group were in the subset in which prolongation of life was achieved by surgery. I have long suspected there may be considerably less to coronary bypass surgery than meets the eye.—J.M. Porter, M.D.

Combined Epidural and General Anesthesia Versus General Anesthesia for Abdominal Aortic Surgery

Baron J-F, Bertrand M, Barré E, Godet G, Mundler O, Coriat P, Viars P (Hôpital Pitié-Salpétrière; Hôpital Lariboisiére, Paris)
Anesthesiology 75:611–618, 1991   5–9

Objective.—It was recently shown that the use of epidural anesthesia combined with postoperative epidural analgesia in high-risk surgical patients significantly reduced postoperative mortality and morbidity compared with general anesthesia. However, the isolated effects of the primary anesthetic technique per se on the postoperative outcome in high-risk patients have not been studied. High-risk surgical patients were studied to determine whether intraoperative thoracic epidural anesthesia combined with light general anesthesia alters postoperative morbidity when compared with a standard technique of balanced general anesthesia.

Patients.—Of 173 patients undergoing elective abdominal aortic reconstruction for aneurysm or aortoiliac occlusive disease, 86 (mean age, 62 years) were given balanced general anesthesia and 87 (mean age, 61 years) received thoracic epidural anesthesia combined with light general anesthesia. The preoperative evaluation included dipyridamole thallium gammatomography and radionuclide angiography. During the postoperative period, patients in either group received analgesia of subcutaneous morphine, epidural fentanyl, or epidural bupivacaine.

Results.—Twenty-two patients who were given balanced general anesthesia and 19 patients who received combined anesthesia had a major postoperative cardiac event, including myocardial infarction, congestive heart failure, and prolonged myocardial ischemia. Respiratory complications developed in 61% of patients who had general anesthesia and in 55% of patients who had combined anesthesia. The major part of this respiratory morbidity consisted of minor atelectasis. Of the patients who received general anesthesia, 8 had acute respiratory failure and 4 died. Among those who received combined anesthesia, 4 had respiratory failure and 3 died. The differences between the 2 groups were not statistically significant for any of the outcome parameters.

Conclusion.—Thoracic epidural anesthesia in combination with light general anesthesia offers no major advantage over general anesthesia in high-risk surgical patients. However, the results do not exclude the possibility that postoperative epidural analgesia exerts a beneficial influence on cardiac and respiratory morbidity during the postoperative period.

▶ This prospective randomized study leads to the conclusion that epidural anesthesia conveys no unique benefits to the patient. I continue to be concerned by continuous epidural anesthesia because of the possibility of narcotic overdose resulting from the fact many people have postoperative access to the intrathecal catheter. We do not permit the use of continuous epidural anesthesia on our vascular surgical service. See also the commentary for Abstract 5–13.—J.M. Porter, M.D.

Analysis of Risk Factors for Surgical Wound Infections Following Vascular Surgery

Richet HM, Chidiac C, Prat A, Pol A, David M, Maccario M, Cormier P, Ber-

nard E, Jarvis WR (Ctr for Disease Control, Atlanta; Groupe d'Etude et Recherche en Antibioprophylaxie, Nice, France)
Am J Med 91:170S–172S, 1991   5–10

Introduction.—Surgical wound infection (SWI) after placement of a prosthesis can be catastrophic, and it frequently requires removal of the device. Nevertheless, few attempts have been made to identify the risk factors for these infections.

Methods.—A prospective, multicenter study was undertaken in 561 patients who underwent vascular surgery in 1988–1989. In 23 (4.1%) patients, SWI developed.

Results.—Of the patients, 2 died of SWI, 11 required reoperation, and the prostheses were removed in 5. On stepwise logistic regression analysis, the independent risk factors for SWI included surgery on the lower extremity, delayed operation, insulin-dependent diabetes, previous vascular surgery, and brief antimicrobial prophylaxis with 3 doses of cefamandole. Diabetes was a risk factor only for those patients given brief prophylaxis, and the same was true for delayed surgery and a history of vascular surgery.

Conclusion.—Brief antimicrobial prophylaxis may suffice in patients with no more than 1 risk factor for SWI; otherwise, a 48-hour course is preferable. A multivariate risk index is helpful for identifying patients who are at high risk of SWI.

▶ This study reinforces our practice of routinely using multiday cefamandole prophylaxis in patients receiving vascular prostheses. It is gratifying to have one's empiric prejudices confirmed scientifically.—J.M. Porter, M.D.

Conserving Resources After Carotid Endarterectomy: Selective Use of the Intensive Care Unit
O'Brien MS, Ricotta JJ (State Univ of New York at Buffalo)
J Vasc Surg 14:796–802, 1991   5–11

Objective.—Seventy-three patients having carotid endarterectomy in 1986—half the total number of patients operated on—were reviewed in an attempt to determine whether routine intensive care unit (ICU) admission is appropriate after this procedure.

Methods.—The severity of illness was estimated using the Acute Physiology Score of the APACHE II system. The Therapeutic Index Scoring system served to quantify the postoperative services used.

Results.—The mean length of stay in the ICU was 24.5 hours. Only 18% of the patients actually required ICU services, and in 6 of these 13 patients, treatment began in the recovery room and ended within 3 hours of ICU admission. Only 2 patients required ICU services for as long as 16 hours after surgery. The frequency with which various moni-

Frequencies of Monitoring Services and Active Therapy
Used by Patients After Carotid Endarterectomy ($n = 73$)

Service	No.	Percentage
* ECG monitoring	71	97%
* Hourly vital signs	68	93%
* Systemic arterial monitoring	65	89%
* Hourly neurologic checks	55	75%
+ Vasoactive drug infusion	9	12.3%
+ Active diuresis	2	2.7%
+ Intermittent mandatory ventilation	1	1.4%
+ Emergency operative procedure	1	1.4%

* Monitoring services.
+ Active ICU therapy.
(Courtesy of O'Brien MS, Ricotta JJ: *J Vasc Surg* 14:796–802, 1991.)

toring services and active treatments was necessary is shown in the table. The APACHE II scores did not identify the patients who required ICU services.

Fiscal Aspects.—Observing patients in the recovery room and transferring those who were stable would have precluded the need for ICU admission in 82% of these cases. Intensive care unit charges represented 12.5% of the total hospital charges for carotid endarterectomy.

Conclusion.—Relatively few patients require unique ICU services after carotid endarterectomy. The need usually is apparent shortly after surgery. Prolonged observation in the recovery room or the use of intermediate-care units will help conserve ICU services for those who truly require them.

▶ Changing circumstances have forced us all to closely reexamine the use of expensive hospital resources. Clearly, a large majority of vascular surgery patients do not require ICU care; however, they certainly require an intensive observation unit for at least the first 25 hours after surgery. I suspect the "step-down" acute care unit will result in considerable cost savings without compromise of patient care.—J.M. Porter, M.D.

Preoperative Optimization of Cardiovascular Hemodynamics Improves Outcome in Peripheral Vascular Surgery: A Prospective, Randomized Clinical Trial
Berlauk JF, Abrams JH, Gilmour IJ, O'Connor SR, Knighton DR, Cerra FB
(Univ of Minnesota, Minneapolis)
Ann Surg 214:289–299, 1991   5–12

Objective.—Whether optimizing hemodynamic function by pulmonary artery catheterization will improve the outcome of limb salvage arterial surgery was determined.

Complication Summary

Characteristic	Group 1 (n = 45)	Group 2 (n = 23)	Group 3 (n = 21)
Intraoperative event (arrhythmia, tachycardia or hypotension)	30*	15*	22*
Postop cardiac morbidity	3*	2*	5
Early graft thrombosis (<36 hr)	1*	1*	4
Death†	1 (2.2%)	0	2 (9.5%)

* $P < .05$ compared with group 3.
† 1.5% for groups 1 and 2 vs. group 3 ($P = .08$).
(Courtesy of Berlauk JF, Abrams JH, Gilmour IJ, et al: *Ann Surg* 214:289–299, 1991.)

Methods.—Eighty-nine patients were randomized to undergo a preoperative "tune-up" 12 hours before surgery in the surgical intensive care unit (group 1) or less than 3 hours before surgery in a preinduction room (group 2), or to receive no tune-up (group 3). Fluid loading, afterload reduction, and inotropic support were used as needed to produce a pulmonary arterial wedge pressure between 8 and 15 mm Hg, a cardiac index of 2.8 L/min/m² or greater, and a systemic vascular resistance of 1,100 dyne-sec cm⁻⁵ or lower.

Results.—Patients with a pulmonary artery catheter in place had fewer adverse intraoperative events, less cardiac morbidity postoperatively, and less early graft thrombosis than did control patients (table). Mortality was 1.5% in the catheterized groups and 9.5% in the control patients. Catheterization did not affect the length of stay in the intensive care unit or hospital, or the overall operative costs.

Conclusion.—Optimizing hemodynamics by pulmonary artery catheterization improved the outcome in this series of patients undergoing limb salvage surgery.

▶ This article suggests that there is something about a pulmonary artery catheter that improves the outcome in peripheral vascular surgery. Although there is no question that clinically useful information can be obtained from the pulmonary artery catheter, it is likely that the improved results were the result of better patient care and more intense physician involvement and treatment. There was no increased benefit from a preoperative intensive care "tune-up" using a pulmonary artery catheter to optimize hemodynamics compared with simply placing the pulmonary artery catheter in the preoperative holding area. This was at least as effective—and perhaps more effective, and it reduced the stay in the intensive care unit by one day. Randomization of patients to *not* use a PA catheter (when it might, in fact, have been useful) may have contributed to the high mortality rate in this group. Good clinical judgement and patient care should supersede rigid protocols concerning whether to use a pulmonary artery catheter in high-risk patient populations.—C. Zarins, M.D.

Epidural Versus General Anesthesia for Infrainguinal Arterial Reconstruction

Rivers SP, Scher LA, Sheehan E, Veith FJ (Albert Einstein College of Medicine, Montefiore Med Ctr, New York)
J Vasc Surg 14:764–770, 1991   5–13

Introduction.—Epidural anesthesia is often the preferred approach for patients undergoing infrainguinal bypass surgery, especially those at risk of cardiovascular and pulmonary complications from general endotracheal anesthesia.

Methods.—A total of 174 consecutive patients who underwent 213 infrainguinal bypass operations in 1986–1990 were studied prospectively. The mean patient age was 69 years. More than 90% of the operations were performed for limb salvage. Nearly one third of the patients had secondary revascularization. Epidural anesthesia was used in 96 procedures, and general endotracheal anesthesia was used in 117.

Results.—Cardiac complications were not substantially less frequent in patients who had epidural anesthesia (Table 1). Other systemic complications were more frequent in the epidural group (Table 2). In 69 patients at especially high risk (American Society of Anesthesiologists class IV and V or a Goldman score above 10), there was no significant difference in outcome in the 2 anesthetic groups (Table 3).

Conclusion.—If infrainguinal arterial reconstruction is indicated, it should not be postponed or avoided when a patient requires or requests general anesthesia.

▶ What seems intuitively correct does not always withstand scientific scrutiny. These prospective studies (Abstracts 5–9 and 5–13) show that, despite theoretical advantages, neither epidural anesthesia for leg bypass, nor epidural in combination with light general anesthesia for aortic reconstruction, is superior to general anesthesia alone. Nevertheless, epidural anesthesia may be preferable in select patients with severe pulmonary insufficiency (1). A reduction in postoperative hypercoagulability associated with epidural anesthesia had recently been described in vascular surgical patients; this interest-

TABLE 1.—Cardiac Complications

	30-day mortality rate	Nonfatal postoperative MI	Reversible cardiac events*	Total
EPI n = 96	5 (5%)	6 (6%)	13 (14%)	24 (25%)
GET n = 117	4 (3%)	8 (7%)	21 (18%)	33 (28%)

Abbreviations: MI, myocardial infarction; EPI, epidural; GET, general epidural intubation.
* Includes angina, arrythmia, and pulmonary edema that resolved without sequelae.
(Courtesy of Rivers SP, Scher LA, Sheehan E, et al: *J Vasc Surg* 14:764–770, 1991.)

TABLE 2.—Miscellaneous Systemic Complications

	EPI	GET
Venous thromboembolic	1	2
Renal failure	2	0
Stroke	2	0
Spinal headache	1	N/A
	6 (6%)	2 (2%)

Courtesy of Rivers SP, Scher LA, Sheehan E, et al: *J Vasc Surg* 14:764–770, 1991.)

ing observation requires confirmation (2). The potential benefits of *postoperative* epidural analgesia were not addressed in either report and deserve further study.—J. Mills, M.D.

References

1. Mason RA, et al: *J Cardiovasc Surg* 31:442, 1990.
2. Tuman K J, et al: *Anesth Analg* 73:696, 1991.

TABLE 3.—Results

Patients at high risk

	30-day mortality rate	Nonfatal postoperative MI	Reversible cardiac events	All systemic complications
EPI n = 31	1	5	5	15
GET n = 33	3	1	9	15
Total n = 64	4	6	14	30
				(47%)

Abbreviations: MI, myocardial infarction; *EPI*, epidural; *GET*, general intubation.
(Courtesy of Rivers SP, Scher LA, Sheehan E, et al: *J Vasc Surg* 14:764–770, 1991.)

6 Thoracic Aorta

The Prevalence of Ulcerated Plaques in the Aortic Arch in Patients With Stroke

Amarenco P, Duyckaerts C, Tzourio C, Hénin D, Bousser M-G, Hauw J-J (Hôpital de la Salpêtrière, Paris; Hôpital Saint-Antoine, Paris; Univ Pierre et Marie Curie, Paris; Institut Natl de la Santé et de la Recherche Médicale, Villejuif, France)

N Engl J Med 326:221–225, 1992
6–1

Background.—No cause is apparent in as many as 40% of patients with cerebral infarction who are evaluated prospectively. The frequency of ulcerated plaques in the aortic arch in patients with cerebrovascular disease was determined, and the role they may play in the formation of cerebral emboli was studied.

Methods.—An autopsy databank supplied information on 500 consecutive patients with cerebrovascular and other neurologic disorders. All patients were autopsied between December 1983 and August 1983.

Results.—Ulcerated plaques were found in 26% of 239 patients with cerebrovascular disease and in 5% of the 261 with other neurologic dis-

		PATIENTS WITH ULCERATED
PATIENT GROUP	PATIENTS	PLAQUES
	no.	*no. (%)*
Cerebrovascular disease	239	62 (26)
Other neurologic diseases	261	13 (5)*
Cerebral hemorrhage	56	11 (20)
Cerebral infarction	183	51 (28)
Identified cause†	155	34 (22)
No identifiable cause	28	17 (61)‡

Prevalence of Ulcerated Plaques in Aortic Arch of 500 Patients Examined at Autopsy

* P < .001 for comparison with patients with cerebrovascular disease.

† Atherosclerosis, cardiac emboli, or both, or other causes.

‡ P < .001 for comparison with patients with an identified cause of infarction.

(Courtesy of Amarenco P, Duyckaerts C, Tzourio C, et al: N Engl J Med 325:221–225, 1992.)

orders, a significant difference. Ulcerated plaques were more prevalent in patients with cerebral infarcts than in those with cerebral hemorrhage (table). After adjustment was made for covariate factors, ulcerated plaques were present in 58% of patients with no other known cause of cerebral infarction compared with 20% of those with a known cause. The presence of ulcerated plaques in the aortic arch was not correlated with the presence of extracranial internal carotid artery stenosis.

Conclusion.—Ulcerated plaques in the aortic arch may account for some cerebral infarcts of unknown origin.

▶ Organ infarction or severe dysfunction resulting from embolism of a diseased aorta is being recognized with increasing frequency. This study indicates a remarkable prevalence of ulcerated plaques in the aortic arch in patients with stroke.—J.M. Porter, M.D.

"Shaggy" Aorta Syndrome With Atheromatous Embolization to Visceral Vessels

Hollier LH, Kazmier FJ, Ochsner J, Bowen JC, Procter CD (Ochsner Clinic and Alton Ochsner Med Found, New Orleans; Mayo Clinic Scottsdale, Scottsdale, Ariz)

Ann Vasc Surg 5:439–444, 1991   6–2

Background.—"Shaggy" aorta syndrome involves spontaneous peripheral and visceral embolization from diffuse aortic atherosclerotic disease. This unusual and poorly understood condition results from multiple, recurrent microembolizations resulting from the extensive atheromatous

List of the 28 Operative Procedures Performed on 27 Patients

Operative procedure	No. of operations
Suprarenal endarterectomy (SRE) or graft	2[†]
SRE or graft and infrarenal graft	11
plus lumbar sympathectomy ‡	10
Infrarenal graft	8
plus lumbar sympathectomy ‡	5
Axillobifemoral bypass with external iliac artery ligation	7
artery ligation and lumbar sympathectomy‡	5

Some patients in each group had concomitant lumbar sympathectomy performed.
† One patient had a previous infrarenal graft.
‡ Lumbar sympathectomy was performed on patients who exhibited pain or cutaneous ischemia caused by atheromatous embolization to the toes.
(Courtesy of Hollier LH, Kazmier FJ, Ochsner J, et al: *Ann Vasc Surg* 5:439–444, 1991.)

ulcerations in the aorta. Thirty-six patients with renal or visceral atheromatous embolization from a "shaggy" aorta were studied.

Patients.—During a 27-year period, 36 patients showed evidence of diffuse renal or visceral microembolization from a "shaggy aorta." All but 2 also had diffuse peripheral embolization. Thirty-three patients were men and 3 were women (median age, 69 years). The initial signs were diffuse lower abdominal, buttock, or lower extremity emboli in 32 patients. The precipitating event appeared to be invasive arteriographic studies in 10 patients.

Outcome.—Treatment was nonoperative in 9 patients; 3 died within a week, and 5 of the others died of continuing renal and intestinal embolization within 5 years. The other 27 patients underwent a total of 28 operative procedures (table). Visceral infarction and renal failure were not necessarily prevented by endarterectomy or aortic graft replacement. The procedure with the best morbidity and mortality was extra-anatomical bypass with ligation of the distal external iliac arteries.

Conclusion.—Atheromatous embolization is an uncommon but dangerous event in patients with atherosclerotic vascular disease. Embolization is not prevented by anticoagulation, which may be contraindicated. For patients with suprarenal lesions and visceral emboli, the best approach appears to be axillobifemoral bypass with ligation of the external iliac arteries.

▶ The perioperative mortality in these 27 patients was 22%, which indicates the serious nature of these lesions as well as the frequent debilitation of the patient by the time the diagnosis is made. I am certain we will see more of these patients, especially with improved diagnostic technique (see Abstract 6–3). Once discovered, formulation of optimal treatment recommendations is difficult. Direct surgical approach clearly carries a significant mortality.—J.M. Porter, M.D.

Protruding Atheromas in the Thoracic Aorta and Systemic Embolization
Tunick PA, Perez JL, Kronzon I (New York Univ)
Ann Intern Med 115:423–427, 1991   6–3

Introduction.—Echocardiography is often done in patients with unexplained stroke, transient ischemic attack, or peripheral embolus to determine whether there is a cardiac source of embolization. Four patients whose transesophageal echocardiograms showed large, protruding atheromas in the aortic arch were examined. Whether these protruding atheromas constitute a risk factor for systemic embolization was determined in a case-control study.

Methods.—A total of 122 transesophageal echocardiograms that were done to search for a possible cardiac source of embolization were evalu-

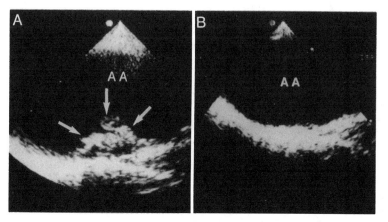

Fig 6–1.—Protruding atheroma as shown by transesophageal echocardiography. **A,** a protruding atheroma (*arrows*) located in the aortic arch of a man, 75, who had had a stroke. **B,** for comparison, a transesophageal echocardiogram showing the aortic arch with no protruding atheroma. *Abbreviation:* AA, aortic arch. (Courtesy of Tunick PA, Perez JL, Kronzon I: *Ann Intern Med* 115:423–427, 1991.)

ated. The patients were matched for age and sex to 122 patients who underwent the same examination for cardiac, rather than embolic, indications.

Findings.—Thirty-three of the patients with emboli had protruding atheromas (Fig 6–1). According to matched logistic regression, the presence of this finding was strongly related to the occurrence of embolic symptoms; the odds ratio was 3.2. The atheroma had a mobile component in 11 patients, but in no controls. In 88% of the patients, the atheroma was located in the aortic arch. Atheroma remained an independent risk factor, even after hypertension and diabetes were factored in. Hypertension itself was an independent predictor (odds ratio, 2.7), but diabetes was not.

Conclusion.—Transesophageal echocardiography may detect protruding atheromas of the thoracic aorta, and these lesions may be considered a cause of stroke, transient ischemic attacks, and peripheral emboli. Some lesions may be missed because of masking of the ascending aorta by the trachea. The importance of the composition of the atheromatous material is unknown.

▶ A total of 27% of the 122 patients with clinical arterial emboli had protruding atheromata in the thoracic aorta (as detected by transesophageal echocardiography). This is almost identical to the percent detected in Abstract 6–1.—J.M. Porter, M.D.

Transesophageal Echocardiography: Preliminary Results in Patients With Traumatic Aortic Rupture
Sparks MB, Burchard KW, Marrin CAS, Bean CHG, Nugent WC Jr, Plehn JF

(Dartmouth-Hitchcock Med Ctr, Hanover, NH)
Arch Surg 126:711–714, 1991   6–4

Objective.—Transesophageal echocardiography was used to image the descending aorta in 11 patients with blunt chest trauma who were at risk of aortic rupture. The findings were compared with those of radiographic studies.

Results.—Ten patients had arch aortography, and 6 of the 10 had positive findings. In 1 case, the CT findings were thought to be consistent with aortic rupture. Transesophageal echocardiography demonstrated aortic rupture in 3 of the 6 patients with positive aortographic findings (Fig 6–2). The findings were negative in the other 8 patients. All 3 patients with positive echocardiographic findings had aortic rupture confirmed at operation. Three of the positive aortographic diagnoses proved incorrect.

Conclusion.—Transesophageal echocardiography is a useful means of diagnosing rupture of the descending aorta in patients with blunt chest trauma.

▶ In this small but important study, transesophageal echocardiography proved to be 100% sensitive and specific in the diagnosis of traumatic thoracic aortic rupture. The test can be performed at the bedside without compromising patient care. Perhaps with increasing experience this will become the procedure of choice for the diagnosis of traumatic aortic rupture.—J.M. Porter, M.D.

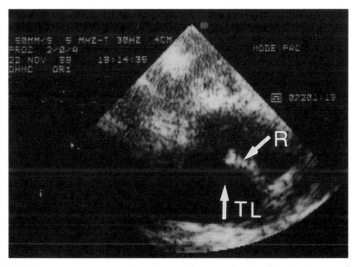

Fig 6–2.—Representative transesophageal echocardiogram of ruptured aorta at region of isthmus. *Abbreviations: TL,* true aortic lumen; *R,* site of rupture. (Courtesy of Sparks MB, Burchard KW, Marrin CAS, et al: *Arch Surg* 126:711–714, 1991.)

Usefulness of Transesophageal Echocardiography in Assessment of Aortic Dissection

Ballal RS, Nanda NC, Gatewood R, D'Archy B, Samdarshi TE, Holman WL, Kirklin JK, Pacifico AD (Univ of Alabama at Birmingham
Circulation 84:1903–1914, 1991   6–5

Introduction.—Acute proximal aortic dissection is a life-threatening emergency. Both aortography and CT have drawbacks, and 2-dimensional echocardiography is not very sensitive or specific. Recent studies have suggested that transesophageal echocardiography is helpful in diagnosing aortic dissection.

Methods.—Transesophageal echocardiography was performed in 34 patients with proved aortic dissection and in 27 others in whom dissection was excluded by aortography. Some studies were performed with the patient awake; others were found intraoperatively. Both 2-dimensional and color-coded Doppler images were acquired. Some patients had biplane examinations. Aortic dissection was diagnosed when a linear echo appeared within the aortic lumen.

Results.—Transesophageal echocardiography correctly diagnosed aortic dissection in 97% of the patients. In 14 patients, thrombi were seen in the nonperfusing lumen (Fig 6–3). Dissection was correctly ruled out in all patients. The various types of dissection were accurately distinguished. In 6 of 7 patients with coronary artery involvement, the dissection flap clearly extended into the ostium and lumen of the coronary artery. Some, but not all, luminal communications were identified by transesophageal echocardiography. Although CT was specific, it was only 67% sensitive in detecting aortic dissection. Aortography was 93% sensitive.

Conclusion.—Transesophageal echocardiography accurately diagnoses aortic dissection and demonstrates involvement of the coronary arteries.

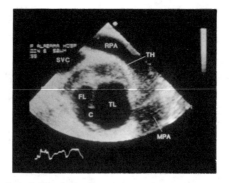

Fig 6–3.—Transesophageal echocardiograms in aortic dissection. Aortic short-axis view shows a thrombus (*TH*) in false lumen (*FL*). C indicates communication between true and false lumens: *MPA*, main pulmonary artery; *RPA*, right pulmonary artery; *SVC*, superior vena cava; *TL*, true lumen. (Courtesy of Ballal RS, Nanda NC, Gatewood R, et al: *Circulation* 84:1903–1914, 1991.)

It also can detect mild aortic regurgitation and is helpful in detecting and localizing intra-aortic thrombi. However, it does not always agree with aortography or surgery in identifying communications between the true and false lumens. The procedure is safe and can be performed when the patient is conscious.

▶ Transesophageal echocardiography appears to be a highly useful procedure in the detection of thoracic aorta atheromata, traumatic thoracic aortic rupture, and aortic dissection, as well as in the detection of cardiac sources of peripheral emboli. With increasing operator experience, additional uses will probably be described. This is clearly an important new diagnostic modality.—J.M. Porter, M.D.

Thoracoabdominal Aneurysm Resection After Previous Infrarenal Abdominal Aortic Aneurysmectomy
Fox AD, Berkowitz HD (Hosp of the Univ of Pennsylvania, Philadelphia)
Am J Surg 162:142–144, 1991   6–6

Introduction.—Some patients undergoing abdominal aortic aneurysm reconstruction will require remedial operations years after the original procedure for the treatment of a recurrent aneurysm proximal to the infrarenal graft. It is not certain whether mortality is higher for such a second procedure than it is for primary thoracoabdominal repair.

Methods.—The results in 51 patients undergoing thoracoabdominal aneurysm resection, 14 of whom had a previous infrarenal aneurysmectomy, were compared.

Patients.—The 51 patients had a mean age of 70.5 years. Those who had a previous infrarenal aneurysmectomy were slightly younger (mean age, 67 years), and all were smokers. The average aneurysm was 8.6 cm; the mean interval of time between initial surgery and resection for thoracoabdominal aneurysm was 8.5 years.

Results.—The overall mortality with thoracoabdominal aneurysm resection in patients with previous infrarenal aneurysm resection was 28%, whereas the mortality was 25% in patients without prior infrarenal aneurysm resection. Age (72 years or older), proximal extent of the aneurysm, a ruptured aneurysm, and a history of myocardial infarction, congestive heart failure, or arrhythmia showed a significant relationship with early mortality (30 days) in those patients who had a previous infrarenal aneurysm resection. These factors, with the exception of the proximal extent of the aneurysm, were also related to mortality in the entire group of patients.

Conclusion.—Patients with a previous infrarenal aneurysm resection should be treated in the same way as those who have not had previous aneurysm surgery, because the risk factors for early mortality are similar in both groups. Multivariate analysis identified age, rupture, and the presence of congestive heart failure as significant predictors of early death.

▶ The progression of atherosclerotic arterial disease does not cease after an operation. An increasing number of patients are being detected with aneurysms occurring above their previous infrarenal aneurysm graft, a certain number of which extend into the thoracoabdominal region. All patients with an infrarenal aortic graft should undergo imaging of the thoracic and super renal aorta at intervals during extended follow-up.—J.M. Porter, M.D.

Selective Deep Hypothermia of the Spinal Cord Prevents Paraplegia After Aortic Cross-Clamping in the Dog Model

Berguer R, Porto J, Fedoronko B, Dragovic L (Wayne State Univ, Detroit)
J Vasc Surg 15:62–72, 1992   6–7

Background.—Paraplegia is a major complication in surgery of the aorta. Both experimental and clinical findings suggest that its prevention requires protection of the spinal cord from ischemia during clamping of the aorta, and reattachment of the intercostal artery that supplies the greater radicular artery.

Methods.—The value of selective deep hypothermia (19°C to 12°C) of the cord was examined in dogs with double aortic cross-clamping below the left subclavian artery and above the diaphragm for 45 minutes. In experimental animals, cord hypothermia was initiated 50 minutes before cross-clamping by using an extracorporeal perfusion system to infuse saline solution at 5°C into the subarachnoid space and to drain it through the cisterna magna.

Results.—Control animals were consistently paraplegic and had histologic evidence of cord infarction. All experimental animals had intact hindlimb function and normal appearance of the spinal cord.

Conclusion.—In this canine model, deep hypothermia of the spinal cord avoids ischemic injury that occurs after aortic cross-clamping.

▶ This innovative study demonstrates a distinct benefit of spinal cord hypothermia in reducing the incidence of paraplegia after thoracic aortic cross-clamping. Whether this methodology will ever be relevant to patient care is unknown.—J.M. Porter, M.D.

Treatment of Aortic Coarctation by Axillofemoral Bypass Grafting in the High-Risk Patient

Connery CP, DeWeese JA, Eisenberg BK, Moss AJ (Univ of Rochester, NY)
Ann Thorac Surg 52:1281–1284, 1991   6–8

Background.—Aortic coarctation has been corrected operatively for nearly 50 years, but as many as 5% to 10% of patients still require reoperation for recurrent coarctation. These operations have a mortality rate as high as 10%, especially in the oldest patients and in those with congestive heart failure or lung disease.

Patients.—Axillofemoral bypass surgery was performed in 3 high-risk patients with coarctation of the aorta. Two of them had undergone repair previously and also had serious medical problems. One patient had had 3 myocardial infarctions and had disabling congestive heart failure.

Results.—All 3 patients had an immediate and marked reduction in the peak systolic pressure gradient across the coarctation. Systemic hypertension decreased, and the symptoms of congestive heart failure improved in all patients. The patients were followed for periods of 15 months to 10½ years. Segmental pressure studies indicated no recurrence of a pressure gradient.

Conclusion.—Axillofemoral bypass should be considered for high-risk adults with coarctation of the aorta.

▶ Older patients undergoing operation or reoperation for thoracic aortic coarctation present significant risk for morbidity and mortality. These authors wisely note that axillofemoral bypass should be considered in these patients only as a reasonable alternative to direct thoracic repair.—J.M. Porter, M.D.

Penetrating Atherosclerotic Aortic Ulcer With Dissecting Hematoma: Control of Bleeding With Percutaneous Embolization
Williams DM, Kirsh MM, Abrams GD (Univ Hosps, Ann Arbor, Mich)
Radiology 181:85–88, 1991   6–9

Background.—Some elderly patients with atherosclerotic disease of the aorta have penetrating aortic ulceration with perforation and pseudoaneurysm. Percutaneous management of symptomatic ulcers would be advantageous because of the high morbidity accompanying interposition grafting in the descending aorta. Percutaneous embolization of a dissecting hematoma and pseudoaneurysm accompanying a penetrating aortic ulcer led to hemodynamic stabilization.

Case Report.—Man, 83, was hypertensive and had a history of emphysema and chronic congestive heart failure. He had intermittent abdominal pain, vague pain in the left chest, and a left apical chest mass; his hematocrit decreased. A chest radiograph showed mediastinal widening and an elevated left hemidiaphragm. Aortography demonstrated a penetrating ulcer and a pseudoaneurysm communicating with the descending aorta just above the diaphragm (Fig 6–4).

The pseudoaneurysm was embolized with 3 Gianturco coils and multiple smaller coils, and thrombin then was injected. Thrombus formation took place immediately. The arterial pressure was controlled with nitroprusside. Hematocrit

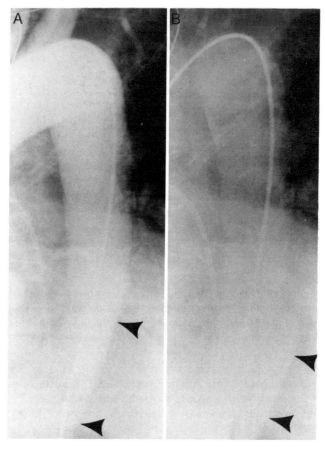

Fig 6–4.—Images produced from an anteroposterior thoracic aortogram show (**A**) a subtle contour deformity in the lower descending aorta (*arrows*), which is caused by (**B**) the intramural dissecting hematoma and adjacent pseudoaneurysm (*arrows*). (Courtesy of Williams DM, Kirsh MM, Abrams GD: *Radiology* 181:85–88, 1991.)

and vital signs stabilized. Purulent pneumonia developed, and the patient died 6 days later.

Autopsy showed 1,800 mL of bloody effusion and clot in the left pleural cavity and 900 mL of clotted blood in the right cavity. Right lower lobe pneumonia was noted. A 2.5-cm tear was found in the descending aorta nearly 4 cm proximal to the celiac origin. The tear led into a dissecting medial hematoma with the spring coils embedded in clot, and from there it led into a pseudoaneurysmal collection of blood beneath the left pleura. A subadventitial dissecting hematoma extended to the aortic arch and the celiac artery.

Conclusion.—Unlike medial degeneration with dissection, a penetrating ulcer lacks an intimal flap and false lumen. Transcatheter embolization may temporarily thrombose the ulcer, allowing surgery to be delayed until the patient is in better condition hemodynamically and biochemically.

▶ This interesting condition has only recently been recognized, and it doubtless will be seen with increasing frequency in our aging population. Although this article clearly does not prove the benefit of catheter embolization, it does raise an interesting point. Perhaps this method of treatment should be considered in sick, elderly patients, because direct aortic surgery with grafting has significant associated mortality and morbidity, including paraplegia.—J.M. Porter, M.D.

Management of Thoracoabdominal Malperfusion in Aortic Dissection
Laas J, Heinemann M, Schaefers H-J, Daniel W, Borst H-G (Hannover Med School, Hannover, Germany)
Circulation 84:20III–24III, 1991   6–10

Background.—Malperfusion of the thoracoabdominal aorta or its branches is a frequent complication of aortic dissection, and it often is fatal. A lack of distal reentry may lead to distention and eventual thrombosis of the false lumen, and the large blind sac compromises the true lumen. Urgent surgery is necessary to restore adequate circulation.

Patients.—Thirteen patients seen since 1985 with aortic dissection had thoracoabdominal aortic malperfusion. In 4 patients undergoing repair of an acute type A aortic dissection, the intimal flap was fenestrated. Two patients with acute type B dissection had fenestration at the level of the aortic bifurcation; in one, the descending aorta was replaced. Six patients had a chronically dilated false lumen without distal reentry, with resultant malperfusion of the viscera, kidneys, and lower extremities.

Management.—All patients with acute type A dissection had emergency repair of the ascending aorta before the fenestration procedure. In most patients with chronic dissection, the affected segment was replaced. Two patients in poor condition underwent extra-anatomical biaxillobifemoral bypass with ringed PTFE prostheses.

Results.—Adequate perfusion of the distal aorta and its branches was restored in 12 of the 13 patients. One patient died during surgery. All 8 long-term survivors, who were followed for a mean of 2½ years, exhibited good restitution of the previously malperfused aortic segment.

Conclusion.—Fenestration of the intimal flap is an effective approach to acute aortic dissection, which causes thoracoabdominal malperfusion. Pseudocoarctation secondary to chronic dissection (usually at the diaphragm) is best managed by replacing the affected aortic segment.

▶ The pattern of visceral and lower extremity malperfusion associated with aortic dissection may be extraordinarily complex. Excision and grafting of a dissection site in the thoracic aorta with obliteration of the distal false lumen does not always eliminate the malperfusion problem. These patients must be very carefully evaluated, and one must be willing to undertake a variety of innovative surgical approaches to revascularization (as necessary). We have found axillofemoral grafting—sometimes accompanied by visceral and renal grafting, usually from the iliacs—to be useful in a number of these patients. We have no experience with aortic fenestration.—J.M. Porter, M.D.

7 Aortic Aneurysm

An Evaluation of New Methods of Expressing Aortic Aneurysm Size: Relationship to Rupture

Ouriel K, Green RM, Donayre C, Shortell CK, Elliott J, DeWeese JA (Univ of Rochester, Rochester, NY)

J Vasc Surg 15:12–20, 1992   7–1

Objective.—Aortic aneurysmal diameter was standardized to measures of patient size and normal aortic size in an attempt to find indices that will predict aneurysmal rupture more accurately than aneurysmal diameter alone.

Methods.—Data on normal aortic diameter were acquired from 100 patients having abdominal CT examination for other reasons. The study also included 100 patients having elective aneurysmal resection and 286 admitted with a ruptured abdominal aortic aneurysm. Accurate measurements of aneurysmal diameter were available in 214 of the latter cases.

Results.—The average normal infrarenal aortic diameter was 2.1 cm, ranging from 1.7 cm in younger women to 2.85 cm in men older than 70 years of age. Five percent of ruptures were in aneurysms less than 5 cm in diameter, and 1.9% of ruptures were in aneurysms less than 4 cm in size. No threshold diameter was found that accurately distinguished between rupture and nonrupture. Standardizing aneurysmal diameter to the transverse diameter of the third lumbar vertebral body (L3) did provide an accurate predictor of rupture. No aneurysm below a ratio of 1 ruptured, whereas 29% of aneurysms removed electively were smaller than L3.

Conclusion.—Aneurysmal diameter alone is not adequate as a sole indicator for elective resection of an abdominal aortic aneurysm.

▶ These authors have commendably attempted to determine the CT characteristics of infrarenal aneurysms that may be predictive of rupture. Not surprisingly, in nonaneurysmal patients, infrarenal aortic size is greater in men than in women. Because small aneurysms rupture in occasional patients, the size of the aneurysm by itself cannot be critically related to rupture. However, these authors found that standardization of the transverse diameter of the aneurysm to the diameter of the L3 body yielded an index that was an accurate predictor of rupture. No aneurysm ruptured when this ratio was less than 1. It is noteworthy that these authors treated a remarkable 286 patients with ruptured aneurysm over the course of 10 years.—J.M. Porter, M.D.

The Relationship Between Aortic Diameter and Body Habitus

Liddington MI, Heather BP (Gloucestershire Royal Hosp, Gloucester, England)
Eur J Vasc Surg 6:89–92, 1992   7–2

Introduction.—Past studies have failed to demonstrate a consistent relationship between abdominal aortic diameter (AD) and body size. The ultrasonographic findings in 906 men, aged 65–74 years, were examined.

Methods.—Correlations were sought between AD and height, weight, age, the Ponderal index, the Quatelet index, and body surface area. Men with an AD greater than 25 mm were restudied after 6, 18, 24, and 30 months.

Results.—Aortic diameter correlated significantly with both age and height in men whose diameters were within the normal range (table). Aortic diameter did not correlate with body weight, the Ponderal or Quatelet indices, or body surface area. It increased with advancing age and increasing height.

Conclusion.—Normal AD in men ranges from 15 to 25 mm, with the sporadic occurrence of an enlarged or aneurysmal aorta independent of age and build. The increase in AD with advancing age probably reflects dilatation secondary to muscular and collagenous degeneration of the aortic wall.

▶ Based on ultrasound-derived data, infrarenal aortic diameter appears unrelated to body weight or obesity, but it does correlate significantly with height and age. We are left to conclude from this abstract and Abstract 7–1 that infrarenal aortic diameter is directly related to male sex, height, and increasing age, but not to body habitus, body weight, or obesity.—J.M. Porter, M.D.

Mean and Median Values for the Group				
	Mean	s.d.	Median	Range
Age (years)	68.9	2.9	68	65–74
Height (cm)	173.1	6.6	173	147–193
Weight (kg)	77.0	11.4	76	40–124
Aortic diameter (mm)	20.1	5.1	19	12–59

(Courtesy of Liddington MI, Heather BP: *Eur J Vasc Surg* 6:89–92, 1992.)

Prevalence of Abdominal Aortic Aneurysm in Patients With Occlusive Peripheral Vascular Disease

Galland RB, Simmons MJ, Torrie EPH (Royal Berkshire Hosp, Reading, England)
Br J Surg 78:1259–1260, 1991   7–3

Introduction.—The advent of modern imaging techniques has led to increasing numbers of abdominal aortic aneurysms (AAAs) being diagnosed and treated. Approximately 5% of asymptomatic men aged 65–74 years have been shown to have an AAA by abdominal ultrasonography, and half of these AAAs are more than 4 cm in diameter. An increased risk for AAA has been demonstrated in patients with hypertension, coronary artery disease, peripheral vascular disease, other aneurysms, or a positive family history. The prevalence of AAA was examined in patients with occlusive vascular disease, and the presence of AAA was correlated with clinical findings.

Patients.—During a 1-year period, 165 men and 77 women with peripheral vascular disease of the lower extremities underwent abdominal US to detect the presence of an AAA, which was defined as a localized aortic dilatation. A diagnosis of AAA was made when the maximum diameter of the infrarenal aorta was either greater than 3.5 cm or 1.5 times that of the aorta at the level of the renal arteries. The aorta was defined as ectatic if it was diffusely and irregularly dilated, with a minimum diameter of 3 cm.

Results.—An AAA was detected in 34 patients (14%), and 17 of these AAAs were more than 4 cm in diameter. Of the 34 AAAs identified, 28 were found in men (17%) and 6 were found in women (8%). In addition, 16 patients had ectatic aortas. Patients with claudication were as likely to have an AAA as those with rest pain or gangrene. The presence of aortoiliac occlusive disease further increased the chance of an AAA being present.

Conclusion.—Patients with occlusive peripheral vascular disease are at high risk for an AAA developing, and they should be carefully assessed by abdominal ultrasonography. Older men with proximal occlusive disease are at even higher risk.

▶ A critically important question: Just how much screening for occult arterial disease should be performed in patients who are seen with symptomatic lower extremity arterial disease? It is my impression that these patients have between a 5% to 10% prevalence of high-grade asymptomatic carotid artery stenosis, as well as a 5% to 10% prevalence of AAA, as confirmed by this study. I continue to believe that all patients with symptomatic lower extremity arterial occlusive disease should have carotid duplex and abdominal ultrasonography done as part of their initial evaluation. Interestingly, a number of leading American academic vascular surgeons who I have quizzed do not share this opinion. Despite considerations of cost-effectiveness, for the present, I will continue with our current policy (1).—J.M. Porter, M.D.

Reference

1. Taylor LM, Porter JP: *Ann Vasc Surg* 4:502, 1986.

Abdominal Aortic Aneurysm in the Patient Undergoing Cardiac Transplantation
Piotrowski JJ, McIntyre KE, Hunter GC, Sethi GK, Bernhard VM, Copeland JC (Univ of Arizona, Tucson)
J Vasc Surg 14:460–467, 1991   7–4

Introduction.—Many survivors of cardiac transplantation for ischemic cardiomyopathy can have other manifestations of atherosclerosis, including aortic aneurysm. Abdominal ultrasonography was used to document the incidence, time of occurrence, and rate of expansion of abdominal aortic aneurysms in 130 cardiac transplant survivors during a 3-year period.

Methods.—The operative indication was ischemic cardiomyopathy in 38% of patients, idiopathic cardiomyopathy in 32%, viral cardiomyopathy in 6.9%, pulmonary hypertension in 6%, and graft atheroslcerosis in 1.5%. Routine preoperative abdominal ultrasonography was performed in 98 patients. In 93 there was specific visualization of the abdominal aorta.

Results.—Abdominal aortic aneurysms were found in 4 patients who were undergoing transplantation for ischemic heart disease (table). All of

Incidence of Abdominal Aortic Aneurysms in the Population
Undergoing Transplantation

Indications for treatment	No.	Aortic size (cm)	Aorta >2.5 cm No.	(%)
Ischemic heart disease	38	1.8 ± 0.7	4	(10.5%)*†
Idiopathic cardiomy-opathy	34	1.7 ± 0.3	0	
Miscellaneous car-diomyopathy	21	1.5 ± 0.5	0	
	93	1.7 ± 0.5	4	(4.3%)

* $P = .025$; Fischer's exact test.
† Does not include an additional patient in whom aneurysmal disease developed despite an initially normal ultrasound finding. If included, the incidence would be 13.2% ($P = .0096$; Fischer's exact test).
(Courtesy of Piotrowski JJ, McIntyre KE, Hunter GC, et al: *J Vasc Surg* 14:460–467, 1991.)

these aneurysms were infrarenal. Despite emergency surgery, one patient died of a ruptured aneurysm 2 months after transplantation. The aneurysms rapidly expanded by as much as 2.1 cm in the other 3 patients who underwent successful repair of their aneurysms at 5, 20, and 33 months respectively. A symptomatic aneurysm developed postoperatively in another patient with an initially normal aorta; the lesion, which measured 4.1 cm, was successfully repaired. The average aneurysm expansion was .74 cm per year.

Conclusion.—Aneurysms may occur in cardiac transplant patients with ischemic heart disease. Preoperative ultrasonography may be appropriate, and careful postoperative surveillance is vital. The combination of hemodynamic stress and steroid therapy may predispose the patient to rapid aneurysm expansion; cyclosporine may play a role in increasing blood pressure.

▶ We, too, are encountering aortic aneurysms in cardiac transplant patients. The Arizona group indicates that aneurysm occurrence in these patients appears limited to those undergoing cardiac transplantations for ischemic cardiomyopathy. These aneurysms are subject to rapid expansion and may rupture at a small size. One obviously wonders whether the vigorous immunosuppressive therapy after cardiac transplantation may be casually related to both expansion and rupture. Interestingly, AAA appears to be more frequent after cardiac transplantation than after renal transplantation.—J.M. Porter, M.D.

High Coincidence of Inguinal Hernias and Abdominal Aortic Aneurysms
Lehnert B, Wadouh F (Hannover Med School; Klinik Heidehaus, Hannover, Germany)
Ann Vasc Surg 6:134–137, 1992   7–5

Introduction.—It has been proposed that a collagen disorder may be responsible for inguinal herniation. Collagen metabolism is increased in aortic aneurysms. Fibrous tissue irregularities in the rectus sheath in patients with inguinal hernias suggest a breakdown of protein fibers by systemic enzymatic attack. If inguinal hernias and abdominal aneurysms are linked by increased systemic fiber metabolism, the disorders should occur within a short time.

Methods.—Patients scheduled to undergo repair of an infrarenal aortic aneurysm were assessed prospectively for a history of inguinal hernia, as were patients with aortic occlusive disease or coronary artery disease.

Results.—Inguinal hernias were found in 41% of patients with abdominal aortic aneurysms, which was significantly more often than in the comparison groups, which had 18% incidence in patients with aortic occlusive disease and 18% incidence in patients with coronary artery disease. Of 119 patients with aneurysms, 19 recently underwent hernia repair and 11 were awaiting repair. Smoking habits were comparable in the different groups.

Conclusion.—The finding that inguinal hernia is more prevalent in patients with aortic aneurysms than in those with peripheral or coronary artery disease supports a role for systemic fiber degeneration.

▶ Although this paper abounds with speculation, I am fascinated by the observation that patients with aortic aneurysms have twice the incidence of inguinal hernia as patients with either aortic occlusive disease or coronary artery disease.—J.M. Porter, M.D.

Abdominal Aortic Aneurysm as an Incidental Finding in Abdominal Ultrasonography
Akkersdijk GJM, Puylaert JBCM, de Vries AC (Westeinde Hosp, The Hague, The Netherlands)
Br J Surg 78:1261–1263, 1991   7–6

Background.—An abdominal aortic aneurysm is a potentially lethal occurrence that apparently is increasing in prevalence, even after allowing for increased life expectancy. Early detection and elective repair, when indicated, obviously could much improve the chance of a patient surviving.

Methods.—The prevalence of aneurysms was determined in a series of 1,687 patients aged 50 years and older who had undergone initial abdominal ultrasonography. Those patients suspected of having an aneurysm were excluded. An aneurysm was defined as a local dilatation with an anteroposterior diameter exceeding 30 mm or more than 1.5 times that of the proximal aorta.

Results.—An abdominal aortic aneurysm was found in 82 patients—8.8% of the men and 2.1% of the women. The prevalence of ab-

The Prevalence of Abdominal Aortic Aneurysm, According to Age, as an Incidental Finding in Abdominal Ultrasonography

Patients	Age (years)				
	50–59	60–69	70–79	80–89	All
Men	2·5	9·7	11·8	14·3	8·8
Women	0·8	0·6	2·7	6·4	2·1
All	1·5	4·2	6·6	9·2	4·9

The values are percentages.
(Courtesy of Akkersdijk GJM, Puylaert JBCM, de Vries AC: *Br J Surg* 78:1261–1263, 1991.)

dominal aortic aneurysm in men age ≥ 60 years was 11.4%. The prevalence increased with advancing age (table). In men 60 years and older, prevalence was 11.4%. The mean diameter of the aneurysms was 35 mm; aneurysmal diameter did not correlate significantly with patient age.

Conclusion.—The incidence of abdominal aortic aneurysm appears to be increasing, possibly because of better methods of detection. It also is possible that reported cases are increasing because effective treatment with acceptable risk has become more widely available.

▶ It is said that, in America, two thirds of unruptured abdominal aortic aneurysms are discovered during abdominal imaging studies performed for other reasons. In a large number of patients undergoing abdominal ultrasound testing for other reasons, these authors observed an overall prevalence of aneurysm of 8.8% in men and 2.1% in women. Admittedly, their definition of aneurysm was quite inclusive but, nevertheless, this is an important study. Primary care physicians should be oriented toward obtaining routine abdominal ultrasound for aortic size in all men older than 60 years of age. I suspect, however, that this recommendation may run afoul of cost-benefit analysis.—J.M. Porter, M.D.

Increasing Prevalence of Abdominal Aortic Aneurysms: A Necropsy Study

Bengtsson H, Bergqvist D, Sternby N-H (Lund Univ, Malmö Gen Hosp, Malmö, Sweden)
Eur J Surg 158:19–23, 1992   7–7

Introduction.—Deaths from abdominal aortic aneurysm have increased in the United States and Western Europe in recent decades, as have the number of operations.

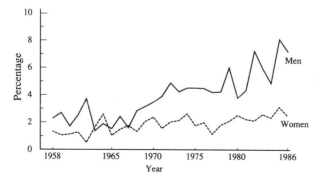

Fig 7–1.—Age-standardized, sex-specific percentages of patients with abdominal aortic aneurysms confirmed at autopsy, Malmö, 1958–1986. (Courtesy of Bengtsson H, Bergqvist D, Sternby N-H: *Eur J Surg* 158:19–23, 1992.)

Methods.—The prevalence of abdominal aortic aneurysm in Malmö, Sweden was estimated by reviewing 45,838 autopsy reports from 1958 to 1986. Data on all patients with aneurysm or surgery for aortic aneurysm below the diaphragm were included.

Results.—Abdominal aortic aneurysms were present in 4,300 per 100,000 men and in 2,100 per 100,000 women. The mean annual age-standardized rates increased by 4.7% in men and by 3% in women (Fig 7-1). The prevalance of aneurysms in men increased rapidly after 55 years of age and peaked at 5.9% at age 80 years. In women, the prevalence increased after 70 years of age and peaked at 4.5% after age 90 years.

Conclusion.—The prevalence of abdominal aortic aneurysmal disease has increased during the past 3 decades.

▶ Sweden has a remarkable state system of mandatory autopsies and medical record keeping. This system provides data for an unlimited number of retrospective studies. The authors of this article conclude that, during the past 30 years, the age-standardized annual increase of abdominal aortic aneurysmal disease discovered at autopsy was 4.7% among men and 3% among women. Despite studies such as this, I continue to wonder whether the apparent increase in aneurysm occurrence is not more a phenomenon of our improved discovery of aneurysms rather than an actual increase.—J.M. Porter, M.D.

Age-Standardized Incidence of Ruptured Aortic Aneurysm in a Defined Swedish Population Between 1952 and 1988: Mortality Rate and Operative Results
Drott C, Arfvidsson B, Örtenwall P, Lundholm K (Central Hosp, Borås, Sweden; Sahlgrenska Hosp, Göteborg, Sweden; Ostra Hosp, Göteborg, Sweden)
Br J Surg 79:175–179, 1992   7–8

Objective.—The incidence and mortality from ruptured aortic aneurysms were estimated for the period 1952–1988 for a stable population in Sweden. In this country, autopsy is required for patients who die outside of hospital.

Findings.—The annual rate of rupture of abdominal aneurysms increased significantly, from .9 per 100,000 population in the 1950s to 6.9 per 100,000 in the 1980s (Fig 7-2). After controlling for age, mortality increased by 2.4% per year between 1960 and 1988. Figures 2 to 3 times higher were reported from the United Kingdom in the 1980s. In Sweden, mortality from ruptured thoracic aneurysms did not increase after adjusting for age. The overall mortality from ruptured abdominal aneurysms in the 1980s was 85%. The rupture rates in Sweden and the United Kingdom are compared in the table. In Sweden, half the patients

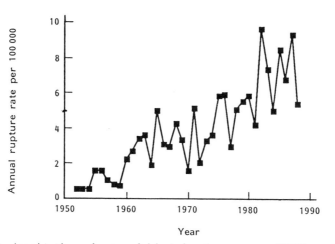

Fig 7–2.—Annual incidence of rupture of abdominal aortic aneurysm per 100,000 population of Göteborg during 1952–1988. The incidence increased significantly. (Courtesy of Drott C, Arfvidsson B, Örtenwall P, et al: *Br J Surg* 79:175–179, 1992.)

died outside surgical clinics, and only 30% underwent aortic reconstruction.

Vascular surgeons completed reconstruction more frequently than general surgeons, had lower blood losses, and performed surgery more rapidly. Mortality was lower for patients treated by vascular surgeons.

Conclusion.—Age-adjusted rupture rates for abdominal aortic aneurysms have increased in Sweden, despite impressive technical improve-

Annual Rupture Rate of Abdominal Aortic Aneurysms in Sweden and the United Kingdom

Place	Study period	Annual rupture rate per 100 000
Göteborg* (Sweden)	1952–1959	0·9
	1960–1969	3·2
	1970–1979	4·1
	1980–1988	6·9
Stockholm (Sweden)	1980	6
London (UK)	1981	13
	1986	21
Worthing (UK)	1979	9·2
	1986	17·5
Swansea (UK)	1974	7
	1980	10
	1983	17

* Present study.
(Courtesy of Drott C, Arfvidsson B, Örtenwall P, et al: *Br J Surg* 79:175–179, 1992.)

ments. Whether more frequent elective repair will reduce the overall mortality can only be learned through a prospective population study.

▶ In another Swedish population cohort, a different group of authors show a marked increase in the annual incidence of ruptured abdominal aortic aneurysms (Abstract 7–7). This study indicates an overall mortality from ruptured aneurysm of nearly 85%, a figure which I believe is also true for America.—J.M. Porter, M.D.

The Selective Management of Small Abdominal Aortic Aneurysms: The Kingston Study

Brown PM, Pattenden R, Gutelius JR (Queen's Univ, Kingston, Ont)
J Vasc Surg 15:21–27, 1992   7–9

Background.—The correct management of abdominal aortic aneurysms with a maximal diameter less than 5 cm remains uncertain, especially in those patients who are medically fit. The Kingston Abdominal Aortic Aneurysm Study, unlike other studies, is prospective, and it includes all patients seen with small aneurysms.

Methods.—A total of 268 patients entered the study between 1976 and 1988 and were monitored through 1990 (mean, 42 months). The criteria for surgery included an increase in aneurysm size to 5 cm, expansion of more than .5 cm in 6 months, and the development of aneurysmal symptoms or significant aortoiliac occlusive disease.

Results.—Surgery was done on 114 patients, in whom the aneurysm increased by a mean of .9 cm annually. The remaining 154 patients were

TABLE 1.—Deaths in the Aneurysm Study Group
Follow-up Patients

Myocardial infarction	15
Respiratory failure	8
Stroke	5
Malignancy	5
Renal failure	3
Suicide	1
Unknown	1
Rupture	1

(Courtesy of Brown PM, Pattenden R, Gutelius JR: *J Vasc Surg* 15:21–27, 1992.)

TABLE 2.—Comparison of Surgical Rates Related to Size at Entry

Aneurysm size	Surgery	Continued follow-up
Less than 4.0 cm at entry	31 patients (24%)	98 patients (76%)
4.0 cm or greater at entry	83 patients (60%)	56 patients (40%)

(Courtesy of Brown PM, Pattenden R, Gutelius JR: *J Vasc Surg* 15:21-27, 1992.)

monitored without operation. There was 1 rupture in this group. The average annual increase in aneurysmal diameter in unoperated patients was .24 cm. Myocardial infarction was the most common cause of death in the monitored group (Table 1). Aneurysms measuring 4 cm or more at the outset more often required surgical treatment (Table 2). Men and women had comparable expansion rates (Table 3).

Recommendation.—These findings support a policy of observation for abdominal aortic aneurysms that have a maximum diameter less than 5 cm.

▶ We are beset on one side by the apparent increase in the incidence of aneurysms, the increased incidence of ruptured aneurysms, and a very high death rate from ruptured aneurysms. On the other side, we are told that small aneurysms less than 5 cm in maximum diameter should not be operated on. Clearly, every ruptured aneurysm population study done to date has shown that nearly 5% of ruptures occurred in aneurysms with a diameter less than 5 cm. Elective aneurysm mortality in America is probably between 3% and 5%. If we operated on 100 patients with small aneurysms to prevent rupture

TABLE 3.—Expansion Rates Stratified to Sex of Patient

Surgical group	Follow-up group	Overall mean expansion
Men		
0.88 cm/yr	0.25 cm/yr	0.53 cm/yr
(98 patients)	(121 patients)	(219 patients)
Women		
0.80 cm/yr	0.24 cm/yr	0.42 cm/yr
(16 patients)	(33 patients)	(49 patients)

(Courtesy of Brown PM, Pattenden R, Gutelius JR: *J Vasc Surg* 15:21-27, 1992.)

in 5, 3–5 patients would not survive aneurysm surgery; therefore, there would be no net gain. These are important numbers with which every vascular surgeon should be familiar.—J.M. Porter, M.D.

The Natural History of Abdominal Aortic Aneurysms
Guirguis EM, Barber GG (Univ of Ottawa, Ottawa, Ont, Canada)
Am J Surg 162:481–483, 1991   7–10

Introduction.—The reported rates of rupture of small abdominal aortic aneurysms (AAAs) vary widely, from as much as 6% per year to a 5-year risk of 0.

Methods.—Data were reviewed on 300 patients, consecutively treated for AAA during a 6-year period, who were initially treated nonoperatively. Men constituted 70% of the patients, 68% of the patients were smokers, and 23% were receiving medication for hypertension. Almost half the aneurysms were discovered on physical examination, and more than 40% were discovered on abdominal ultrasonography.

Results.—The mean initial aneurysmal diameter was 4.1 cm. In 208 patients who had more than 1 ultrasound or CT study, the mean rate of change in aneurysmal diameter was .36 cm per year; 25% of these patients had an increase of .3–.6 cm per year, and 15% had an increase in diameter of .6 cm or greater per year. During a mean follow-up of 34 months, 14 patients had a rupture, 4 of whom survived emergency repair. All but 2 of the 14 patients had an aneurysm 5 cm or larger before rupture. The risk of rupture at 10 months was 1% for patients with aneurysms less than 4 cm in diameter, and 8% in those with aneurysms 5 cm or more in diameter. The cumulative rate of rupture at 6 years was 1% to 2% in patients with aneurysms less than 4 cm diameter and 20% in those with aneurysms 5 cm or larger.

Conclusion.—Referral-based studies may have overestimated the growth rate of AAAs. The rate of aneurysmal expansion increases as the lesion becomes larger. Ultrasonography or CT should be performed every 6 months in patients with aneurysms less than 5 cm in diameter. Larger aneurysms should be considered for early elective repair.

▶ One is left to conclude that Canadians have historically been very conservative when it comes to operating on small aneurysms. See Abstract 7–9.—J.M. Porter, M.D.

Surgery for Abdominal Aortic Aneurysms: A Survey of 656 Patients
Olsen PS, Schroeder T, Agerskov K, Røder O, Sørensen S, Perko M, Lorentzen JE (Rigshospitalet, Copenhagen, Denmark)
J Cardiovasc Surg 32:636–642, 1991   7–11

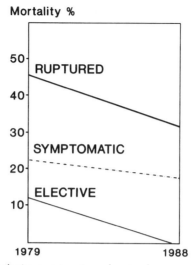

Fig 7–3.—Mortality for elective, symptomatic, and ruptured aneurysms, 1979-1988. (Courtesy of Olsen PS, Schroeder T, Agerskov K, et al: *J Cardiovasc Surg* 32:636-642, 1991.)

Introduction.—Surgery for abdominal aortic aneurysm was carried out in 656 patients in 1979-1988. The aneurysmal sac was partially resected, and a prosthesis was implanted using the in-lay technique. Surgery was acute in 56% of the cases and elective in 44%.

Results.—A ruptured aneurysm was present in 33% of patients. Half these patients and 5% of the others were in shock. Postoperative mortal-

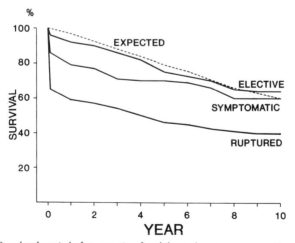

Fig 7–4.—Cumulated survival after operation for abdominal aortic aneurysm. After 5 years, there was no statistically significant difference in survival between symptomatic and elective cases. The survival for patients with ruptured aneurysm was significantly lower (P < .01, log-rank test). (Courtesy of Olsen PS, Schroeder T, Agerskov K, et al: *J Cardiovasc Surg* 32:636-642, 1991.)

ity was 5% after elective surgery and 37% in patients with ruptured aneurysms, with a significant decrease during the study period (Fig 7–3). After 6 months, survival of electively operated patients did not differ from that of an age- and sex-matched control population (Fig 7–4). Symptomatic patients had a 5-year survival of 70%, and those with rupture had a 5-year rate of 48% compared with 80% for control subjects. Of the patients with a ruptured aneurysm, 40% remained alive after 10 years, at which time symptomatic patients were doing as well as the control population.

Conclusion.—Further improvement in survival of patients operated on for abdominal aortic aneurysm should come from limiting intraoperative and postoperative mortality, as well as from increasing the number of patients who are operated on electively.

▶ There are few surprises in this large retrospective study of aortic aneurysms by excellent surgeons in Copenhagen. Of note is that only 44% of the 656 operations took place electively. A ruptured aneurysm was seen in 33% of the patients, which indicates a significant failure of their aneurysm detection network, such as we have in America. Of concern is that 23% of the aneurysms in this series were operated on emergently and found to be nonruptured. The death rate in this group was 17.2% compared with an elective mortality of 4.8%. We continue to use the CT scan to differentiate between ruptured and unruptured symptomatic aneurysms. We do not perform emergency surgery for the symptomatic unruptured aneurysm, but we do perform urgent elective surgery at the next opening in our operating schedule, usually within 12–24 hours. I continue to believe that emergency surgery should be avoided (if at all possible) for symptomatic unruptured aneurysms, because of the striking increase in mortality that has been reported in this group by every series to date.—J.M. Porter, M.D.

Late Iliac Artery Aneurysms and Occlusive Disease After Aortic Tube Grafts for Abdominal Aortic Aneurysm Repair: A 35-Year Experience
Calcagno D, Hallett JW Jr, Ballard DJ, Naessens JM, Cherry KJ Jr, Gloviczki P, Pairolero PC (Mayo Med School and Mayo Med Ctr, Rochester, Minn)
Ann Surg 214:733–736, 1991   7–12

Background.—It remains unclear whether patients with Dacron aortic tube grafts meant to replace an abdominal aortic aneurysm are at significant risk of having either an iliac artery aneurysm or occlusive disease develop.

Methods.—A total of 432 patients with a diagnosis of abdominal aortic aneurysm were studied in the period 1951–1984. The aneurysm was eventually repaired in 206 patients. Thirty-nine patients having successful repair with a straight graft were compared with the same number of patients treated with a bifurcated graft.

Complications Related to Graft Among Rochester, Minnesota, Residents Who Underwent Tube ($n = 39$) and Bifurcated ($n = 39$) Aortic Graft Placement, 1951–1984

Complications Related to Graft	Type of Graft	
	Tube	Bifurcated
Rupture of proximal anastomosis	1 (1 mo)	1 (6 yr)
Rupture of distal anastomosis	0	1 (16 yr)*
False aneurysm of proximal anastomosis	1 (15 yr)	0
False aneurysm of distal anastomosis	0	2 (4, 8 yr)†
Lymphocele	0	1 (2 mo)†

* Iliac.
† Femoral.
(Courtesy of Calcagno D, Hallett JW Jr, Ballard DJ, et al: *Ann Surg* 214: 733–736, 1991.)

Results.—During a mean follow-up of 6 years, graft-related complications developed in 13% of the patients with a bifurcated graft and 5% of those with a straight graft (table). New aneurysms were comparably frequent in the groups.

Conclusion.—Use of a straight tube graft to repair an abdominal aortic aneurysm provides reliable late patency with a minimal risk that an iliac artery aneurysm will develop. Long-term follow-up is necessary, because some of the complications that occur are seen 5 years or more postoperatively.

▶ Isn't there a remarkable difference in the incidence of tube grafting performed for aortic aneurysm disease at various centers? Our experience has been that less than 5% of our patients seem appropriate for a tube graft, whereas other centers have an incidence of tube grafting as great as 50%. This series had a 19% incidence rate. This study and others indicate a gratifyingly low incidence of iliac aneurysm development after use of a tube graft for aortic aneurysm surgery.—J.M. Porter, M.D.

Transfemoral Intraluminal Graft Implantation for Abdominal Aortic Aneurysms
Parodi JC, Palmaz JC, Barone HD (Instituto Cardiovascular de Buenos Aires; Univ of Texas, San Antonio)
Ann Vasc Surg 5:491–499, 1991   7–13

Experimental.—Animal experiments have been done to determine the feasibility of excluding an abdominal aortic aneurysm by placing an intraluminal, stent-anchored knitted Dacron graft (Fig 7–5). The graft is in-

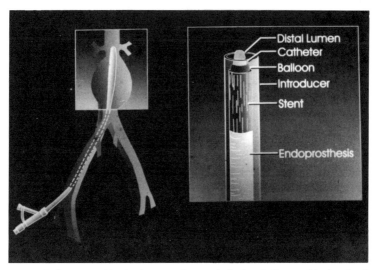

Fig 7–5.—Graft-stent combination is mounted on a valvuloplasty balloon and is placed under fluoroscopy through a sheath introduced through femoral arteriotomy. (Courtesy of Parodi JC, Palmaz JC, Barone HD: *Ann Vasc Surg* 5:491–499, 1991.)

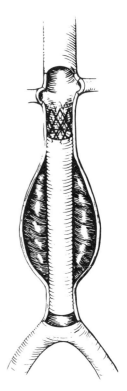

Fig 7–6.—Graft-stent combination with cephalic stent. (Courtesy of Parodi JC, Palmaz JC, Barone HD: *Ann Vasc Surg* 5:491–499, 1991.)

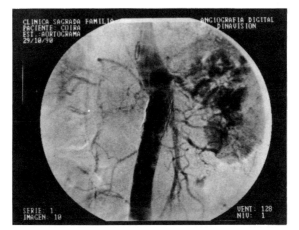

Fig 7–7.—Aortography 53 days after implantation of graft-stent combination. (Courtesy of Parodi JC, Palmaz JC, Barone HD: *Ann Vasc Surg* 5:491-499, 1991.)

troduced by retrograde cannulation of the common femoral artery under either local or regional anesthesia. When the balloon-expandable stent was sutured to the partly overlapping ends of the tubular graft, friction seals resulted, fixing the graft ends to the vessel wall and excluding the aneurysm from the circulation.

Clinical.—Five patients with serious co-existing conditions received an individually tailored graft. In 3 cases, only a cephalic stent was used (Fig 7–6). In the 2 other patients, both ends of the tubular stent were joined to other stents with a one-third overlap. One patient required conventional abdominal aortic aneurysm surgery because of stent misplacement. Four of the 5 patients had heparin reversal when the procedure was completed. The early results have been encouraging (Figs 7–7). In 3 cases, the excluded aneurysm has decreased in size.

▶ This paper probably attracted more attention among vascular surgeons than any paper published in America during the past year, with the possible exception of the NASCET North American Symptomatic Carotid Endarterectomy Trial Collaborators' report (see Abstract 12–1). Burning questions remain: For how many patients with aneurysms is this type of intraluminal grafting feasible? Is it safe? Is it effective? All vascular surgeons will follow developments in this field with considerable interest.—J.M. Porter, M.D.

Isolated Testicular Pain: An Unrecognized Symptom of the Leaking Aortic Aneurysm
Cawthorn SJ, Giddings AEB, Taylor RS, Thomas MH (St George's Hosp, London; The Royal Surrey County Hosp, Guildford, England; St Peter's Hosp, Chertsey, England)
Br J Surg 78:886–887, 1991   7–14

Introduction.—Delay in diagnosis continues to be a significant factor in the high mortality associated with ruptured abdominal aortic aneurysm where as ruptured aortic aneurysms may frequently present with collapse and severe hypotension, posterior rupture may present with such confusing symptoms as severe backache or renal colic, which frequently obscure the accurate diagnosis. In 3 patients, severe testicular pain was found as a previously unrecognized symptom of a leaking or rapidly expanding abdominal aortic aneurysm.

Patients.—The 3 male patients were examined because of isolated severe bilateral or unilateral testicular pain. In each patient, the testes were normal and not tender. In 1 patient, abdominal examination revealed a tender aortic aneurysm near rupture. In the second patient, the aneurysm had leaked posteriorly. The third patient collapsed and was admitted to the hospital with an unrecordable blood pressure and distended abdomen. Laparotomy confirmed an anterior rupture of an aortic artery. All patients underwent grafting and had uneventful recoveries. The mechanism for referred pain to the testes may be the sudden posterolateral expansion of the aneurysm pressing on the visceral afferent pain fibers of the testes. Severe back pain often develops when an aneurysm starts to rupture, and it may mask testicular pain.

Conclusion.—Although testicular pain has been previously described as a symptom of an iliac aneurysm, it has not been described as the presenting symptom of an abdominal aortic aneurysm. In these 3 patients, severe testicular pain with a finding of normal testes was the initial symptom of a leaking or ruptured aortic aneurysm. All admitting staff should be aware of unusual symptoms of aneurysms to reduce delay in diagnosis of aneurysm and referral of the patient to a vascular surgeon.

▶ The abrupt onset of peculiar pain almost anywhere in the general abdominal region must be considered as a possible indicator of rupture in a patient with a known aortic aneurysm. In addition to testicular pain, we have seen an occasional ruptured aneurysm present with femoral triangle pain, and, even occasionally, with severe hip pain. Significant localized pain felt anywhere around the abdomen in a patient with aneurysm indicates the need for a well-performed CT scan.—J.M. Porter, M.D.

Aortic Dissection With the Entrance Tear in Abdominal Aorta
Roberts CS, Roberts WC (Natl Heart, Lung, and Blood Inst, Bethesda, Md)
Am Heart J 121:1834–1835, 1991   7–15

Background.—In a series of 182 necropsies of patients with spontaneous aortic dissection, only 2 had the entrance tear in the abdominal aorta.

Case 1.—Man, 30, "wrenched" his back while swimming. He collapsed from pain the next morning. His systolic blood pressure was 60 mm Hg, which increased to 90 mm Hg after he received 2 L of lactated Ringer's solution. He was resuscitated from cardiac arrest in the emergency department; a peritoneal tap showed gross blood, whereas a previous tap had been clear. Exploratory laparotomy showed a rupture in the abdominal aorta nearly 2 cm from the aortic bifurcation. The infrarenal abdominal aorta was replaced, but the patient died of left colonic ischemia and renal failure. Necropsy disclosed an aortic intimal tear connected to a false channel that extended to the proximal graft anastomosis.

Case 2.—Woman, 78, with a history of systemic hypertension was admitted 2 days after a fall. Computed tomography showed subdural hematomas that were evacuated by craniotomy. However, reaccumulated hematomas required another operation 9 days later. She became comatose and died 5 days postoperatively. A healed dissection of the abdominal aorta was found at necropsy, with an entry tear just caudal to the renal arteries and a reentry tear 8 cm distal. The 6-cm false channel was filled almost completely with organized thrombus.

Discussion.—In a series of 182 patients with spontaneous aortic dissection studied at autopsy, only 2 (1%) originated in the abdominal aorta. Limited available information suggests that nearly 50% of these rare aneurysms may rupture. Early operative intervention appears reasonable when these are detected.

▶ Aortic dissection occasionally begins in the infrarenal aorta, but not very often. The vascular surgeon must have a clear concept of aortic dissection, false lumen, and branch artery occlusion caused by malperfusion. Graft replacement, with or without fenestration, extra-anatomical bypass, and visceral grafting are all occasionally required in the treatment of patients with malperfusion and complications associated with aortic dissection.—J.M. Porter, M.D.

Replacement of the Abdominal Aorta With an Aortic Homograft in a Patient With an Aortic Dissection
Steinberg JB, Nickell SA, Jacocks MA, Stelzer P (Univ of Oklahoma; Health Sciences Ctr, Oklahoma City,; Lenox Hill Hosp, New York)
Ann Vasc Surg 5:538–541, 1991   7–16

Background.—The availability of synthetic substitutes has largely replaced the use of aortic and femoral homografts. Recently reported improved methods of homograft cryopreservation may have resulted in the availability of an improved homograft.

Case Report.—Man, 40, with a DeBakey type I aortic dissection had the aortic root replaced by a pulmonary homograft. Subsequent intra-abdominal infection was complicated by progressive ischemia in the mesenteric region and lower extremities. The abdominal aorta was then replaced by an aortic homograft. After 3 years, the patient had good gastrointestinal function and no evidence of vascular insufficiency in the lower extremities.

Conclusion.—Laboratory studies are needed to evaluate newer cryopreserved homografts for use in the presence of infection, or where the potential for intra-abdominal infection exists.

▶ Are aortic homografts going to made a comeback? Other investigators reported interesting preliminary experience with the new generation of homografts.—J.M. Porter, M.D.

Salmonella Infection of the Aorta
Edwards PR, Moody P, Harris PL (Broadgreen Hosp, Liverpool, England)
J R Coll Surg Edinb 36:181–183, 1991   7–17

Background.—As many as 10% of individuals who ingest nontyphoidal *Salmonella* species develop systemic infection, and nearly 10% of them will have metastatic infection, often involving the cardiovascular system. Lesions usually develop on preexisting disease, such as damaged valve tissue. Mortality can be as high as 80% when the aorta is involved.

Patients.—Two patients with acute abdominal aortic aneurysm after *Salmonella* species infection of the gastrointestinal tract were recently encountered. Woman, 72, who was previously well, had back pain, dysuria, nausea, and diarrhea. She improved rapidly with antibiotics, and *Salmonella* species were isolated from the blood. Periumbilical pain was noted 5 weeks later. An abdominal aortic aneurysm 6 cm in diameter was confirmed. The saccular aneurysm was resected from the infrarenal aorta and revascularization was performed with extra-anatomical bypass grafting; the patient did well. Man, 56, was seen with severe colicky lower abdominal pain, which was present intermittently for 8 weeks after an episode of diarrhea. Ultrasonography showed slight aortic enlargement, and *Salmonella typhimurium* was isolated from the blood. The patient collapsed and died 9 days after admission. Massive intraperitoneal bleeding was caused by a 4-cm disruption of a severely atheromatous lower abdominal aorta. Postmortem cultures yielded *S. typhimurium*.

Conclusion.—Older patients with atheromatous disease are those most likely to have endovascular *Salmonella* species infection develop. Antibiotics may reduce the risk in older patients who have nontyphoidal *Salmonella* species gastroenteritis, negative blood cultures, and mild systemic symptoms. Regular outpatient screening is recommended for at least 3 months after presumed uncomplicated *Salmonella* gastroenteritis to detect endovascular infection.

▶ I am impressed that *Salmonella* species aortic infection is occurring with increasing frequency. I note with fascination that some primary care physicians do not advocate antibiotic treatment of apparently uncomplicated *Salmonella* gastrointestinal infection. This interesting policy may well lead to an increased incidence of *Salmonella* species arteritis.—J.M. Porter, M.D.

The Retroperitoneal Approach to Aortic Surgery Associated With Horseshoe Kidney
Mason RA, Kvilekval KHV, Hartman A, Giron F (State Univ of New York at Stony Brook)
J Cardiovasc Surg 32:763–766, 1991   7–18

Introduction.—A horseshoe kidney can impede the repair of an abdominal aortic aneurysm. The left retroperitoneal approach sufficiently exposes the abdominal aorta while avoiding structures that may be associated with a horseshoe kidney.

Case Report.—Man, 70, had unstable angina and marked triple-vessel coronary disease; however, before open heart surgery, he was found to have both an asymptomatic abdominal aortic aneurysm measuring 6.5 cm and a horseshoe kidney. Renal function was reduced, with the left kidney contributing 75% of total function. Coronary artery bypass surgery was completed uneventfully. Subsequent angiography showed reduced perfusion of the isthmus part of the horseshoe kidney. A left retroperitoneal approach allowed the aneurysm to be opened along its left lateral border after cross-clamping the aorta. A Dacron tube graft was inserted, and the aneurysm was closed over the graft. The patient recovered well and maintained baseline renal function.

Advantages.—This approach provides ready access to the lower abdominal aorta without dividing the renal isthmus. Single or multiple anomalous renal arteries arising from the aorta can be managed endovascularly, and ureteral injury is avoided.

▶ The retroperitoneal approach to aortic surgery in patients with horseshoe kidney is probably the approach of choice.—J.M. Porter, M.D.

CT of Inflammatory Abdominal Aortic Aneurysm: Development From an Uncomplicated Atherosclerotic Aneurysm
Latifi HR, Heiken JP (Washington Univ, St Louis)
J Comput Assist Tomogr 16:484–486, 1992   7–19

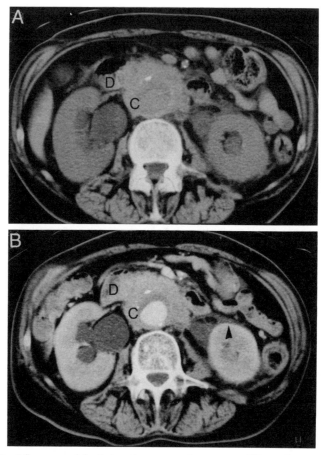

Fig 7–8.—Inflammatory abdominal aortic aneurysm. **A,** precontrast CT scan demonstrates soft tissue mass anterior and lateral to abdominal aortic aneurysm with a partially calcified wall. There is a lack of fat planes between the mass and adjacent duodenum (D) and inferior vena cava (C). Bilateral hydronephrosis is present. **B,** after administration of intravenous contrast material, the periaortic soft tissue mass enhances moderately. The fluid adjacent to the left kidney is part of small urinoma (*arrowhead*). (Courtesy of Latifi HR, Heiken JP: *J Comput Assist Tomogr* 16:484–486, 1992.)

Introduction.—The term "inflammatory aneurysm" has been given to abdominal aortic aneurysms with a thickened aortic wall, dense perianeurysmal fibrosis, and adhesions. In 1 case, such an aneurysm developed over 6½ months.

Case Report.—Woman, 58, was seen with pain in the left flank and upper abdominal quadrant, as well as anorexia and vomiting of 5 days' duration. She was anemic and had a pulsatile abdominal mass. Abdominal CT showed a 3.8-cm aneurysm with a 1.5-cm mantle of soft tissue density material abutting its anterior and lateral walls (Fig 7–8). A CT study done 6 months earlier had demonstrated the aneurysm, but not the periaortic soft tissue (Fig 7–9). Exploration

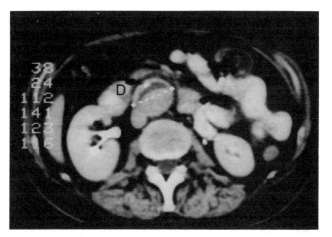

Fig 7–9.—A CT scan obtained 6½ months earlier shows an abdominal aortic aneurysm but no surrounding soft tissue mass. The anterior wall of the aneurysm is thick. There is a fat plane between the aneurysm and duodenum (D). (Courtesy of Latifi HR, Heiken JP: *J Comput Assist Tomogr* 16:484–486, 1992.)

revealed a thick fibrotic mass extending cephaled to the renal arteries. A biopsy specimen indicated fibrosis without malignant change. An aortoiliac Y-graft was placed, with implantation of the left renal artery into the graft. The patient had small bowel obstruction, left renal infarction, and an enterocutaneous fistula, but she recovered.

Conclusion.—An inflammatory abdominal aortic aneurysm can develop from an uncomplicated aneurysm in as little as 6½ months. The CT findings are characteristic and can alert the surgeon to the possibility of intraoperative complications.

▶ These authors put forward the interesting hypothesis that inflammatory aneurysms are not inflammatory from the beginning, but may develop from previously noninflammatory aneurysms. Based on sequential CT scans in a single patient, they further state that changes can occur in as few as 6 months. On balance, I am impressed by the large volume of our literature directed toward inflammatory aneurysms. The number of publications may exceed the number of patients.—J.M. Porter, M.D.

Human Immunodeficiency Virus and Infected Aneurysm of the Abdominal Aorta: Report of Three Cases
Gouny P, Valverde A, Vincent D, Fadel E, Lenot B, Tricot J-F, Rozenbaum W, Nussaume O (Hôpital Rothschild, Paris; Hôpital André Mignot, Versailles, France)
Ann Vasc Surg 6:239–243, 1992   7–20

Background.—Infected abdominal aortic aneurysm has rarely been found in patients with AIDS or in those who are positive for HIV. Three patients who were seropositive for HIV underwent surgery for such an aneurysm in 1989 and 1990.

Cases.—In these patients, fever and abdominal pain were the chief clinical features. None of the patients had opportunistic infection or endocarditis. In 2 patients, radiography demonstrated a ruptured aneurysm. The causative organisms were *Salmonella, Haemophilus,* and *Mycobacterium tuberculosis.*

Treatment and Outcome.—All patients had placement of an in situ prosthetic graft protected by omentum. Antibiotics were continued for several weeks. All 3 were well when last seen at 10–21 months after surgery.

Conclusions.—Bacterial invasion of an atheromatous aorta may occur in an HIV-seropositive patient. Surgery is warranted when rupture is imminent.

▶ We shall surely see more of this in the future.—J.M. Porter, M.D.

Abdominal Aortic Aneurysm in 4237 Screened Patients: Prevalence, Development and Management Over 6 Years
Scott RAP, Ashton HA, Kay DN (St Richard's Hosp, Chichester, England)
Br J Surg 78:1122–1125, 1991   7–21

Background.—Abdominal aortic aneurysm (AAA) is not reliably detected clinically, and it may rupture without previous symptoms. Planned surgery is far safer than emergency treatment. Detection of AAA by ultrasonographic screening may well reduce overall mortality. Ultrasound follow-up of small aneurysms will detect expansion and may allow treatment before rupture occurs.

Methods.—Of 7,200 individuals aged 65–80 years who were contacted by letter in a community project, 4,237 agreed to ultrasonographic

| | \multicolumn{5}{c}{Aortic Size (≥ 3 cm) in 179 Patients at Initial Scan} |
| | \multicolumn{5}{c}{Aortic size (cm)} |

	3–3·9	4–4·9	5–5·9	>6	Total
Men	101	27	8	12	148
Women	23	3	4	1	31
Total	124	30	12	13	179

(Courtesy of Scott RAP, Ashton HA, Kay DN: *Br J Surg* 78:1122–5, 1991.)

screening. In 4,122 of these subjects, it was possible to measure the aorta.

Results.—A total of 179 aneurysms that were 3 cm or larger in diameter were detected, for a prevalence of 4.3% (table). Thirteen patients had an aortic diameter of 6 cm or more on initial screening, and 14 had expansion of this degree on follow-up. Fourteen other patients had a 1-cm or greater increase in aortic diameter in 1 year, but diameter did not reach 6 cm. Two patients became symptomatic.

Conclusion.—Fewer than 10% of patients with an ultrasonographically detected AAA required surgery, assuming ultrasound follow-up was assured to detect subsequent AAA changes. A total of 4.3% of a large group of unselected patients between 65 and 80 years of age had an AAA by screening abdominal ultrasonography.

▶ This is an important epidemiologic study indicating that, in a very large population of elderly patients, duplex screening for AAA revealed that 4.3% of the patients had an AAA greater than 3 cm in diameter. Using the criteria of a diameter greater than 6 cm, an annual increase in aortic diameter of greater than 1 cm, or the development of symptoms, these authors conclude that less than 10% of the aneurysms detected in the population require surgery. The importance of this study lies in its basic epidemiologic data and in the size distribution of detected aneurysms.—J.M. Porter, M.D.

8 Aorto-Iliac Disease

Acute Aortic Occlusion Presenting With Lower Limb Paralysis
Meagher AP, Lord RSA, Graham AR, Hill DA (Univ of New South Wales, Sydney, Australia)
J Cardiovasc Surg 32:643–647, 1991   8–1

Introduction.—Acute aortic occlusion is a rare but serious vascular emergency; mortality rates as high as 50% have been reported. Data on 8 patients treated for acute occlusion of the aorta during a 2-year period were reviewed. The mean diagnostic delay was 24 hours, resulting in a poor outcome in 7 of the patients.

Clinical Features and Course.—All patients had some degree of paralysis at presentation, as well as findings of acute ischemia, including pain, absent pulses, color change, and anesthesia. Even after diagnosis, a mean of 13 hours passed before revascularization was undertaken. Unnecessary aortography was the cause of this delay in 4 patients. In 3 of 6 patients who were operated on, an aortic bifurcation graft was placed. Aortic occlusion was caused by thrombosis of an atherosclerotic aorta in 5 patients, aneurysmal thrombosis in 2, and embolism in 1 patient who had heparin-induced thrombocytopenia. Five patients died, 1 was left paraplegic, 1 had amputation, and 1 recovered.

Conclusion.—Immediate operation is necessary in patients with acute aortic occlusion. If the diagnosis is in doubt, it can be rapidly confirmed by Doppler examination. The patient in this series who recovered had surgery after only 2¼ hours.

▶ Acute aortic occlusion with lower extremity paralysis is one of the most profound emergencies in vascular surgery. Immediate revascularization, although usually resulting in limb survival, by no means always reverses the neurologic deficit. The extremely adverse outcome in this series, which is attributable to a remarkable delay in diagnosis and treatment, is sobering and indicates an area where we all need to make considerable improvement.—J.M. Porter, M.D.

Aortic Mural Thrombus in Young Women: Premature Arteriosclerosis or Separate Clinical Entity?
Perler BA, Kadir S, Williams GM (Johns Hopkins Hosp, Baltimore)
Surgery 110:912–916, 1991   8–2

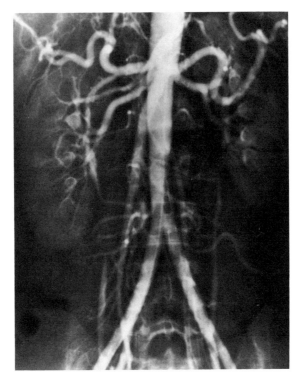

Fig 8–1.—Aortogram in patient 1. Note the distal aortic lesion. (Courtesy of Perler BA, Kadir S, Williams GM: *Surgery* 110:912–916, 1991.)

Introduction.—Arteriosclerotic peripheral artery disease typically occurs in older individuals, although arteriosclerosis remains the most common cause of limb ischemia in young adults. These patients tend to have focal lesions in the aortoiliac segment, and a disproportionate number of them are women. Smoking is frequent, and oral contraceptive use has also been implicated.

Patients.—Woman, 28, was seen with ischemic symptoms in her left foot and absent distal pulses. Angiography demonstrated a filling defect at the left aortic wall just above the bifurcation (Fig 8–1), and there were abrupt occlusions of several arteries in the calf. Organized thrombus was found adhering to a thickened aortic intima, and thromboendarterectomy was done. Oral contraception was withdrawn, and the patient did well when given warfarin treatment, with normal perfusion to the left lower extremity. Woman, 34, who was a heavy smoker and received steroids for Crohn's disease, was seen with unilateral claudication and had a similarly placed aortic filling defect with presumed embolism to the left internal iliac artery. She did well after aortic thromboendarterectomy and left popliteal thromboembolectomy. The aortic intima appeared thickened but not arteriosclerotic.

Discussion.—Nearly all premenopausal women with aortic thrombosis are heavy smokers. Some have used anovulatory steroids, suggesting that they may have a distinct clinical disorder rather than premature arteriosclerosis. The disorder is characterized by intimal hyperplasia and thromboses.

Recommendations.—Distal embolization should be considered in a young woman who smokes and is seen with peripheral arterial insufficiency. Aortography is in order and, if indicated, aortic thromboendarterectomy is an effective and safe approach. In a patient who has aortic mural thrombus but no underlying arteriosclerotic disease, intra-arterial thrombolysis might be equally effective.

▶ What is going on in these patients? In the past, we have occasionally operated on young females with this finding, have removed the thrombus, and have performed a localized thromboendarterectomy with restoration of normal appearing aorta and normal peripheral pulses. We have been very disappointed to have the patient return with recurrent thrombosis within 30–60 days. In our patients, we did not use warfarin. It is my belief that these patients generally have a hypercoagulable disorder (in our recent experience, lupus anticoagulant), and that long-term administration of postoperative warfarin is mandatory. The excellent results obtained in these 2 patients, both of whom were followed with long-term warfarin, are noteworthy.—J.M. Porter, M.D.

The Retroperitoneal, Left Flank Approach to the Supraceliac Aorta for Difficult and Repeat Aortic Reconstructions
Mills JL, Fujitani RM, Taylor SM (Wilford Hall United States Air Force Med Ctr, Lackland Air Force Base, Tex)
Am J Surg 162:638–642, 1991   8–3

Patients.—Eleven patients with aortoiliac occlusive disease for whom standard infrarenal reconstruction was contraindicated underwent supraceliac aortofemoral bypass. In 4 patients, multiple infrarenal attempts had failed; whereas in 5 others, an infected aortofemoral bypass graft had been removed and an extra-anatomical bypass had failed. One patient had had para-aortic lymph node dissection and had received radiotherapy. Another patient had aortic aneurysmal disease proximal to the renal arteries.

Procedure.—A left-flank incision extending into the 11th intercostal space was made, and retroperitoneal and extrapleural dissection were carried out (Fig 8–2). Conduits included either a bifurcated Dacron graft or a tube graft to the left femoral artery combined with a femorofemoral crossover graft. Three patients had left renal artery reconstruction at the same time.

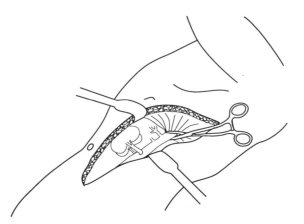

Fig 8–2.—After medial rotation of the intraperitoneal viscera and the left kidney, the left diaphragmatic crus is partially divided, exposing the supraceliac aorta and allowing proximal clamp placement. A second, more distal clamp placed just above the celiac artery, not shown here, is used to control backbleeding. (Courtesy of Mills JL, Fujitani RM, Taylor SM: *Am J Surg* 162:638–642, 1991.)

Results.—One patient had transient postoperative acute tubular necrosis. The mean cross-clamp time was 24 minutes, and there were no operative deaths. The rate of graft limb patency was 95% after a mean follow-up of 17 months.

Conclusion.—In difficult cases of aortoiliac occlusive disease—including repeat procedures—the supraceliac aorta is a useful inflow source. This bypass appears more durable than inflow reconstruction based on the axillary artery.

▶ Repeated infrarenal aortic operations are hazardous and have a diminishing likelihood of success. I always prefer extra-anatomical bypass in patients with multiple, failed, infrarenal operative procedures. In the older patient group, my first choice is axillobifemoral bypass, and in the younger patient group, my first choice is supraceliac-aortofemoral bypass (as described in this paper). I strongly prefer to route the supraceliac graft to the left femoral artery and then perform a femorofemoral bypass. Efforts to route the right limb of a bifurcated supraceliac graft, either retroperitoneally or retrorectus, to the femoral artery have both been met with complications in my experience.—J.M. Porter, M.D.

Unilateral Iliofemoral Occlusive Disease: Long-Term Results of the Semiclosed Endarterectomy With the Ringstripper

van den Dungen JJAM, Boontje AH, Kropveld A (Univ Hosp Groningen, The Netherlands)

J Vasc Surg 14:673–677, 1991   8–4

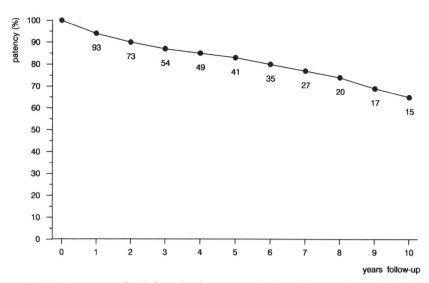

Fig 8–3.—Patency rate after iliofemoral endarterectomy. Numbers indicate patients at risk during the time interval. (Courtesy of van den Dungen JJAM, Boontje AH, Kropveld A: *J Vasc Surg* 14:673–677, 1991.)

Introduction.—Fewer endarterectomies are performed for the treatment of occlusive arterial disease; more often, bypass procedure is performed. To determine whether the results of the semiclosed endarterectomy for unilateral iliofemoral occlusive disease indicate a wider use of bypass procedures for such short obstructions, data were reviewed on 94 patients who underwent 101 operations for extensive obstructions of 1 external iliac and common femoral artery in 1971–1989. In 7 patients, surgery was performed for occlusive disease on the contralateral side at a later stage. A total of 93 endarterectomies were performed; an iliofemoral bypass graft was used in 8 patients when endarterectomy was not possible. Of the procedures, 62 were for disabling claudication and 39 were for limb-threatening ischemia.

Results.—Of the patients who underwent endarterectomy for disabling claudication, 85% became asymptomatic; 80% who underwent endarterectomy for limb-threatening ischemia became asymptomatic or improved to claudication. No one died after endarterectomy. There also were no false aneurysms or infections after the procedure. The patency rates were 94% at 1 year, 83% at 5 years, and 65% at 10 years (Fig 8–3).

Conclusion.—The semiclosed endarterectomy with the ringstripper of a unilateral obstruction of 1 external iliac and common femoral artery can be performed with no mortality, low morbidity, and good long-term results. The best results were in patients with an open superficial femoral artery, which indicates that associated distal disease is of prognostic value.

▶ The technique of extensive aortoiliac endarterectomy is slipping into the past, much like the dinosaurs. Although occasional good results are still reported (as in this abstract) I wonder how representative they are. I find very few occasions on which I am even remotely tempted to consider using extensive aortoiliac endarterectomy.—J.M. Porter, M.D.

Simultaneous Revascularization for Critical Coronary and Peripheral Vascular Ischemia
Carrel T, Niederhäuser U, Pasic M, Gallino A, von Segesser L, Turina M (Univ Hosp, Zurich, Switzerland)
Ann Thorac Surg 52:805–809, 1991   8–5

Background.—As many as 15% of patients who have myocardial revascularization reportedly have severe peripheral vascular ischemia as well. As many as half the patients who require peripheral revascularization have serious coronary artery disease. When disease is severe at both sites, it would be advantageous to perform a single operation if feasible, avoiding the added risk from waiting for the second part of staged procedures.

Methods.—Thirty-two patients with strong indications for operative treatment of both coronary disease and critical peripheral vascular ischemia underwent simultaneous coronary and peripheral surgery (table). A single team performed both operations, with coronary bypass grafting being performed first under cardiopulmonary bypass with moderate hypothermia and blood cardioplegia. Low-level systemic heparinization was done before clamping the aorta or the peripheral arterial segment. The patients were monitored with Swan-Ganz catheters. If necessary, platelet inhibitors were given after surgery.

Operative Procedures					
	Number of Bypass Grafts				
Vascular Procedure	1	2	3	4	5
Aortoiliac endarterectomy	. . .	1	1	2	. . .
Iliacofemoral endarterectomy	3	5	2	3	2
Bifurcation prosthesis	. . .	2	1	2	1
Aortofemoral bypass	. . .	2	1	1	. . .
Femoropopliteal bypass	. . .	1	1	1	. . .

(Courtesy of Carrel T, Niederhäuser U, Pasic M, et al: *Ann Thorac Surg* 52:805-809, 1991.)

Results.—Hospital mortality was 3.1%, but no patient died early after elective operation. The actuarial survival at 8 years was 87.5%, and the risk factors included incomplete revascularization, age, ejection fraction, and preoperative renal failure.

Conclusion.—Coronary artery disease and peripheral arterial disease may be operated on simultaneously with encouraging long-term results and an acceptable risk. Simultaneous operations are recommended when both disorders are symptomatic and when the peripheral vascular surgery is imperative in the presence of significant coronary artery disease.

▶ This paper introduces an interesting topic. We all accept that some patients are optimally served by a combination of coronary and carotid surgery, although the number probably is very small. I am sure that there are also a few patients with sufficiently severe coronary disease, as well as leg ischemia, to warrant combined treatment. I am equally sure, however, that these patients are extraordinarily uncommonly encountered, and that this will be a most infrequently performed combined procedure.—J.M. Porter, M.D.

Pentoxifylline in the Treatment of Vascular Impotence: Case Reports
Allenby KS, Burris JF, Mroczek WJ (Cardiovascular Ctr of Northern Virginia, Alexandria)
Angiology 42:418–420, 1991   8–6

Introduction.—Pentoxifylline is a methylxanthine for the treatment of intermittent claudication caused by chronic arterial disease. Although the mechanisms of action are unclear, pentoxifylline has the potential for improving blood flow to other organs with stenotic vascular compromise. In 3 patients with occlusive vascular disease and impotence, there was an improvement in sexual function after initiation of pentoxifylline therapy.

Results.—The 3 male patients underwent angiography because of claudication of the lower extremities, not because of sexual dysfunction. Pentoxifylline was prescribed for its rheologic effects. The patients spontaneously reported improvement of sexual function. Because pentoxifylline administration improves arterial blood flow, it may also improve any area of impaired perfusion caused by a stenotic vascular lesion.

Conclusion.—Three patients who were treated with pentoxifylline for occlusive vascular disease reported improved sexual function. Based on these interesting anecdotal results, a controlled trial of pentoxifylline for vascular impotence appears warranted.

▶ Pentoxifylline is not the valueless drug that many vascular surgeons assume it to be. It obviously does not cure claudication, but it has objectively improved claudication in many randomized, well-conducted prospective studies. It appears to have important actions in venous ulcer healing and, perhaps, in the treatment of impotence. In my opinion, this drug should be regarded as important, not only for its intrinsic pharmacologic actions, but as a milestone in our quest for pharmacologic agents that favorably affect the course of arterial and venous disease.—J.M. Porter, M.D.

Clinical Implications of Combined Hypogastric and Profunda Femoral Artery Occlusion
Cikrit DF, O'Donnell DM, Dalsing MC, Sawchuk, AP, Lalka SG (Indiana Univ Med Ctr, Indianapolis)
Am J Surg 162:137–141, 1991   8–7

Objective.—A study was conducted to examine the potential complications of combined hypogastric and profunda femoral artery occlusion.

Methods.—The courses of 9 patients seen in 1983–1990 with combined occlusive disease of the hypogastric artery (HA) and profunda femoral artery (PFA) were reviewed. Five patients had non healing hip disarticulations, and 3 had above-knee amputations that were not healing. Six of the patients exhibited perineal necrosis, and 4 had necrosis of the buttock. Two patients had visceral ischemia, and 1 had changes of lumbosacral spinal ischemia.

Outcome.—Five patients died of ischemic complications. Two patients who survived required hemipelvectomy, and another required an axillary-to-hypogastric artery bypass graft for stump salvage. One patient survived despite lumbosacral paralysis and total cystectomy.

Conclusion.—Attempts should be made to preserve or restore the HA and PFA circulation when possible. If the local circulation is inadequate in a patient with an above-knee amputation and revascularization is not feasible, then hemipelvectomy should be considered.

▶ The authors very appropriately call attention to the effects of combined occlusion of the hypogastric and profunda arteries. Early revascularization or hip disarticulation is the most appropriate therapy. The mortality is extremely high, especially if one procrastinates in the removal of the ischemic tissue. It would appear that several areas of collateral circulation are evolving as being important for the vascular surgeon to remember: colonic, hip, and knee. With refined techniques, we are able to revascularize distal circulations, but we may forget the intermediate circulation.—G. Johnson, Jr., M.D.

Ischemic Injury to the Spinal Cord or Lumbosacral Plexus After Aorto-Iliac Reconstruction
Gloviczki P, Cross SA, Stanson AW, Carmichael SW, Bower TC, Pairolero PC, Hallett JW Jr, Toomey BJ, Cherry KJ Jr (Mayo Clinic and Found, Rochester, Minn)
Am J Surg 162:131–136, 1991   8–8

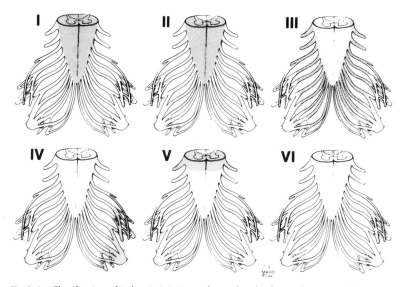

Fig 8–4.—Classification of ischemic injuries to the cord or lumbosacral roots or plexus. Type I, complete infarction of the distal spinal cord; type II, infarction of anterior two thirds of the cord (anterior spinal artery syndrome); type III, infarction of the lumbosacral roots with or without patchy infarcts in the cord; type IV, unilateral lumbosacral plexus infarction; type V, segmental infarction of the spinal cord; type VI, infarction of the posterior third of the cord (posterior spinal artery syndrome). (Reproduced by permission of the Mayo Foundation.) (Courtesy of Gloviczki P, Cross SA, Stanson AW, et al: Am J Surg 162:131–136, 1991.)

Introduction.—Paraplegia is a very serious and unpredictable complication of aortoiliac reconstruction. Mechanisms of neurologic injury were identified in a series of 3,320 abdominal aortic reconstructions, according to a classification scheme (Fig 8–4).

Findings.—Nine patients (.3%) had ischemic injury to the cord or lumbosacral plexus. The incidence was highest (1.4%) after emergency aortic aneurysm repair. Eight of the 9 patients received a bifurcated graft. In only 2 patients was supraceliac aortic cross-clamping done. Four of the 9 patients were hypotensive. Two patients died, and 7 had severe perioperative complications which, for the most part, were related to visceral and somatic ischemia and sepsis. Patients with ischemic injury of the lumboscral roots or plexus did better than those with cord injury.

Prevention.—The risk of paraplegia may be minimized by using gentle operative technique and by avoiding hypotension and prolonged supraceliac cross-clamping of the aorta. At least 1 internal iliac artery should be revascularized. Particular care is needed in patients who have a ruptured aortic aneurysm or shaggy aorta syndrome.

▶ There is only 1 legitimate conclusion that is possible regarding the development of spinal cord ischemia after infrarenal aortic reconstruction: this rare complication is more likely to occur after a difficult operation or after an operation performed under difficult circumstances. As a result, it is often associated with other complications as well. All other conclusions, including those in this paper, are actually only speculation.—G.L. Moneta, M.D.

9 Visceral Artery Disease

Renovascular Hypertension: Predicting Surgical Cure With Exercise Renography

Hupp T, Clorius JH, Allenberg JR (Univ of Heidelberg, Heidelberg, Germany)
J Vasc Surg 14:200–207, 1991   9–1

Background.—Ergometric exercise can lead to disordered transrenal hippurate transport; this abnormality reverses when exercise ends. The disorder presumably indicates abnormal renal cortical perfusion, and it has been demonstrated only in hypertensive patients. Affected patients may have a form of renal hypertension that is not curable by either operation or angioplasty.

Methods.—A group of 31 hypertensive patients with documented unilateral or bilateral renovascular stenosis was studied prospectively. Rest and exercise hippurate scintigrams were recorded preoperatively (table).

Results.—A total of 19 patients (61%) had abnormal transrenal hippurate transport during exercise. Twenty-six patients subsequently had renovascular surgery, and 5 underwent percutaneous transluminal angioplasty. Of the 12 hypertensive patients with normal exercise renograms, 10 were cured. Hypertension persisted after therapy in 17 of the 19 patients with an abnormal preoperative exercise scintigram.

Conclusion.—Exercise scintigraphy may help to identify those patients with curable renovascular hypertension and those who may benefit most from surgery.

▶ These authors make the empiric observation that patients with apparent renovascular hypertension have a far better blood pressure response to reno-

Preoperative Exercise Response vs. Postoperative BP Status in 23 Patients With Unilateral Stenosis		
	Hypertension cured	*Hypertension not cured*
Normal scintigram (*n* = 11)	9	2
Abnormal scintigram (*n* = 12)	0	12

(Courtesy of Hupp T, Clorius JH, Allenberg JR, et al: *J Vasc Surg* 14:200–207, 1991.)

vascular surgery when they do not have an exercise-induced abnormality of cortical renal perfusion as determined by isotope tracing. I have no idea whether this observation is either real or important. It is, however, sufficiently interesting that those performing renovascular surgery should be aware of it and pay careful attention to future developments in this area.—J.M. Porter, M.D.

A Preliminary Study of the Role of Duplex Scanning in Defining the Adequacy of Treatment of Patients With Renal Artery Fibromuscular Dysplasia

Edwards JM, Zaccardi MJ, Strandness DE Jr (Univ of Washington, Seattle)
J Vasc Surg 15:604–611, 1992   9–2

Background.—Fibromuscular dysplasia (FMD) of the renal arteries is a recognized cause of hypertension that has a characteristic arteriographic appearance. It often is difficult to determine the functional significance of FMD lesions, particularly when both renal arteries are involved. Duplex scanning is an accurate means of detecting and quantifying renal artery stenosis.

Methods.—Nine patients with FMD of the renal artery were managed by either angioplasty or surgery. Eighteen arteries were treated, 4 of them more than once. Transluminal angioplasty was done 16 times, and 2 arteries that failed to improve underwent bypass surgery.

Results.—Fourteen of 18 treatments led to a reduction in blood pressure. In all these cases, the renal-aortic ratio decreased below the level at which greater than 60% stenosis is diagnosed. In the failures, velocity at the site of narrowing did not improve after intervention. Hemodynamic improvement was noted in patients who improved clinically.

Conclusion.—Duplex scanning is able, along with the clinical response, to help determine the cause of failure when a patient with FMD fails to improve after angioplasty or operative treatment.

▶ Well-performed duplex scanning can provide important information about visceral artery stenosis, both before and after surgery. It has become the initial diagnostic test of choice in centers with experienced and skilled vascular laboratory technologists.—J.M. Porter, M.D.

Renal Revascularization for Recurrent Pulmonary Edema in Patients With Poorly Controlled Hypertension and Renal Insufficiency: A Distinct Subgroup of Patients With Arteriosclerotic Renal Artery Occlusive Disease

Messina LM, Zelenock GB, Yao KA, Stanley JC (Univ of Michigan, Ann Arbor)
J Vasc Surg 15:73–82, 1992   9–3

Background.—Recurrent pulmonary edema in a patient with refractory hypertension and renal insufficiency appears to be a marker for the presence of bilateral renal artery occlusive disease. The efficacy of renal revascularization was examined in 17 such patients treated between 1984 and 1990.

Patients.—The mean preoperative blood pressure was 207/110 mm Hg, and the mean serum creatinine clearance was 3.8 mg/dL. Pulmonary edema occurred despite normal ventricular function in two thirds of the patients. More than half the patients had an occluded renal artery.

Management.—Renal revascularization was achieved most often by iliorenal bypass, aortorenal bypass, or endarterectomy. Forty percent of patients had the other kidney removed, and 24% had concomitant aortic reconstruction.

Results.—There were no postoperative deaths, and hypertension was more readily controlled in all patients. Dialysis was discontinued in 2 of 3 patients. Hypertension was improved in 16 patients and cured in 1 at a mean follow-up of 2½ years. Only 1 patient had pulmonary edema during late follow-up. Renal function improved after surgery in 77% of the patients, and it became worse in 2, 1 of whom required dialysis.

Conclusion.—Renal revascularization can prevent recurrent pulmonary edema in patients with bilateral renal arterial occlusive disease, renal insufficiency, and poorly controlled hypertension.

▶ I was unaware of the association between bilateral renal artery disease and recurrent pulmonary edema. It is primarily important for our internists and cardiologists to become familiar with this entity, because I suspect there have been far more of these patients on the medical services than any of us realize.—J.M. Porter, M.D.

Hepato-Left Renal Artery Bypass
Sharp WJ, Shamma AR, Hoballah JJ, Kresowik TF, Corson JD (Univ of Iowa Hosps and Clinics, Iowa City)
Ann Vasc Surg 6:193–194, 1992   9–4

Introduction.—The splenic artery has been used as an inflow source as an alternative to aortorenal reconstruction to revascularize the left renal artery; however, the procedure is not simple, and the splenic artery may itself be affected by atherosclerotic disease. A common hepatic-to-left renal artery bypass using autogenous saphenous vein has been found to be an acceptable alternative to splenorenal bypass.

Technique.—After an aortogram excludes significant celiac artery stenosis, the proximal aorta is dissected and the left renal artery is exposed. The gastrohepatic omentum is incised to expose the common hepatic artery. A segment of greater saphenous vein is taken from either proximal thigh and is prepared as a reversed

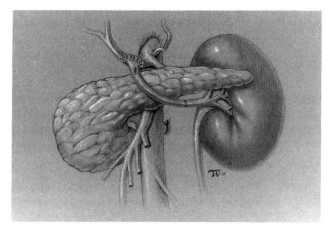

Fig 9–1.—The spatulated renal artery is anastomosed to the saphenous vein graft with fine, monofilament suture. (Courtesy of Sharp WJ, Shamma AR, Hoballah JJ, et al: *Ann Vasc Surg* 6:193–194, 1992.)

bypass graft. Under systemic heparinization, the spatulated end of the vein is joined end-to-side to the common hepatic artery using a T-junction technique. The vein graft is passed through a hole in the base of the transverse mesocolon. The origin of the left renal artery is suture-ligated and divided, and the spatulated renal artery is joined to the vein graft with a fine monofilament suture (Fig 9–1).

Results.—This procedure was performed electively in 3 patients, with good short-term results. A fourth patient underwent emergent renal revascularization with this method for renal salvage in the presence of renal artery thrombosis and recent myocardial infarction, but renal function did not return.

Conclusion.—This bypass technique is quite short, and it may be efficiently performed with minimal surgical dissection. It is useful in patients with difficult aortic problems, in high-risk patients, and in patients with staged renal revascularization. Pancreatic-splenic artery dissection is avoided.

▶ There clearly are many ways to remove the integument from a feline (skin a cat). This is another innovative approach to renal revascularization, this time using the relatively accessible and generally atherosclerotic, uninvolved, proximal visceral vessels. In more and more patients requiring renal revascularization, the abdominal aorta and the iliac arteries are simply too diseased to serve as the origin for a bypass graft.—J.M. Porter, M.D.

Renal Artery Stenosis Caused by Nonspecific Arteritis (Takayasu Disease) Results of Treatment With Percutaneous Transluminal Angioplasty

Sharma S, Saxena A, Talwar KK, Kaul U, Mehta SN, Rajani M (All India Inst of Medical Sciences, New Delhi)
AJR 158:417–422, 1992

9–5

Background.—Renovascular hypertension is frequent in patients with nonspecific aortoarteritis. Percutaneous transluminal renal angioplasty is a comparatively infrequent means of treatment.

Methods.—The results of renal angioplasty were reviewed in 20 patients with Takayasu disease in whom a total of 33 stenoses were treated. All patients had severe hypertension that was unresponsive to single-drug treatment and at least 70% stenosis of the renal artery, with a pressure gradient exceeding 20 mm Hg. The sedimentation rate was normal. All stenoses were treated via the transfemoral route.

Results.—Angioplasty was technically successful in treating 85% of the lesions and the same proportion of patients (Fig 9–2). All failures were in patients who had tight proximal stenosis of the renal artery and coexisting abdominal aortic disease. Some patients with a tough, noncompliant stenosis felt back pain and had a decrease in blood pressure during balloon inflation. One patient required surgery for injury to the renal vein during angioplasty. The clinical success rate of 82% (of patients achieving technical success) included 6 cures. Six of 28 lesions restenosed after a mean follow-up of 8 months.

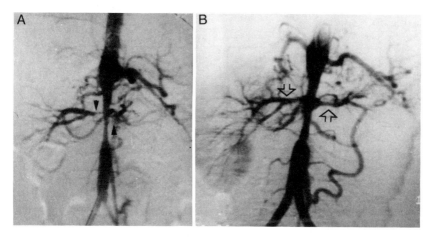

Fig 9–2.—Boy, 10 years, with severe uncontrolled hypertension. **A,** an anteroposterior intra-arterial digital subtraction angiogram of abdominal aorta shows a long segment narrowing in its perirenal segment and light proximal stenosis of both renal arteries (*arrowheads*). **B,** after angioplasty, an intra-arterial digital subtraction angiogram shows normal diameter of both renal arteries and brisk antegrade flow (*arrows*). (Courtesy of Sharma S, Saxena A, Talwar KK, et al: *AJR* 158:417–422, 1992.)

Conclusion.—Renal angioplasty may be technically difficult in patients with nonspecific arteritis, but reliable short-term results are achieved at an acceptable rate of complications.

▶ After a mean follow-up of only 8 months, there was a considerable recurrence of stenosis and hypertension in a large number of these young patients. This is another disturbing example of interventional radiologists refusing to display their data in life-table format. I am hard-pressed to understand the long-term benefit of balloon dilatation of collagenous or fibrous stenosis. Successful dilatation appears to require plaque fracture with medial stretching. This is not the case in this type of disease. The reader must decide for himself how to interpret these data. I am unimpressed.—J.M. Porter, M.D.

Duplex Ultrasonography in the Diagnosis of Celiac and Mesenteric Artery Occlusive Disease

Bowersox JC, Zwolak RM, Walsh DB, Schneider JR, Musson A, LaBombard FE, Cronenwett JL (Dartmouth-Hitchcock Med Ctr, Hanover, NH)
J Vasc Surg 14:780–788, 1991   9–6

Background.—There is a need for agreed-on criteria to diagnose celiac and superior mesenteric arterial occlusive disease by duplex ultrasonography. In a blinded, retrospective study, duplex findings were compared with the arteriographic appearances in 24 consecutive patients having both studies.

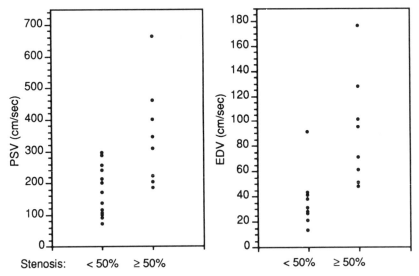

Fig 9–3.—Scatter plots of fasting superior mesenteric artery (peak systolic velocity, **A**) and (end-diastolic velocity, **B**) in 13 normal or minimally stenotic arteries, and 8 severely stenotic (≥ 50%) arteries. (Courtesy of Bowersox JC, Zwolak RM, Walsh DB, et al: *J Vasc Surg* 14:780–788, 1991.)

Methods.—Mesenteric duplex scans were acquired using a Diasonics DRF-400 instrument with a 3-MHz imaging probe and a 2.25-MHz pulsed Doppler. Biplane arteriograms were interpreted by observers who were unaware of the duplex scan findings. Severe stenosis was defined as a reduction of 50% or more in arterial diameter on an arteriogram.

Results.—Eight patients had severe stenosis, and 3 had occlusion of the superior mesenteric artery. Peak systolic velocity (PSV) was less in patients with minimal or no stenosis than in patients with severe stenosis. The best indicator of severe stenosis was an end-diastolic velocity (EDV) exceeding 45 cm/sec (Fig 9–3). Although a PSV exceeding 300 cm/sec was less sensitive, it was highly specific. No particular value of celiac PSV or EDV distinguished clearly between minimal and severe stenosis.

Conclusion.—Specific velocity criteria remain lacking, but severe superior mesenteric artery stenosis is suggested by the absence of a triphasic waveform, a fasting EDV more than 45 cm/second, and a fasting PSV more than 300cm/sec.

▶ See also Abstract 3–4. These authors believe that the EDV is the best indicator of stenosis in the visceral vessels, whereas Dr. Greg Moneta has stated that an increase in PSV is best. Moneta's data have the advantage of prospective validation.—J.M. Porter, M.D.

Atherosclerotic Occlusive Disease of the Superior Mesenteric Artery: Late Results of Reconstructive Surgery
Cormier JM, Fichelle JM, Vennin J, Laurian C, Gigou F (Hôpital Saint Joseph, Paris)
Ann Vasc Surg 5:510–518, 1991   9–7

Introduction.—Late outcomes for 103 patients undergoing an isolated superior mesenteric artery (SMA) revascularization were assessed.

Methods.—Of 200 patients who underwent an SMA revascularization procedure between 1975 and 1988, 103 had a direct SMA revascularization for atherosclerotic occlusive disease, but did not have associated intestinal resection. There were 14 women and 89 men, with a mean age of 57.2 years. Those patients with symptoms (groups I, II, and III) usually required revascularization of the splanchnic bed; asymptomatic patients (groups IV and V) had prophylactic SMA revascularization. The revascularization techniques that were used depended on the location of the lesion and evolved over time (table).

Results.—Four deaths occurred among the 103 patients, for a postoperative mortality of 4%. Complications and secondary deaths occurred in 5 patients; 4 arterial occlusions were observed in these patients. The 98 surviving patients had a mean follow-up of 69 months, during which 5 patients did not return for reexamination. During the follow-up period,

Revascularization Techniques in 103 Patients

Bypass	Antegrade	Retrograde	Total
Saphenous vein	8	9	17
PTFE	45	17	62
Dacron	0	4	4
Reimplantation	**Supraceliac**	**Infrarenal**	**Total**
PTFE	2	2	4
Dacron	1	4	5
Aorta	0	5	5
Endarterectomy	6	0	6

Abbreviation: PTFE, polytetrafluoroethylene.
(Courtesy of Cormier JM, Fichelle JM, Vennin J, et al: *Ann Vasc Surg* 5:510–518, 1991.)

18 patients died. Four cases of asymptomatic vascular problems occurred. The vascular complications were more frequent and serious in those patients having the initial surgery for severe intestinal ischemia. Patients receiving vein grafts had a high rate of complications of 22%. The type of revascularization procedure did not influence the occurrence of the complications.

Conclusion.—Superior mesenteric artery revascularization plays an important role in the treatment for and the prevention of intestinal ischemia and infarction. Failure of the SMA revascularization procedure occurs more often and produces more serious complications when severe intestinal ischemia is seen initially.

▶ I am fascinated that one third of these patients underwent SMA surgery prophylactically. On balance, the surgical results were excellent during a prolonged follow-up period.—J.M. Porter, M.D.

Splenic Artery Aneurysms Occurring in Liver Transplant Recipients
Bronsther O, Merhav H, Van Thiel D, Starzl TE (Univ of Pittsburgh)
Transplantation 52:723–724, 1991   9–8

Background.—Splenic artery aneurysms (SAAs) are reported in .1% of large autopsy series and much more frequently in patients with portal hypertension. A high mortality rate is associated with rupture of an SSA.

Findings.—A review of 1,311 liver transplant operations revealed 5 patients with a ruptured SAA, 4 of whom died. An additional patient was found to have an SAA after a second orthotopic liver transplant, and this aneurysm was removed electively.

Factors.—Increased splenic and splanchnic blood flow secondary to arteriovenous shunting and collateral vessel formation may explain the more frequent and larger SAAs found in patients with chronic liver disease and portal hypertension. The hormonal changes in vessels and increased cardiac output secondary to hyperglucagonemia also could be factors.

Management.—The splenic artery should be ligated on both sides of the aneurysm, and the lesion should be resected if feasible. Both splenic artery ligation without splenectomy and therapeutic embolization carry a risk of splenic infarction with abscess formation.

▶ The estimated incidence of SAAs in unselected aortograms is .8%. The incidence of SAA is much higher in patients with portal hypertension, in whom it is estimated to range between 8.8% and 50% of all patients. In this article, the authors have found an incidence of 6 SAAs among 1,311 liver transplant recipients. Apparently, no routine screening tests were done. The authors conclude that their data indicate a high incidence of SAA in liver transplant patients, but I am hard-pressed to understand the basis for their conclusion, because 6 of 1,311 is an incidence of only .4%. Perhaps routine screening would have revealed a much higher incidence, but this information is not available in the present study.—J.M. Porter, M.D.

Routine Reimplantation of Patent Inferior Mesenteric Arteries Limits Colon Infarction After Aortic Reconstruction

Seeger JM, Coe DA, Kaelin LD, Flynn TC (Univ of Florida, Gainesville; VA Med Ctr, Gainesville)
J Vasc Surg 15:635–641, 1992   9–9

Background.—Ischemic colitis leading to colonic infarction after reconstructive surgery on the aorta carries a high mortality. Reimplanting all patent inferior mesenteric arteries should lessen mortality, but it is justified only if it is both effective and safe.

Methods.—Data were reviewed on 337 aortic reconstructive procedures performed between July 1982 and May 1989. In 151 operations done in the last 3 years of this period, patent inferior mesenteric vessels were reimplanted when possible. These vessels had previously been selectively ligated on the basis of the appearance of the bowel, colonic mesenteric Doppler signals, and stump pressures in the inferior mesenteric arteries.

Results.—No patient in the latter part of the review period had colonic infarction. Five earlier patients (2.7%) had colonic infarction and perforation, and 4 of them died. Operative mortality was 14.5% earlier in the series and 4% when the mesenteric arteries were reimplanted, if possible. Transfusion requirements did not differ significantly in the 2 periods.

Conclusion.—Routine reimplantation of patent inferior mesenteric arteries reduces the risk of colonic infarction after reconstruction of the aorta.

▶ Should all inferior mesenteric arteries be implanted? Considering time and possible surgical complications, I do not think so. The nonrandomized patient cohorts compared in this study prove nothing, but the findings do indicate the need for a prospective randomized trial, which should be considered by these authors.—J.M. Porter, M.D.

10 Leg Ischemia

Causes of Primary Graft Failure After In Situ Saphenous Vein Bypass Grafting
Donaldson MC, Mannick JA, Whittemore AD (Harvard Med School, Boston)
J Vasc Surg 15:113–120, 1992   10–1

Introduction.—Of 455 consecutive patients undergoing in situ saphenous vein bypass graft surgery, 92 were primary failures. Seventy of these patients had occlusion, and 22 had nonocclusive stenosis.

Causes.—In 7 grafts, the cause of failure could not be determined. Nearly two thirds of the identified causes of failure were intrinsic to the graft itself (table). Perianastomotic stenosis was the most frequent intrin-

104 Causes Contributing to Primary Failure of 85 In Situ Saphenous Vein Grafts	
Intrinsic	
Perianastomotic stenoses	18
Vein stricture	14
Focal vein stenosis	10
Valvulotome injury	9
Kink	6
Retained valve leaflet	4
Arteriovenous fistula	2
Intimal flap	3
Total	66 (63%)
Extrinsic	
Compromised outflow	19
Compromised inflow	2
Hypercoagulability	9
Hypotension	6
Graft sepsis	2
Total	38 (37%)

(Courtesy of Donaldson MC, Mannick JA, Whittemore AD: *J Vasc Surg* 15:113–120, 1992.)

sic factor. The most frequent extrinsic causes of graft failure were compromised outflow and hypercoagulability.

Conclusion.—Improved techniques, better patients selection, and more effective perioperative management might have eliminated as many as 44% of the causes of primary graft failure in this series. Delayed graft stenosis and late progression of outflow disease remain difficult treatment problems.

▶ Despite the uncertainty of this retrospective data, it is interesting to note that nearly two thirds of graft failures are attributable to factors intrinsic to the graft, and almost one third are attributable to factors extrinsic to the graft. It is especially noteworthy that approximately one third of the intrinsic causes were directly related to the in situ technique. Despite my best efforts, I simply cannot understand the widespread uncritical preference for the in situ graft configuration.—J.M. Porter, M.D.

Wound Complications of the In Situ Saphenous Vein Bypass Technique
Reifsnyder T, Bandyk D, Seabrook G, Kinney E, Towne JB (Med College of Wisconsin, Milwaukee)
J Vasc Surg 15:843–850, 1992   10–2

Background.—Wound complications are frequent after in situ saphenous vein bypass surgery. They may lengthen hospitalization and threaten the viability of the graft.

Series.—A total of 126 in situ operations were done in 117 consecutive male patients in 1981–1991. They included 45 femoropopliteal by-

TABLE 1.—Classification of Wound Complications After In
Situ Saphenous Vein Bypass

Class	Wound characteristics	Treatment
Class 1	Skin edge necrosis Lymphatic leak	Empiric antibiotics
Class 2	Wound infection or necrosis involving subcutaneous tissue	Culture specific antibiotics
		Wet to dry dressing changes
Class 3	Invasive wound infection to depths of wound about graft	Operative debridement Graft coverage
		Culture specific antibiotics

(Courtesy of Reifsnyder T, Bandyk D, Seabrook G, et al: *J Vasc Surg* 15:843–850, 1992.)

TABLE 2.—Wound Complications in In Situ Saphenous Vein Bypass Grafts—Degree of Severity, Anatomical Distribution, Type of Treatment, and Time of Onset

Class	No.	Primary location			Operative debridement	Mean time to presentation
		Groin	Thigh	Leg		
1	19	13	2	4	1	10.7 days
2	12	3	5	4	4	18.9 days
3	13	3	0	10	12*	31.2 days

Note: Graft coverage: sartorious flap (n = 2), calf muscle apposition (n = 3), slip thickness skin graft (n = 2).
(Courtesy of Reifsnyder T, Bandyk D, Seabrook G, et al: J Vasc Surg 15:843–850, 1992.)

passes, 75 femorotibial bypasses, and 6 grafts to the dorsal pedal artery. Sixty-nine procedures were done for ulceration or gangrene, 54 for rest pain, and 3 for claudication. The wound complications were classified as shown in Table 1.

Results.—Wound complications developed in 44% of the grafts and included 13 infections that threatened the graft (Table 2). The risk factors for wound infection included lymph leakage and early graft revision for thrombosis, hematoma, retained valve, or arteriovenous fistula. Graft-threatening infections developed a mean of 1 month postoperatively. Most infections were in the distal graft limb. All but 1 of the 13 deep infections required surgical débridement, and 7 required coverage by a flap or split-thickness skin graft. No grafts were lost, and no patient died.

Conclusion.—Wound complications have been frequent after in situ saphenous vein bypass surgery, but aggressive management has resulted in the salvage of all grafts.

▶ A disturbing 44% of patients who underwent in situ saphenous vein bypass performed by this very experienced group had significant wound complications develop. Despite successful outcome in the treatment of these patients, their hospitalization was significantly prolonged, and expenses increased. We continue to believe that lower extremity wounds should be closed with a fine subcuticular suture technique; in our experience with reverse vein grafts, this has virtually eliminated skin edge necrosis and localized lymphatic leak.—J.M. Porter, M.D.

Cephalic Vein Grafts for Lower Extremity Revascularization

Sesto ME, Sullivan TM, Hertzer NR, Krajewski LP, O'Hara PJ, Beven EG
(Cleveland Clinic Found; Cleveland Clinic Florida, Fort Lauderdale)
J Vasc Surg 15:543–536, 1992   10–3

Introduction.—The graft material used for arterial bypass in the lower extremity significantly affects the outcome.

Methods.—Infrainguinal revascularization using cephalic vein grafts was performed in 34 consecutive patients in 1980–1989. Saphenous veins in the 35 operated extremities either were inadequate or had been harvested for coronary or lower-limb bypass. Ischemic rest pain or focal tissue necrosis was the indication for surgery in 71% of the extremities. The other patients had disabling claudication, popliteal aneurysm, or an infected prosthetic femoropopliteal graft.

A preliminary arteriovenous fistula was constructed in the arm in two thirds of the patients to increase the diameter of the cephalic vein. Cephalic vein alone was used in 69% of the procedures. The distal popliteal artery was used for the outflow anastomosis in 10 extremities, a tibial vessel was used in 12, and the peroneal artery was used in 13.

Results.—During a mean follow-up of 28 months, there were 14 graft occlusions, and 6 amputations were necessary. The cumulative primary and secondary patency rates at 3 years were 40% and 46%, respectively, and the limb salvage rate was 82%.

Conclusion.—Cephalic vein grafts, although relatively inconvenient, appear preferable to prosthetic materials for infrainguinal revascularization below the knee.

▶ In our experience, arm veins are the second best conduit after the greater saphenous vein. Lower extremity grafts, which can be fashioned from an intact arm vein, appear to be nearly as good in our experience as a saphenous vein graft. However, arm vein grafts that have been pieced together are clearly inferior, and they appear little better than a prosthetic graft, at least to the popliteal artery.—J.M. Porter, M.D.

Unsuspected Preexisting Saphenous Vein Disease: An Unrecognized Cause of Vein Bypass Failure
Panetta TF, Marin ML, Veith FJ, Goldsmith J, Gordon RE, Jones AM, Schwartz ML, Gupta SK, Wengerter KR (Montefiore Med Ctr/Albert Einstein College of Medicine, New York; Mt Sinai Med Ctr, New York)
J Vasc Surg 15:102–112, 1992   10–4

Background.—Previous experience with unsuspected, preexisting saphenous vein disease prompted a study of 513 infrainguinal arterial bypasses performed with the use of saphenous veins in 1984–1990. Sixty-three diseased saphenous veins were identified. Fifty veins or vein segments with minimal or unsuspected disease were used for the bypasses.

Results.—The lesions found in the 63 cases (12%) included thick-walled veins, varicose veins, and postphlebitic sclerotic veins with occlusion or recanalization. Severe changes precluded the use of the vein in 13 cases. Ten of the 50 veins that were used failed at an early stage. At 30 months, the cumulative primary patency rate for these 50 cases was only 32% (Fig 10-1). A review of 21 preoperative duplex ultrasound studies revealed vein abnormalities in 62% of the cases. The histologic findings

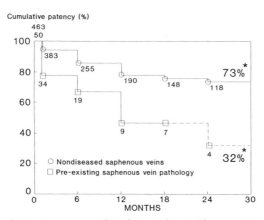

Fig 10–1.—Cumulative primary patency for infrainguinal arterial bypasses with autogenous saphenous vein. Vein grafts with preexisting venous disease had significantly decreased patency at all time intervals (* *P* ≤ .001). (Courtesy of Panetta TF, Marin ML, Veith FJ, et al: *J Vasc Surg* 15:102–112, 1992.)

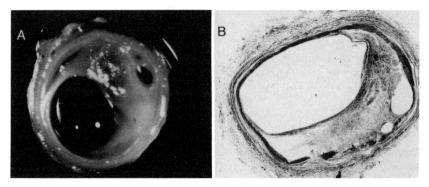

Fig 10–2.—Recanalized saphenous vein segment. **A,** this vein would irrigate normally and allow passage of the catherer, thereby allowing recanalized disease to go undetected, although the vein is markedly thickened. **B,** this section clearly demonstrates the thick wall of the vein composed of abundant connective tissue surrounding several recanalized channels. Trichrome stain; original magnification, ×10.) (Courtesy of Panetta TF, Marin ML, Veith FJ, et al: *J Vasc Surg* 15:102–112, 1992.)

in diseased veins included intimal and medial thickening, calcification of the vein wall, and luminal recanalization (Fig 10–2).

Conclusion.—Unsuspected saphenous vein disease is not infrequent and can cause early or late graft failure. Some cases are detectable by duplex ultrasonography. A thick-walled, calcified, or recanalized vein should not be used if an alternative is available.

▶ Diseased veins unquestionably form very poor bypass conduits. We are readily able to detect a thick-wall, nondistensible segment of vein during hydrostatic dilatation of a reversed vein, which we perform with chilled, autologous heparinized blood. We are in total agreement with the authors that recanalized or thick-walled sclerotic veins give such poor results that they should not be used. These veins should be discarded, and alternate autogenous veins should be used for bypass. I do not identify any need for angioscopy to assist in vein evaluation.—J.M. Porter, M.D.

Is Long Vein Bypass From Groin to Ankle a Durable Procedure? An Analysis of a Ten-Year Experience
Shah DM, Darling RC III, Chang BB, Kaufman JL, Fitzgerald KM, Leather RP (Albany Med College, Albany, NY)
J Vasc Surg 15:402–408, 1992   10–5

Background.—Long vein bypasses from the femoral artery to the ankle level may be done with good initial results, despite limited outflow; however, the long-term performance of these bypasses remains uncertain.

Methods.—Two hundred seventy patients who had single, greater saphenous vein in situ bypass procedures to the ankle level were studied. Most of the patients had diabetes. Half the bypasses originated from the proximal superficial femoral artery, and most of the rest originated from the common or deep femoral artery. The bypasses ended in the distal peroneal, distal posterior tibial, distal anterior tibial, or dorsal pedal artery. The mean patient age was 69 years.

Results.—The perioperative mortality rate was 3.7% in this series. The life-table cumulative primary patency rate was 61% at 5 years, and the secondary patency rate was 73%. The cumulative limb salvage rate at 5 years was 89%. Patency rates did not differ substantially with the particular inflow artery or the outflow tract.

Conclusion.—Long in situ vein bypass grafts may be done with the same expectation of success and durability as with a more proximal infrainguinal bypass procedure. The concept of bypassing all occlusive disease to a distal open artery is a sound one.

▶ This experienced group presents convincing evidence that a well-performed long vein bypass from groin to ankle is a very durable procedure, with a primary patency of 61% at 5 years and a secondary patency of 73%. As a matter of convenience, we continue to use as short a vein graft as possible, and in many patients (such as those described herein), we electively originate our vein graft from the superficial femoral artery to shorten its length.—J.M. Porter, M.D.

Popliteal-to-Distal Bypass for Limb-Threatening Ischemia
Marks J, King TA, Baele H, Rubin J, Marmen C (Mt Sinai Med Ctr and Case Western Reserve Univ, Cleveland)
J Vasc Surg 15:755–760, 1992   10–6

Background.—It may be feasible to use the popliteal artery for inflow in some patients who require lower limb revascularization, thereby minimizing the extent of dissection and the length of vein needed for bypass.

Patients.—Twenty-nine patients had 32 popliteal-to-distal bypass procedures in 1986–1990. The mean patient age was 68 years; two thirds were diabetics. Most patients had more than 1 indication for surgery, and 29% had gangrene.

Surgery.—Arterial bypass using the popliteal artery for the proximal anastomosis was performed with in situ saphenous vein in 50% of the cases; reversed saphenous vein in 41%; and orthograde autologous vein in 9%. Distal anastomoses were to the posterior or anterior tibial arteries, the peroneal artery, or the dorsal pedal artery.

Results.—The perioperative mortality was 7%. Life-table analysis showed cumulative graft patency rates of 97% at 1 year, 97% at 2 years, and 63.5% at 4 years (table). Four patients required below-knee amputation, 2 because of persistent pedal sepsis in the perioperative period, and 2 because of graft failure and subsequent ischemia late in the follow-up period.

Cumulative Graft Patency and Limb Salvage

Time period	Grafts at risk	Thrombosed grafts	Cumulative graft patency	Limbs at risk	Limbs amputated	Cumulative limb salvage, %	Standard error
0 - 1 mo	32	1	96.8%	32	1	96.8%	0.0308
1 - 3 mo	29	0	96.8%	29	2	90.1%	0.0308
3 - 6 mo	24	0	96.8%	24	0	90.1%	0.0308
6 - 12 mo	21	0	96.8%	21	0	90.1%	0.0308
12 - 24 mo	16	0	96.8%	16	0	90.1%	0.0308
24 - 36 mo	9	1	84.7%	9	1	78.8%	0.0368
36 - 48 mo	6	1	63.5%	6	0	78.8%	0.2030

(Courtesy of Marks J, King TA, Baele H, et al: J Vasc Surg 15:755–760, 1992.)

Conclusion.—Selective use of the popliteal artery for proximal inflow is warranted in patients requiring lower limb reconstruction. Excellent limb salvage and long-term patency rates may be expected.

▶ I believe a leg bypass graft should originate as distally as possible to keep the graft length as short as possible. Of course, one must document an absence of stenosis proximal to the site of graft origin. See also Abstract 10–5.—J.M. Porter, M.D.

The Lesser Saphenous Vein: An Underappreciated Source of Autogenous Vein
Chang BB, Paty PSK, Shah DM, Leather RP (Albany Med College, Albany, NY)
J Vasc Surg 15:152–157, 1992   10–7

Background.—An intact ipsilateral greater saphenous vein may not be available for vascular reconstruction. Use of the lesser saphenous vein (LSV) as an alternative has received little attention.

Methods.—Duplex scanning was carried out in 311 instances to map the LSV, and correlation with the actual surgical anatomy was excellent. Harvest of the LSV was facilitated by using a medial subfascial approach (Fig 10–3), which does not require special positioning of the extremity.

Results.—Ninety-one LSVs were used for arterial bypass; 66 were repeat cases. In 40 cases, the LSV served as the entire conduit. In 18 of those 40 cases, the LSV was used in the reversed position for coronary artery bypass. In 33 cases, the LSV was spliced to another vein to complete a bypass procedure. The overall patency was 77% at 2 years (table).

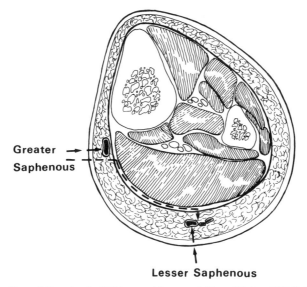

Fig 10–3.—Plane of dissection for LSV harvest. (Courtesy of Chang BB, Paty PSK, Shah DM, et al: *J Vasc Surg* 15:152–157, 1992.)

Primary Bypass Patency Rates With Lesser Saphenous Vein

Interval	No. at risk	Occlusions	Interval patency	Cumulative patency
1 mo	69	6	0.897	0.897
3 mo	41	2	0.943	0.846
6 mo	27	2	0.911	0.771
1 yr	16	0	1.000	0.771
2 yr	12	0	1.000	0.771
3 yr	8	2	0.714	0.551

(Courtesy of Chang BB, Paty PSK, Shah DM, et al: *J Vasc Surg* 15:152–157, 1992.)

Conclusion.—The high rate of use of the LSV (90% in this study) and its ease of harvesting make this vessel a useful alternative to the greater saphenous vein for arterial bypass procedures.

▶ I have found the LSV to be only occasionally useful as a bypass conduit. This is a vein in which preoperative duplex scanning is especially helpful for planning. I am quite impressed with the authors' harvest technique, which does not require either placing the patient prone or making a separate incision; however, I am a bit concerned by the extensive undermining required.—J.M. Porter, M.D.

Reversed Vein Graft Stenosis: Early Diagnosis and Management
Berkowitz HD, Fox AD, Deaton DH (Hosp of Univ of Pennsylvania, Philadelphia)
J Vasc Surg 15:130–142, 1992   10–8

Background.—As many as 1 in 5 reversed vein grafts may become stenotic, increasing the risk of ultimate graft occlusion. Close surveillance of infrainguinal bypass grafts is necessary to detect vein graft stenosis. It

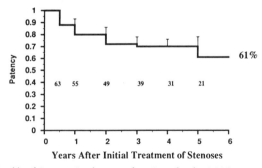

Fig 10–4.—Life table of 5-year assisted patency for vein grafts after initial treatment of graft stenosis. (Courtesy of Berkowitz HD, Fox AD, Deaton DH: *J Vasc Surg* 15:130–142, 1992.)

remains unclear whether balloon angioplasty is an adequate alternative to surgical treatment.

Methods.—The management of 72 stenotic reversed femoropopliteal and femorotibial vein grafts was reviewed. These grafts represented 12% of all bypass grafts at this institution, but prosthetic in-situ, and occluded grafts were excluded. Stenosis was most often found within 4 cm of the proximal anastomosis.

Results.—Fifty-eight of the 72 lesions (81%) were initially treated by balloon angioplasty, and 31% recurred. The recurrence rate in 14 grafts treated by vein patch angioplasty or by short jump grafts was 29%. The 5-year life-table primary patency rate after treatment for stenosis was 61% (Fig 10–4). Lesions in the proximal part of the graft, the proximal anastomosis, or the distal graft had the best outcome.

Recommendations.—Balloon angioplasty is preferred as the primary measure for vein graft stenoses, except those in the midgraft region or distal anastomosis. Stenosis that recurs after angioplasty should be repaired surgically.

▶ I continue to believe that balloon angioplasty makes no sense in the treatment of vein graft stenosis. These stenotic segments are collagenous, and collagen has no ability to stretch. If the balloon dilatation is sufficiently severe, collagen will rupture. I am unable to imagine how ruptured collagen can lead to a permanent increase in the size of vein graft stenosis. We do not recommend the use of balloon angioplasty for vein graft stenosis under any circumstances.—J.M. Porter, M.D.

Aspirin Usage and Its Influence on Femoro-Popliteal Vein Graft Patency

Franks PJ, for the Femoro-Popliteal Bypass Trial (Charing Cross Hosp, London)

Eur J Vasc Surg 6:185–188, 1992   10–9

Background.—Aspirin has been shown to lower rates of cardiovascular events in primary and secondary prevention trials. A sensitive assay for serum level of salicylate was used to monitor aspirin consumption by patients in the multicenter Femoro-popliteal Bypass Trial.

Methods.—Patients scheduled for femoropopliteal vein bypass surgery were randomized to receive either aspirin, 300 mg, and dipyridamole, 150 mg, twice daily, or placebo tablets. The serum level of salicylate was analyzed in 145 patients with a mean age of 66 years who had patent grafts at 6 months.

Results.—More than one fourth of the patients randomized to receive placebo had significant serum levels of salicylate. At the same time, one fourth of those who were randomized to active treatment and were considered to be good compliers, had no evidence of salicylate in their sera.

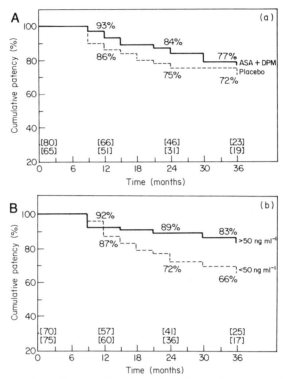

Fig 10–5.—Cumulative graft patency in patients who underwent femoropopliteal vein bypass. **A,** analyzed by "intention to treat": risk in the placebo group was higher but failed to achieve statistical significance (RR, 1.33; 95% CI, .64–2.78; P = .438). **B,** analyzed by serum concentration of salicylate: difference in risk achieved statistical significance (RR, 2.38; 95% CI, 1.08–5.26; P = .024). (Courtesy of Franks PJ, for the Femoro-Popliteal Bypass Trial: *Eur J Vasc Surg* 6:185–188, 1992.)

Patients with serum levels of salicylate that exceeded 50 ng/mL had a significantly higher graft patency rate at 3 years than those without detectable saliclyate (Fig 10–5). The difference persisted after adjusting for a number of possible risk factors, including age, diabetic status, and indication for surgery.

Conclusion.—These findings support the use of aspirin and dipyridamole in patients who have femoropopliteal vein bypass surgery.

▶ These authors bring up the important point that patients who are randomized to a drug cannot be presumed to be actually taking the drug, unless you have some independent confirmation. We presently recommend that our patients with leg bypass take aspirin daily, although I recognize that it probably has no effect on fibrointimal hyperplasia or graft patency. Several studies have indicated that it diminishes the likelihood of myocardial infarction, and this, by itself, appears to be a more-than-adequate reason for drug use. This report suggests that faithful aspirin use may enhance femoropopliteal bypass patency, but this method of data presentation is unorthodox at best.—J.M. Porter, M.D.

Peripheral Vascular Bypass in Juvenile-Onset Diabetes Mellitus: Are Aggressive Revascularization Attempts Justified?
Kwolek CJ, Pomposelli FB, Tannenbaum GA, Brophy CM, Gibbons GW, Campbell DR, Freeman DV, Miller A, LoGerfo FW (Harvard Med School, Boston)
J Vasc Surg 15:394–401, 1992   10–10

Objective.—Individuals with diabetes mellitus account for as many as two thirds of patients having lower limb amputation. The results of 67 bypass procedures in 60 patients with juvenile-onset diabetes mellitus were evaluated. The procedures constituted 5.5% of all bypasses done in patients with diabetes during the 6-year review period. The mean age was 44 years.

Surgery.—All but 9% of the operations were done for limb salvage. Most were primary infrainguinal bypasses using saphenous vein. Six procedures were revision surgery procedures, and 4 were inflow procedures.

Results.—Nearly one third of the patients had morbidity, but there were no postoperative deaths. The actuarial patency rate after primary vein graft surgery was 66% at 2 years, and the limb salvage rate was 83.4%. Seventeen primary infrainguinal bypass grafts that were done using saphenous vein failed, leading to 9 major limb amputations. Five of 8 failed grafts were successfully revised.

Conclusion.—Patients with juvenile-onset diabetes mellitus require arterial bypass surgery at a much younger age than other patients; nevertheless, a successful outcome may be anticipated.

▶ Type I diabetics, especially cigarette smokers, are among the most difficult patients with leg ischemia that we encounter. Although the results obtained by this excellent group are admirable, they are considerably inferior to those obtained by the same group in other patients. It is important for vascular surgeons to recognize the substantial difficulties presented by these patients, and for both the patients and surgeon to have realistic expectations from surgery.—J.M. Porter, M.D.

Intravenous Prostacyclin (PIG₂) Infusion to 108 Patients With Ischaemic Peripheral Vascular Disease: Phase II–Open Study
Virgolini I, Fitscha P, Weiss K, Linet OI, O'Grady J, Sinzinger H (Wilhelm-Auerswald Atherosclerosis Research Group, Vienna; Policlinic, Vienna; Upjohn Co, Kalamazoo, Mich; Univ of Vienna)
Prostaglandins 42:9–14, 1991   10–11

Introduction.—In a double-blind trial, 108 patients with ischemic peripheral vascular disease received either a 5-day infusion of intravenous prostacyclin (PGI_2), no more than 6 ng/kg/min for 8 hours daily, or placebo. Nonresponders and patients treated with placebo then entered a second open trial of the same regimen of PGI_2.

Patients and Methods.—The second infusion was given to 45 patients from the original placebo group and 44 patients from the original treatment group. The patients underwent treadmill testing to determine absolute and relative claudication times.

Results.—In the double-blind trial, 44% of patients receiving the PGI_2 infusion and 15% of the placebo-treated patients were positive responders at 1 month, as scored by an increase in absolute and relative walking times. One month after the second infusion, 52% of the initially placebo-treated patients and 31% of the initially PGI_2-treated patients were positive responders.

Conclusion.—Before the first trial, both groups of patients had similar absolute and relative claudication times. Improvement in walking times was generally sustained for the first 2 months after PGI_2 infusion. This improvement continued among patients from the group originally treated by placebo, but it was not maintained in the nonresponders from the double-blind trial. The latter patients probably represent a group that is relatively nonresponsive to PGI_2.

▶ Are the prostaglandins going to be of significant benefit in the treatment of patients with arterial occlusive disease? Although short-term infusions may be of some benefit in the treatment of selected patients with acute or subacute limb ischemia not amenable to other therapy, I can see no long-term benefits from the prostaglandins.—J.M. Porter, M.D.

Superiority of L-Propionylcarnitine vs L-Carnitine in Improving Walking Capacity in Patients With Peripheral Vascular Disease: An Acute, Intravenous, Double-Blind, Cross-Over Study
Brevetti G, Perna S, Sabbà C, Rossini A, di Uccio VS, Berardi E, Godi L (Univ of Naples, Naples, Italy; Univ of Bari, Italy)
Eur Heart J 13:251–255, 1992   10–12

Background.—Carnitine is a quaternary amine that is necessary for mitochondrial oxidation of long-chain fatty acids and improves stress tolerance of the heart in patients with coronary disease by making needed substrates more available. One of the most potent of the carnitine analogues is L-propionylcarnitine.

Methods.—The effects of L-propionylcarnitine on walking ability were examined in 33 men with peripheral vascular disease and intermittent claudication. A preliminary study showed that a dose of 600 mg, given intravenously, increased initial claudication distance and maximum walk-

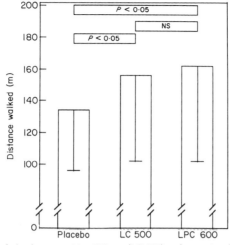

Fig 10–6.—Effect of placebo, L-carnitine 500 mg (LC 500) and L-propionylcarnitine 600 mg (LPC 600) on the initial claudication distance. (Courtesy of Brevetti G, Perna S, Sabbà C, et al: *Eur Heart J* 13:251–255, 1992.)

ing distance, whereas a 300-mg dose was ineffective. The effective dose was then compared with an equimolar dose of L-carnitine (500 mg), using a double-dummy cross-over design.

Results.—Both active treatments improved walking capacity, but L-propionylcarnitine was most effective in enhancing maximum walking distance (Fig 10–6). Neither of the drugs influenced blood velocity or the blood flow rate in the ischemic leg on duplex ultrasonography.

Conclusion.—Administration of L-propionylcarnitine improves walking capacity in patients with peripheral vascular disease, presumably through a metabolic mechanism that increases the energy yield in ischemic muscle.

▶ See also the comment after Abstract 1–9. This study indicates that L-propionylcarnitine clearly improves walking distance in patients with peripheral vascular disease, and that it appears to be more effective than L-carnitine. I continue to believe that carnitine has the greatest promise of any drug currently being evaluated as being effective in the treatment of intermittent claudication. Large-scale, double-blind trials are currently being designed and will soon be implemented in America. The results of these trials are eagerly awaited.—J.M. Porter, M.D.

β-Adrenergic Blocker Therapy Does Not Worsen Intermittent Claudication in Subjects With Peripheral Arterial Disease: A Meta-Analysis of Randomized Controlled Trials

Radack K, Deck C (Univ of Cincinnati)
Arch Intern Med 151:1769–1776, 1991   10–13

Background.—Beta-blockers have been considered relatively contraindicated in peripheral arterial disease, because there is an impression that they may make intermittent claudication worse.

Methods.—A meta-analysis of randomized controlled trials found in the English-language literature was undertaken to determine whether β-blockers exacerbate claudication. Six of the 11 eligible studies included a total of 11 individual controlled treatment comparisons of pain-free exercise capacity.

Results.—Patients taking β-blockers did not have a substantial decrement in walking ability. Only 1 study found that certain β-blockers are associated with worsening of claudication.

Conclusion.—Beta-blockers do not lessen walking capacity in patients with mild-to-moderate peripheral arterial disease, in contrast to uncontrolled studies and clinical impressions. This conclusion does not apply to patients with severe disease, other vasospastic disorders, or Raynaud's phenomenon.

▶ Many vascular surgeons have adopted, as a matter of faith, the proposition that β-adrenergic blocker therapy should not be given to patients with claudication because of a significant likelihood of symptomatic worsening. This important meta-analysis did not confirm this. On critical analysis, β-blockers do not appear to diminish walking capacity in claudicants and can be used safely in these patients.—J.M. Porter, M.D.

Randomized Placebo-Controlled, Double-Blind Trial of Ketanserin in Treatment of Intermittent Claudication

Walden R, Bass A, Rabi I, Adar R (Sheba Med Ctr, Tel Hashomer, Israel; Tel Aviv Univ, Israel)
J Cardiovasc Surg 32:737–740, 1991   10–14

Background.—Ketanserin is a selective antagonist of serotonin (5-HT) at 5-HT2 receptors, which reportedly can improve walking distance and peripheral hemodynamics in patients with intermittent claudication, although the results of trials have been mixed. A double-blind controlled study in 40 patients covered 12 months of treatment.

Methods.—The 35 evaluable patients had typical claudication after walking less than 200 meters, secondary to atherosclerotic disease. Symptoms had been present for 6 months or longer, and the ankle-brachial pressure index (ABPI) in the most severely affected leg was below

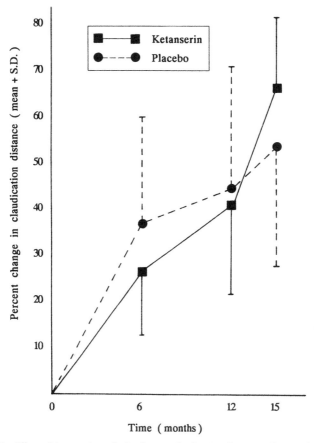

Fig 10–7.—Effect of ketanserin and placebo on claudication distance. Changes from baseline. (Courtesy of Walden R, Bass A, Rabi I, et al: *J Cardiovasc Surg* 32:737-740, 1991.)

.75. Treated patients received ketanserin in an initial dose of 20 mg 3 times daily, which was increased after 1 month to 40 mg of ketanserin 3 times daily.

Results.—Claudication distance improved 42% to 44% after a year of observation, and it improved further to as much as 67% during a 3-month run-out period on placebo. The ketanserin-treated and placebo groups responded similarly (Fig 10-7). There were no significant changes in ABPI or pulse volume recordings during the study period, and there were no significant differences between the 2 groups.

Conclusion.—Ketanserin is not an effective treatment for intermittent claudication of atherosclerotic origin.

▶ Ketanserin has been critically examined for its potential benefit in reducing the incidence of cardiovascular death, improving the symptoms of Raynaud's syndrome, and improving lower extremity claudication. To date, the clinical results have not been encouraging.—J.M. Porter, M.D.

Outcome of Intraarterial Urokinase for Acute Vascular Occlusion
Parent FN III Piotrowski JJ, Bernhard VM, Pond GD, Pabst TS III, Bull DA, Hunter GC, McIntyre KE (Univ of Arizona, Tucson)
J Cardiovasc Surg 32:680–690, 1991   10–15

Objective.—Percutaneous intra-arterial catheter-directed low-dose fibrinolytic therapy is currently recommended for the treatment of thrombotic or embolic occlusion in peripheral arteries and bypass grafts. However, its success is commonly influenced by adjunctive procedures that make it difficult to assess the therapy's true value. The immediate efficacy and long-term results of intra-arterial urokinase (IAUK) and the durability of this technique alone or in combination with adjunctive therapies were determined.

Patients.—During a 3-year period, 33 patients with a mean age of 60.4 years received local infusion of IAUK on 40 occasions for the treatment of acute lower extremity ischemia caused by a thrombotic or embolic event involving a native artery or bypass graft. All patients underwent arteriography before infusion of IAUK. Fibrinolysis was considered successful when the intravascular defect resulting from thrombus was completely eliminated on follow-up arteriography.

Results.—Lysis was successful in 39 of the 40 cases. Occlusive thrombus was cleared in 12 of 13 patients with native artery occlusion, 8 of 9 patients with autologous vein graft occlusion, and in all 18 patients with synthetic graft occlusion. The primary cumulative patency after successful IAUK was 100% for native arteries, 47% for synthetic grafts at 12 months, and 23% for autologous vein grafts at 9 months. The rethrombosis rate was 67% for autologous vein grafts and 63% for prosthetic grafts, but it was 0% for native arteries. Thus, IAUK was most effective in the treatment of occlusion in the native artery, whereas it was significantly less effective for occlusion in autologous vein or synthetic grafts because of the high incidence of reocclusion. Autogenous vein grafts had the lowest immediate success rate and the shortest patency, regardless of adjunctive therapy to relieve the underlying obstruction.

Conclusion.—Intra-arterial urokinase provides the best immediate results and the best long-term patency in the treatment of native artery occlusion. Thrombosed infrainguinal autologous vein grafts and synthetic grafts have a high immediate success rate, but reocclusion is common.

▶ What is the optimal role of intra-arterial lytic therapy for acute vascular occlusion? This paper concludes that such therapy is most effective for native artery occlusion and is much less effective for thrombosed infrainguinal grafts. I concur. Abundant data indicate that, although intra-arterial lytic therapy may successfully reopen infrainguinal bypass grafts, the 1-year patency rates are extraordinarily disappointing, no matter what type of therapy is undertaken once initial thrombolytic opening occurs. In our practice, we do not recommend the use of intra-arterial thrombolytic therapy in graft occlusion patients at all (1, 2).—J.M. Porter, M.D.

References

1. Graor RA, et al: *J Vasc Surg* 7:347, 1988.
2. Belkin M, et al: *J Vasc Surg* 11:289, 1990.

Risk Factors for Early Lower Limb Loss After Embolectomy for Acute Arterial Occlusion: A Population-Based Case-Control Study
Ljungman C, Adami H-O, Bergqvist D, Sparen P, Bergström R (Univ Hosp, Uppsala, Sweden; Malmö Gen Hosp, Sweden; Uppsala Univ, Sweden)
Br J Surg 78:1482–1485, 1991   10–16

Background.—Amputation rates as high as 40% have been reported after conventional embolectomy for acute arterial occlusion. Postoperative mortality has been 15% to 48%.

Methods.—A total of 165 patients (among 1,189 undergoing embolectomy) had major amputation within 30 days of the procedure. One hundred sixty-five age- and sex-matched subjects served as controls.

Results.—The risk of amputation was increased in patients with 2 or more myocardial infarctions, chronic ischemia, symptoms for 25 hours or longer (compared with those having symptoms for 6 hours or less), or postoperative heart failure. Patients with acute infarction and those who were given warfarin after operation had a reduced risk of amputation. Multivariate analysis confirmed that chronic ischemia and the duration of symptoms had independent prognostic value, and that postoperative anticoagulation was beneficial.

Conclusion.—Clinical factors can predict the risk of early amputation after arterial embolectomy or thrombectomy. The anatomical site of the clot is not a major prognostic factor.

▶ This is another retrospective study regurgitated by the remarkable computerized patient registry maintained in Sweden. Studies such as this, although they are of modest interest, appear to provide no concrete data upon which physicians can rely to make difficult decisions concerning treatment choices for specific patients. In my opinion, studies such as this one are not very helpful.—J.M. Porter, M.D.

Surgical Management of Severe Acute Lower Extremity Ischemia
Yeager RA, Moneta GL, Taylor LM Jr, Hamre DW, McConnell DB, Porter JM
(Oregon Health Sciences Univ, Portland)
J Vasc Surg 15:385–393, 1992   10–17

Introduction.—At the Oregon Health Sciences University in Portland, patients with acute limb ischemia have undergone prompt amputation of a nonviable extremity, whereas those with a threatened limb are heparinized and undergo angiography and operative reconstruction.

Methods.—Management was evaluated in 74 patients seen in 1986–1990 with severe, acute lower extremity ischemia. Arterial thrombosis was responsible in 68 patients and embolism was responsible in 6. All patients had absent pedal Doppler signals and were treated within 2 weeks of the onset of ischemic symptoms. If the extremity was potentially salvageable, surgery was done on an emergency or urgent basis. Thrombosed infrainguinal grafts did not undergo thrombectomy but, instead, were redone with a new conduit.

Results.—Limb viability was severely threatened in more than 80% of the patients, and 18% of the patients had major irreversible ischemic limb changes at the time of presentation. Seven patients underwent primary amputation (table). Most of the patients were initially anticoagulated with heparin. The primary patency rate at 3 years was 81% for patients having inflow procedures and 78% for those having outflow procedures. The cumulative limb salvage rate was 68% at 3 years, but patient survival was only 51% at this stage. No deaths were directly related to complications of limb reperfusion.

Surgical Management of 74 Patients With Severe Acute
Lower Limb Ischemia

Procedure	Patients
Amputation without revascularization	7
Inflow reconstructions (9 with amputation)	42
Femorofemoral bypass (16,38%)	
Axillofemoral bypass (13,31%)	
Common femoral repair/profundaplasty (10,24%)	
Aortofemoral bypass (3,7%)	
Outflow reconstructions† (3 with amputation)	20
Femoropopliteal bypass (9,45%)	
Femoroinfrapopliteal bypass (9,45%)	
Superficial femoral endarterectomy (2,10%)	
Simple thrombectomy or embolectomy (3 with amputation)	9

* Four patients underwent combined inflow and outflow procedure.
† Autogenous vein was used in all but 1 case.
(Courtesy of Yeager RA, Moneta GL, Taylor LM Jr, et al: *J Vasc Surg* 15:385–393, 1992.)

Conclusion.—Early amputation or angiography with prompt operative revascularization, when an extremity is threatened but viable, maximizes limb salvage while minimizing morbidity. No thrombolytics were used in these patients.

▶ These authors take the novel position that patients seen with acute lower extremity ischemia are best treated by heparinization and operative reconstruction, not intra-arterial thrombolytic therapy. Life-table primary patency at 36 months was 81% for inflow procedures and 78% for outflow procedures, with limb salvage of 70% at 1 month. Almost all limbs lost were nonviable on presentation. These interesting results will clearly be useful for comparison with comparable groups of patients treated with thrombolysis or endovascular methods. See also the commentary after Abstract 10–15. —J.M. Porter, M.D.

The Distribution of Atherosclerosis in the Lower Limbs
Aston NO, Thomas ML, Burnand KG (St Thomas' Hosp, London)
Eur J Vasc Surg 6:73–77, 1992   10–18

Introduction.—The distribution of occlusive vascular lesions in the lower extremity was examined arteriographically in 67 consecutive nondiabetic patients being considered for arterial reconstruction. Eighteen of 67 patients had symptoms of critical ischemia, the remainder having claudication.

Methods.—Aortograms were reviewed and scored by a vascular radiologist and 2 vascular surgeons.

Results.—Generalized disease, with no critical stenoses or occlusions above the knee but occlusions in the infrapopliteal vessels, was present in 31% of the extremities. Another 11% had aortoiliac disease; 42% had superficial femoral involvement; and 16% had disease in multiple segments. At least 1 calf vessel was occluded in half the extremities, most often the anterior tibial artery. Only one fourth of the extremities had 2 patent ankle arteries, and only 16% had a complete pedal arch. Half the limbs with symptoms of critical ischemia and claudication had disease in the superficial femoral artery. Occlusions were present in 81% of asymptomatic extremities (table).

Conclusion.—Atherosclerosis, rather than a disease mainly limited to large- and medium-sized arteries, is a generalized process that involves small arteries at an early stage. If there is proximal occlusion, the extent of disease in the small arteries of the leg and foot determines the severity of ischemic symptoms.

▶ These authors found that nondiabetic patients in the seventh decade of life who are undergoing arteriography for leg ischemic symptoms show an abundance of stenosis and occlusion in the small vessels of the calf and foot.

Patency Related to Symptoms

Anatomical level	Percentage of total in group			χ^2 $(df = 2)$	p
	Critical ischaemia	Claudication	No symptoms		
Aortic occlusion	5	4	2	0.58	>0.5
Aortic occlusion or >50% stenosis	11	6	9	0.70	>0.5
Iliac occlusion or >50% occlusion	28	32	9	8.84	<0.02*
Profunda occlusion	17	14	11	0.54	>0.5
Superficial femoral occlusion	72	58	32	11.43	<0.01*
Popliteal occlusion	50	22	6	15.61	<0.001*

*Statistically significant.
(Courtesy of Aston NO, Thomas ML, Burnard KG: *Eur J Vasc Surg* 6:73–77, 1992.)

Significant proximal disease did not appear to protect the distal vessel. I suspect these authors are correct when they hypothesize that, in the past, the failure to appreciate the extent of tibial disease in nondiabetic ischemic limbs was related to techniques of arteriography, and not to any particular difference in disease distribution compared with the present time.—J.M. Porter, M.D.

The Natural History of Superficial Femoral Artery Stenoses
Walsh DB, Gilbertson JJ, Zwolak RM, Besso S, Edelman GC, Schneider JR, Cronenwett JL (Dartmouth-Hitchcock Med Ctr, Hanover, NH)
J Vasc Surg 14:299–304, 1991   10–19

Background.—The availability of endovascular treatment for atherosclerotic disease of the superficial femoral artery (SFA) makes it important to acquire knowledge of the natural course of SFA stenosis.

Methods.—The progression of SFA stenoses was monitored in 45 affected lower extremities of 38 patients who had symptomatic atherosclerotic disease in the other leg or in the abdomen. Both arteriography and duplex scanning were used. The mean follow-up interval was slightly more than 3 years.

Results.—Only 28% of the SFA stenoses had progressed at follow-up. Of these vessels, 7 (17% of the total) had become occluded. The patients who reported progressive symptoms were more likely to have worsening of SFA stenosis, as were those patients whose disease in the opposite limb led to occlusion. Smoking history also predicted progression of the disease. In the patients whose stenoses progressed to occlusion, the progression occurred at an average rate of 12% per year.

Conclusion.—Duplex scanning may be used to determine the severity of SFA atherosclerosis. Management can be adequately planned by assuming a maximum rate of progression of 30% per year.

▶ After 3 years' follow-up, almost one fourth of the SFA stenoses progressed, becoming either more stenotic or occluded. Superficial femoral artery stenosis clearly does not warrant treatment in and of itself, but only for associated symptoms. It is inappropriate to direct surgical or endovascular therapy at SFA stenoses in the absence of a vigorous trial of nonoperative treatment of claudication.—J.M. Porter, M.D.

Natural History of Claudicants With Critical Hemodynamic Indices
Fowl RJ, Gewirtz RJ, Love MC, Kempczinski RF (Univ of Cincinnati)
Ann Vasc Surg 6:31–33, 1992   10–20

Background.—Earlier studies lacking hemodynamic data suggested that intermittent claudication of the lower extremity is a benign disorder.

In more recent studies, the prognosis was much worse when ankle/brachial indices were low.

Methods.—An examination of records of nearly 1,500 patients having arterial studies in the lower extremity yielded 23 patients in whom 25 extremities had an ankle/brachial index of .35 or less, an ankle or transmetatarsal pulse volume of 3 mm or less in amplitude, and no history of ischemic rest pain or gangrene. The patients were followed up for a mean of 45.2 months.

Results.—Thirteen of the 25 extremities did not have limb-threatening symptoms, and claudication improved in 3 instances. The other 12 extremities had rest pain, ischemic ulceration or, in 3 extremities, gangrene. Eight of these limbs underwent revascularization, and only 1 ultimately required major amputation. One patient had primary above-knee amputation for extensive gangrene.

Conclusion.—All patients with intermittent claudication and critical ischemia require close follow-up, because perhaps half will have limb-threatening ischemia necessitating surgical treatment. Early surgery may be considered for patients who are considered unlikely to comply with regular follow-up.

▶ This is another important natural history study of claudication, this time in patients with critical hemodynamic indices. Of considerable interest is the observation that, during a mean follow-up of 45 months, half the patients with an initial ankle/brachial index equal to or less than .35 stabilized or improved, whereas half of these patients regressed. Did you know that almost all of the natural history information on claudication obtained before 1980 was based on questionnaires without vascular lab or patient examinations? A widely held belief that 80% to 90% of claudicants stabilize or improve with time and that only 10% to 20% deteriorate is erroneous. Detailed vascular laboratory studies reveal that the behavior of claudication is significantly related to the ankle/brachial index at the time of the initial evaluation. At least 50% of the patients with a claudication ankle/brachial index less than .5 will eventually require interventional therapy (1).—J.M. Porter, M.D.

Reference

1. Cronenwett JL, et al: *Arch Surg* 119:430, 1984.

Isolated Thigh Claudication as a Result of Fibromuscular Dysplasia of the Deep Femoral Artery
Schneider PA, LaBerge JM, Cunningham CG, Ehrenfeld WK (Univ of California, San Francisco)
J Vasc Surg 15:657–660, 1992   10–21

Background.—Isolated claudication in the thigh resulting from fibromuscular dysplasia of the deep femoral artery has not been described. One patient had dysplastic disease of the carotid arteries and also had progressive claudication develop in 1 thigh, despite normal femoral pulses. A common femoral-to-distal deep femoral artery bypass was successful.

Case Report.—Woman, 69, had developed one-block claudication in her left thigh over the 6 months previous to hospitalization. There were no risk factors for atherosclerotic disease, but left hemispheric transient ischemic attacks had appeared 2 months earlier and angiography had shown fibromuscular dysplasia. The left carotid was dilated operatively. A left femoral bruit developed after brief walking, and angiography demonstrated occlusion of the deep femoral artery befond the lateral circumflex origin. Fibromuscular dysplasia was confirmed at exploration, and a 5-mm knitted Dacron flanged graft was placed from the common femoral artery to the distal deep femoral artery. Thigh claudication resolved postoperatively; walking was unlimited after several months. Fibromuscular dysplasia was confirmed histologically.

▶ Thigh and/or buttock claudication is infrequently considered in patients who have normal extremity pulses. In a few patients, some combination of hypogastric and/or profunda femoris disease may cause this symptom. Imaging studies of these vessels is appropriate in selected patients.—J.M. Porter, M.D.

Lymphoscintigraphic Assessment of Leg Oedema Following Arterial Reconstruction Using a Load Produced by Standing
Suga K, Uchisako H, Nakanishi T, Utsumi H, Yamada N, Oohara M, Esato K (Yamaguchi Univ, Yamaguchi, Japan)
Nucl Med Commun 12:907–917, 1991   10–22

Objective.—A lymphoscintigraphic method was developed to assess lymphatic function in the lower extremities in patients in whom lymphedema developed after arterial reconstructive surgery. Eleven patients (mean age, 70.5 years), had undergone arterial reconstructive surgery on 14 legs in the past 3 years.

Methods.—Lymphoscintigraphy is performed in the supine subject after the intradermal injection of 111 MBq of ^{99m}Tc-human serum albumin. A 26.5-gauge needle is used to inject nuclide into the first interdigital space of the foot. After gamma camera recording, the subject stands up slowly over 1–2 minutes, moving the legs as little as possible; imaging is repeated for 15 minutes.

Results.—Time-activity curves normally exhibit a large spiking wave and a rapid stepwise increase in tracer activity on standing (Fig 10–8). The large spiking wave was inconsistently seen in postoperative studies, and a stepwise increase in activity was seen in only 1 instance. A repre-

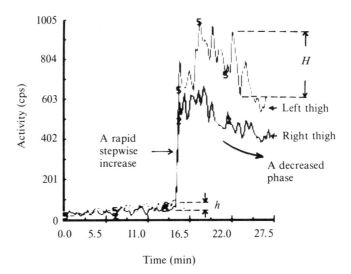

Fig 10–8.—Typical time-activity curve obtained in a normal subject after a load produced by standing from the supine position. The time-activity curves manifest 3 prominent changes: the appearance of a large spiking wave, a rapid stepwise increase of tracer activity immediately after standing, and a phase of decreasing tracer activity. A large spiking wave is defined as a wave whose amplitude (H) is more than threefold that of the wave (h) observed before standing. (Courtesy of Suga K, Uchisako H, Nakanishi T, et al: *Nucl Med Commun* 12:907–917, 1991.)

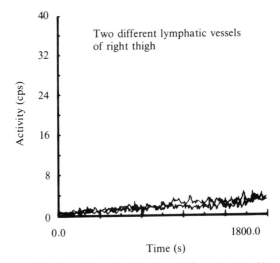

Fig 10–9.—Patient with edema of the right thigh after right femoral-popliteal bypass surgery. Time-activity curves obtained from the 2 regions of interest in 2 different lymphatic vessels observed in the right thigh. These curves show no change after the load produced by standing and only a gradual increase in activity with time. (Courtesy of Suga K, Uchisako H, Nakanishi T, et al: *Nucl Med Commun* 12:907–917, 1991.)

sentative case is illustrated in Figure 10-9. Studies in 11 extremities showed no significant change in supine venous pressure after operation. Peripheral venous pressure increased by more than 10 cm of H_2O on standing.

Conclusion.—It is suggested that lymphatic disruption is the cause of leg edema in patients having arterial reconstructive surgery. This lymphoscintigraphic technique is a technically simple and noninvasive means of assessing lymphatic function after such surgery.

▶ Small-needle injection contrast lymphangiography must be relegated to the historical archives. If one must obtain documentation of lymphatic function, a currently available test is lymphoscintigraphy. This article is included to familiarize vascular surgeons with the appearance of the lymphoscintigraphy examination. As to the content of the article, it hardly seems necessary. We all know that leg edema after limb arterial reconstruction is caused by lymphatic disruption. In fact, we have known this for 20 years (1).—J.M. Porter, M.D.

Reference

1. Porter JM, et al: *Arch Surg* 105:883, 1972.

The Use of Angioplasty, Bypass Surgery, and Amputation in the Management of Peripheral Vascular Disease
Tunis SR, Bass EB, Steinberg EP (Johns Hopkins Univ, Baltimore)
N Engl J Med 325:556–562, 1991   10–23

Introduction.—Although percutaneous transluminal angioplasty has become a popular alternative to peripheral bypass surgery in selected patients with peripheral vascular disease of the lower extremities, its effect on management of peripheral vascular disease and patient outcome has not been clearly defined. The extent to which angioplasty is used and the impact of this procedure on the surgical management of peripheral vascular disease were determined.

Methods.—Study data were derived from the records of hospital discharges in Maryland between 1979 and 1989. Information was obtained on all angioplasty procedures, peripheral bypass operations, and lower extremity amputations performed for peripheral vascular disease during this period.

Findings.—Between 1979 and 1989, the estimated annual rate of angioplasty for peripheral vascular disease of the lower extremities increased from 1 to 24 per 100,000 Maryland residents. The adjusted annual rate of peripheral bypass surgery increased as well, from 32 to 65 per 100,000. The adjusted annual rate of lower-extremity amputation remained stable, at approximately 30 per 100,000. There was a substantial increase in the number of hospital days and in the total charges associated with revascularization procedures. Charges increased from $14.7 million in 1979 (in 1989 dollars) to $30.5 million in 1989.

Conclusion.—The use of percutaneous transluminal angioplasty instead of peripheral bypass surgery in selected patients with peripheral vascular disease was expected to substantially reduce costs and the need for amputation. In Maryland, however, numbers of surgical procedures have increased, costs have risen, and the amputation rate remains unchanged. These findings may reflect more frequent diagnosis and an expansion of the indications for angioplasty and bypass surgery.

▶ Isn't it amazing that the prestigious *New England Journal of Medicine* is so uninformed about peripheral arterial disease? Percutaneous transluminal angioplasty (PTLA) is used in the treatment of claudication; rarely is it used in the treatment of end stage limb ischemia. No vascular surgeon is surprised by the published observation that, although the use of PTLA and leg bypass procedures increased over a period of time, the amputation rate remained stable. In fact, the editors were so shocked by this finding that they produced an editorial on the topic in the same issue of the *New England Journal of Medicine*. It is obvious that we vascular surgeons have a large educational chore ahead of us.—J.M. Porter, M.D.

Long-Term Evaluation of Composite Sequential Bypass for Limb-Threatening Ischemia
McCarthy WJ, Pearce WH, Flinn WR, McGee GS, Wang R, Yao JST (Northwestern Univ Med School, Chicago; Univ of South Alabama, Mobile)
J Vasc Surg 15:761–770, 1992   10–24

Background.—Patients requiring treatment of severe leg and foot ischemia not infrequently lack adequate autogenous vein for use in bypass surgery. In this instance, composite sequential grafting using vein combined with polytetrafluoroethylene (PTFE) is an option.

Methods.—Sixty-two patients received 67 composite sequential bypasses in a 7-year period, 38 for rest pain; 18 for ulceration; and 11 for gangrene. The mean patient age was 66 years. Half the patients were diabetic. Thirty patients had primary bypass procedures, whereas 21 had had multiple failed bypasses. Forty-four femoral-to-above knee popliteal (Fig 10–10) and 23 below-knee (Fig 10–11) PTFE grafts were placed. An extension of greater saphenous vein (or lesser saphenous vein in 10 instances) was then joined to the posterior tibial, anterior tibial, or peroneal artery. Long-term warfarin therapy was given to 53% of patients, and aspirin was given to 33%.

Results.—There were no perioperative deaths, and 72% of patients were alive after 3 years. Cumulative life-table primary patency rates were 72% at 1 year, 64% at 2 years, and 48% at 3 years (table). The limb sal-

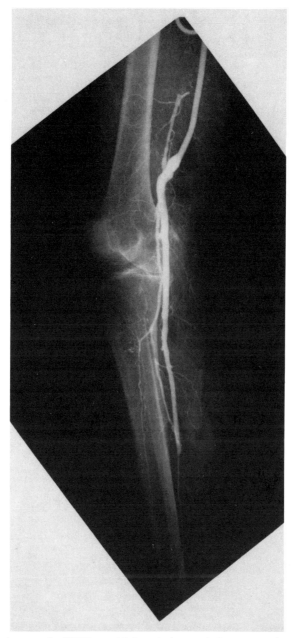

Fig 10–10.—Anastomosis of PTFE material above the knee is ideal. Venous conduit is then used to most proximal tibial vessel providing patency to the foot. (Courtesy of McCarthy WJ, Pearce WH, Flinn WR, et al: *J Vasc Surg* 15:761-770, 1992.)

Life-Table Cumulative Patency

Interval	Bypasses at risk	Failed grafts	No. withdrawn patent because of			Interval patency	Cumulative patency (%)	Standard error (%)
			Duration	Loss to follow-up	Death			
0 - 1	67	1	0	2	0	0.99	100	0
1 - 3	64	1	2	0	1	0.98	99	1.48
3 - 6	60	7	0	2	0	0.88	97	2.13
6 - 9	51	5	2	0	0	0.90	85	4.21
9 - 12	44	3	1	0	0	0.93	77	5.18
12 - 15	40	2	0	0	3	0.95	72	5.75
15 - 18	35	0	0	0	0	1.00	68	6.43
18 - 21	35	0	1	1	1	1.00	68	6.50
21 - 24	32	2	1	0	0	0.94	64	6.78
24 - 27	29	0	1	0	0	1.00	64	7.12
27 - 30	28	1	0	1	2	0.96	61	7.20
30 - 33	24	0	1	0	1	1.00	61	7.78
33 - 36	22	0	2	0	1	1.00	61	8.13
36 - 39	19	4	0	0	0	0.79	48	7.96
39 - 42	15	0	3	0	0	1.00	48	8.96
42 - 45	12	1	1	0	0	0.91	44	9.51
45 - 48	10	1	1	0	0	0.90	40	9.71

(Courtesy of McCarthy WJ, Pearce WH, Flinn WR, et al: J Vasc Surg 15:761–770, 1992.)

vage rate was 84% at 2 years and 70% at 4 years. Five grafts retained a patent venous segment at the time they failed, allowing prompt reconstruction of the proximal portion. Patency at 2 years was better when the popliteal anastomosis was above the knee.

Conclusion.—When femorotibial bypass is necessary to save an extremity, composite sequential PTFE and saphenous vein grafts provide

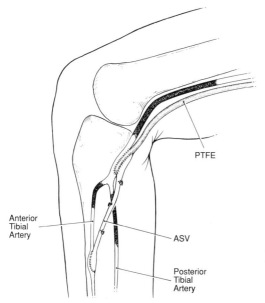

Fig 10–11.—Prosthetic grafting to below-knee popliteal may be necessary because of arterial anatomy or lack of available vein length. Making the middle 2 anastomoses nearly adjacent maximizes flow through entire PTFE graft. (Courtesy of McCarthy WJ, Pearce WH, Flinn WR, et al: *J Vasc Surg* 15:761-770, 1992.)

predictable patency and limb salvage. Patency likely will prove better than when all-prosthetic tibial bypass grafts are used.

▶ The primary patency rate (by life-table methodology) of 72% at 1 year, 64% at 2 years, and 48% at 3 years is remarkable and noteworthy. More than half of these patients were maintained on long-term warfarin anticoagulation. It is interesting to note that these authors used the intermediate anastomosis technique described by DeLaurentis more than 20 years ago.—J.M. Porter, M.D.

European Prospective Randomised Multi-Centre Axillo-Bifemoral Trial
Wittens CHA, van Houtte HJKP, van Urk H (Univ Hosp, Rotterdam, The Netherlands)
Eur J Vasc Surg 6:115–123, 1992   10–25

Background.—The unilateral axillofemoral bypass graft was first used nearly 3 decades ago in patients with unilateral aortoiliac occlusive disease. A newly designed axillobifemoral bypass graft with a flow-splitter

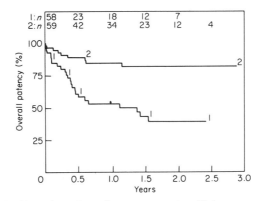

Fig 10–12.—Life-table analysis of overall patency rates. 1 = 90-degree group; 2 = flow-splitter group. (Courtesy of Wittens CHA, van Houtte HJKP, van Urk H: *Eur J Vasc Surg* 6:115–123, 1992.)

at the bifurcation has exhibited superior hemodynamic properties in vitro and in vivo.

Methods.—Patency rates were compared in 59 patients who received an axillobifemoral bypass graft with a flow-splitter and 58 others whose prosthesis had a 90-degree bifurcation. The 2 groups had similar risk factors and similar indications for surgery.

Results.—After a mean follow-up of 1 year, patients given the prosthesis with a flow-splitter had a significantly better patency rate than those whose prostheses had a 90-degree–angled bifurcation (Fig 10–12). The difference remained after controlling for surgical indication, associated risk factors, outflow tract, and anticoagulant therapy. There were no significant differences in graft injection or mortality.

Conclusion.—An axillobifemoral bypass with a flow-splitter is recommended for use in future cases.

▶ This trial involved the use of externally supported gelatin-coated knitted Dacron. After 2 years, the primary patency of the group randomized to an oblique fem-fem configuration was 84%. Although I am not particularly interested in the flow-splitter, I am very interested in the 84% primary patency after 2 years, which is essentially identical to that reported by us and others using externally supported PTFE. The conclusion is inescapable that modern results with axillobifemoral grafting are quite similar (through 3 years) to the results of aortofemoral grafting. This observation should be considered by all vascular surgeons as we encounter an increasnig population of very elderly and infirm patients (1).—J.M. Porter, M.D.

Reference

1. Harris EJ, et al: *J Vasc Surg* 12:416, 1990.

Intermittent Claudication as a Manifestation of Silent Myocardial Ischemia: A Pilot Study

Salmasi A-M, Nicolaides A, Al-Katoubi A, Sonecha TN, Taylor PR, Serenkuma S, Eastcott HHG (St Mary's Hosp, London)
J Vasc Surg 14:76–86, 1991   10–26

Background.—Patients with atherosclerotic disease in a lower extremity have an increased risk of obstructive coronary artery disease. Because peripheral vascular disease often leads to claudication, treadmill testing is not an ideal way of evaluating myocardial ischemia in this setting.

Methods.—One hundred consecutive patients (85 men and 15 women aged 54–74 years) who were being treated for intermittent claudication

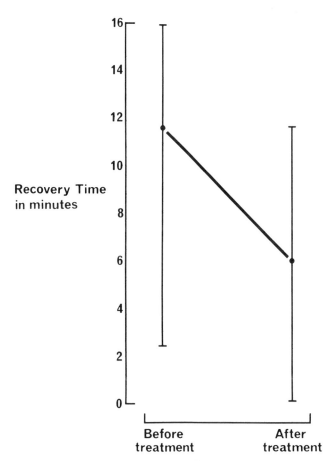

Fig 10–13.—Recovery time in 30 patients before and after treatment. The results are presented as median and 90% tolerance levels (90% range). P < .01, Wilcoxon rank sum test. (Courtesy of Salmasi A-M, Nicolaides A, Al-Katoubi A, et al: *J Vasc Surg* 14:76–86, 1991.)

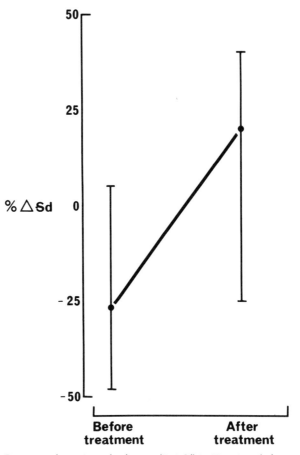

Fig 10–14.—Percentage change in stroke distance (% Δ Sd) in 30 patients before and after treatment. The results are presented as median and 90% tolerance levels (90% range). $P < .01$, Wilcoxon rank sum test. (Courtesy of Salmesi A-M, Nicolaides A, Al-Katoubi A, et al: *J Vasc Surg* 14:76–86, 1991.)

were screened with the ECG chest wall mapping exercise test. A bicycle was pedaled at a constant rate of 60 rpm, with a work load of up to 100 W. Transcutaneous aortovelography also was done.

Results.—The chest wall stress test demonstrated 3-vessel coronary disease in 25 patients and disease of the left anterior descending and circumflex arteries in 7. Aortovelography showed a reduced stroke distance (an index of cardiac stroke volume) in these patients. Claudication distance ranged from 50 to 250 m. The time needed for the pressure index to return to pre-exercise level decreased after myocardial revascularization or medical treatment of heart disease (Fig 10–13), and the stroke distance increased significantly (Fig 10–14). The resting ankle-pressure index did not change. Claudication lessened or disappeared in all but 3 patients.

Conclusion.—Silent myocardial ischemia is frequent in patients with claudication, and it compromises left ventricular function. Stroke volume decreases, promoting an early onset of claudication with exercise. These effects are countered by nitrate treatment or myocardial revascularization.

▶ I am sure we are all vaguely aware that claudication may be a manifestation of cardiac disease and not primarily peripheral vascular disease. These authors have attempted to quantitate this concept, and they observe that, after myocardial revascularization or medical cardiac therapy, a significant improvement occurs in claudication symptoms and vascular lab indices. They conclude that silent myocardial ischemia is a frequent finding in patients with intermittent claudication. Anyone interested in these data must carefully read the erudite discussion of this paper by Dr. Craig Miller, who was the invited discussant of this paper, which was presented at the June 1990 meeting of the Society for Vascular Surgery. Dr. Miller raises a number of interesting and critical points.—J.M. Porter, M.D.

Capillary Recruitment and Pain Relief on Leg Dependency in Patients With Severe Lower Limb Ischemia
Ubbink DT, Jacobs MJHM, Slaaf DW, Tangelder GJWJM, Reneman RS (Academic Hosp, Maastricht; Cardiovascular Research Inst, Maastricht, The Netherlands)
Circulation 85:223–229, 1992   10–27

Background.—Patients with severe lower extremity ischemia typically have less pain during leg dependency, even though dependency ordinarily leads to arteriolar vasoconstriction. This apparent paradox was examined by assessing the microcirculation of the extremity skin in 75 patients with different stages of ischemia and in 12 asymptomatic subjects.

Methods.—Video microscopy of the nailfold was undertaken to determine the density of red blood cell–perfused capillaries, capillary diameter, and red blood cell velocity with the patients sitting and supine.

Results.—Capillary density increased when patients changed from the supine to the sitting position. Those with limb-threatening ischemia had a 4.5-fold increase in capillary density compared with a 1.5-fold increase in asymptomatic subjects. Perfusion was substantially reduced in patients with severe ischemia, but it was slightly greater in the sitting position. Patients whose pain was relieved by sitting had a higher capillary density in this position—but not always greater capillary perfusion.

Conclusion.—The vasoconstrictive arteriolar response to leg dependency is lost in patients with severe ischemic disease. Capillary recruitment may explain why these patients prefer leg dependency.

▶ There is a finely tuned series of microcirculatory physiologic responses in the limbs, one of the more important of which is the venoarterial arteriolar reflex reducing limb arterial pressure while standing (1). This reflex appears to be abolished in advanced ischemia. Detailed studies of phenomena using the innovative technique of capillary microscopy and video microscopy are described in this paper. The question remains as to whether microcirculatory studies are merely interesting, or whether they will have a significant impact on decision-making in the treatment of clinical vascular disease. I suspect the former.—J.M. Porter, M.D.

Reference

1. Eickhoff JH, Henriksen O: *Cardiovasc Res* 19:219, 1985.

Vascular Rehabilitation: Benefits of a Structured Exercise/Risk Modification Program
Williams LR, Ekers MA, Collins PS, Lee JF (Saint Anthony's Hosp, St Petersburg, Fla)
J Vasc Surg 14:320–326, 1991   10–28

Background.—Structured programs of physical reconditioning and risk factor modification have proved helpful in patients with atherosclerotic coronary artery disease, but they have not been widely tried in those who are seen with peripheral arterial insufficiency. This has occurred despite the fact that exercise can improve walking ability. A rehabilitation program was designed for 68 patients who either had claudication or were recovering from lower extremity revascularization or endovascular procedures.

Methods.—After excluding 6 patients with silent myocardial ischemia, the remaining 62 were entered into a program (table) that offered 24 1-hour monitored exercise sessions, 12 personalized education lectures, and a home program for maintaining fitness. The activities included treadmill walking, cycling, walking on steps, and use of a rowing machine and free weights.

Results.—No patient died, and none had major morbidity. Thirty-eight of 45 patients who completed the program more than doubled their walking distances. Nearly 90% of the smokers quit, and most remained off smoking. Improved ambulation generally persisted on follow-up 2 years or more after the start of the program. Levels of cholesterol and triglycerides decreased significantly at 1 year.

Vascular Rehabilitation

Phase I
    Referral by physician
    History and physical examination
    Risk factor profile
    Cholesterol/triglyceride analysis
    Segmental Doppler pressures
    Graded exercise testing (cardiac stress test)
Phase II
    Initial rehabilitation exercise prescription
    12-week program of exercise, education, monitoring
Phase III
    Home maintenance program
    Periodic assessment and modification

(Courtesy of Williams LR, Ekers MA, Collins PS: *J Vasc Surg* 14:320–326, 1991.)

Conclusion.—This type of program not only identifies patients who are at increased cardiovascular risk from independent exercise, but it also improves exercise tolerance and reduces cardiovascular risk factors in those who can participate.

▶ Would you like to have a highly structured program of physical conditioning and risk factor modification available to which you could refer claudicants? Although it may be convenient, programs such as this will certainly be judged by a detailed cost-benefit analysis. It is uncertain whether third-party payers will approve such programs in this era of health care cost containment.—J.M. Porter, M.D.

Use of Lower Extremity Deep Veins as Arterial Substitutes: Functional Status of the Donor Leg
Schanzer H, Chiang K, Mabrouk M, Peirce EC II (Mt Sinai School of Medicine, New York)
J Vasc Surg 14:624–627, 1991   10–29

Background.—Femoropopliteal bypass using the superficial femoropopliteal venous unit reportedly provides excellent long-term results, but there has been a reluctance to remove the deep leg veins for fear of producing severe venous outflow restriction in the donor leg. The sequelae of deep vein donation in 25 extremities undergoing femoropopliteal bypass using the superficial femoropopliteal vein as an arterial substitute were examined.

Methods.—Veins were taken just distal to the confluence with the profunda vein; most of them extended to the distal popliteal-tibioperoneal trunk. Twenty-two limbs of 19 patients served as a control group; most

	Results		
	Deep vein donors extremities	*Saphenous-PTFE bypass extremities*	*p value*
Early swelling	56%	63.6%	NS
Late swelling	40%	40.9%	NS
Difference calf circumference mean ± SD (cm) (operated vs nonoperated side)	1.4 ± 1.8	0.53 ± 0.97	*p* < 0.05
Obstructive plethysmographic pattern	84%	50%	*p* < 0.02

(Courtesy of Schanzer H, Chiang K, Mabrouk M, et al: *J Vasc Surg* 14:624–627, 1991.)

had bypass with the reversed saphenous vein. Strain gauge plethysmography in the foot was used to evaluate function.

Results.—Swelling was no more frequent after removal of the deep veins than when saphenous or synthetic infrainguinal bypass was carried out (table). Plethysmography indicated that venous outflow obstruction was significantly more prevalent in extremities that had provided a deep vein.

Conclusion.—Removing part of the deep venous system of the lower extremity does not necessarily cause severe symptomatic limb enlargement through restricting venous outflow. A deep vein may be considered as a replacement for a large vein, or as an infrainguinal arterial substitute when superficial vein is not available.

▶ Reports of satisfactory results from use of deep leg veins as bypass conduits continue to appear, primarily from the group in New York. I believe the use of such conduits deserves serious consideration in desperate situations, when the only alternative is prosthetic. Our modest experience with the use of deep veins for leg bypasses has generally been satisfactory.—J.M. Porter, M.D.

Structural and Functional Smooth Muscle Injury After Surgical Preparation of Reversed and Non-Reversed (*In Situ*) Saphenous Vein Bypass Grafts

Sayers RD, Watt PAC, Muller S, Bell PRF, Thurston H (Leicester Royal Infirmary, Leicester, England)
Br J Surg 78:1256–1258, 1991   10–30

Background.—In patients undergoing reversed and in situ vein grafting, intimal hyperplasia and isolated stenoses have major effects on long-term patency. Surgical handling is known to cause functional endothelial damage, but there are no data on the use of the valvulotome. The effect of surgical preparation on smooth muscle cell structure and function in saphenous vein grafts was investigated.

Methods.—The study material consisted of 27 samples of saphenous vein from 22 patients undergoing in situ femorodistal or reversed coronary artery bypass. Control samples were taken after minimal dissection, whereas others were taken after saline distention or passage of a valvulotome. Rectangular strips of vein were mounted in an organ bath, and cumulative noradrenaline dose contraction curves were performed. Noradrenaline dose ranged from 10^{-8} to 10^{-5} M.

Findings.—Both the saline-distended and valvulotomized veins showed a significant reduction in contractile response compared with the control veins. Histologically, the distended veins had partial endothelial cell loss, and the valvulotomized veins had total endothelial cell loss with patchy necrosis of the smooth muscle.

Conclusion.—In reversed and in situ saphenous vein grafts, use of the valvulotome appears to not only render the valves incompetent, but to cause serious damage to the smooth muscle function. Smooth muscle function also appears to be damaged by saline distention. More studies of the contribution of smooth muscle injury to the development of intimal hyperplasia are needed.

▶ There can be little doubt that the passage of a valvulotome through the lumen of a vein must cause serious damage. The question, of course, is whether vein damage incurred at the time of surgery is associated with an increased incidence of hyperplasia and graft failure. I conclude that proof of such a relationship is lacking. Clearly, all veins are significantly damaged, at least by electron micrographic studies, incident to preparation for use as a bypass conduit. I find no convincing evidence that the degrees of damage associated with different methods of vein preparation have any influence on long-term graft outcome.—J.M. Porter, M.D.

Muscle Denervation in Peripheral Arterial Disease
England JD, Regensteiner JG, Ringel SP, Carry MR, Hiatt WR (Univ of Colorado, Denver)
Neurology 42:994–999, 1992   10–31

Background.—Atherosclerotic occlusive peripheral arterial disease is frequent in the lower extremities, and muscle function often is markedly impaired. Nevertheless, the precise effects of repeated ischemia on nerve and muscle function are incompletely understood.

Methods.—Electrophysiologic studies were carried out in 6 patients with unilateral peripheral arterial disease and 5 control subjects matched with the patients for age and level of activity. In addition, skeletal muscle samples were examined histologically.

Results.—All ischemic extremities exhibited evidence of chronic partial denervation-reinnervation limited to the distal muscles. Two of the patients had milder distal denervation in their nonischemic extremities. Two control subjects had evidence of denervation in at least 1 leg, but the electrophysiologic findings indicated L-5 or S-1 radiculopathy.

Conclusion.—Denervation of skeletal muscle may be the first neurologic manifestation of peripheral arterial disease and 1 of the factors in decreased muscular function.

▶ Recurrent episodes of ischemia associated with occlusive disease of the lower extremities may result in partial muscle denervation. This muscle denervation may be one of the causes for decreased exercise performance in these patients.—J.M. Porter, M.D.

Unilateral Iliac Artery Occlusive Disease: A Randomized Multicenter Trial Examining Direct Revascularization Versus Crossover Bypass
Ricco J-B (Hospital Jean Bernard, Poitiers, France)
Ann Vasc Surg 6:209–219, 1992   10–32

Introduction.—In a randomized trial patency rates for direct unilateral aortofemoral or iliofemoral prosthetic bypass grafts were compared with those for crossover femorofemoral or iliofemoral bypass grafts in patients with atheromatous occlusive disease of the iliac artery. A total of 143 patients were enrolled in this study.

Methods.—Seventy-four patients had crossover procedures and 69 had direct revascularization between May 1986 and March 1991. The groups were comparable with respect to cardiovascular risk factors, symptoms, and atheromatous lesions. Duplex ultrasonography with systolic pressure index estimates was used to follow the patients. Digital subtraction arteriography was done after operation and when hemodynamic abnormalities developed. The mean follow-up was 22 months.

Results.—One patient died after direct revascularization. The primary patency rate at 3 years was 90% for patients who had direct revascularization and 79% for those who had crossover bypass. Secondary patency rates at 4 years were 93% and 94%, respectively, which was not a significant difference.

Conclusion.—Crossover bypasses may seem to be an attractive approach to unilateral iliac occlusive disease, but direct revascularization is preferred for young patients lacking major surgical risk. The crossover bypass is indicated for patients at risk.

▶ The debate continues as to the optimal repair for the patient with symptomatic unilateral iliac artery occlusive disease. There seems to be no escaping the fact that the femorofemoral bypass is an inferior procedure and simply not comparable to aortofemoral or iliac femoral direct revascularization procedures in terms of patency. Of course, the cross femoral graft is quick and relatively uncomplicated. In the younger patient, however, and especially in the patient with superficial femoral artery occlusion, the femorofemoral bypass appears especially unattractive.—J.M. Porter, M.D.

Limb Salvage vs Amputation for Critical Ischemia: The Role of Vascular Surgery
Taylor LM Jr, Hamre D, Dalman RL, Porter JM (Oregon Health Sciences Univ, Portland)
Arch Surg 126:1251–1258, 1991   10–33

Introduction.—Since 1980, all patients treated for limb-threatening ischemia have been considered for revascularization. A total of 498 patients with 627 critically ischemic legs underwent revascularization in this period.

Methods.—Primary amputation was performed in 14 patients when no graftable distal vessels were identified, and in neurologically impaired patients who had no chance of walking.

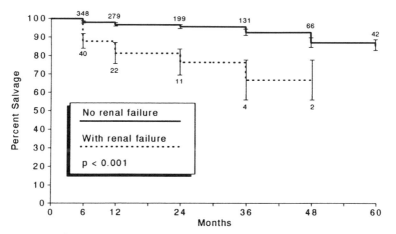

Fig 10–15.—Life-table limb salvage of patients without renal failure compared with limb salvage for patients with renal failure. (Courtesy of Taylor LM Jr, Hamre D, Dalman RL, et al: *Arch Surg* 126:1251-1258, 1991.)

Results.—During follow-up, 41 (7%) extremities were amputated, 31 after revascularization failed. Renal failure increased the need for amputation, even if patent revascularization was achieved (Fig 10–15).

Conclusion.—Aggressive revascularization is possible with low operative morbidity and excellent long-term salvage in patients with critical lower limb ischemia. Patients with renal failure are at an increased risk of losing their extremity. Patients without renal failure have achieved a limb salvage rate of 87% at 5 years.

▶ This large clinical series provides strong justification for the modern approach of aggressive revascularization for all functional patients seen with critical limb ischemia. Primary amputation is rarely indicated; only 2.8% of the patients had no identifiable graftable distal vessels. Mortality was low (2.3%), and limb salvage was durable, with only 7% of revascularized limbs progressing to amputation during long-term follow-up. End stage renal failure adversely affected the limb salvage rate.—J. Mills, M.D.

Atheroembolism Presenting as Selective Muscle Embolization
Adamson AS, Pittam MR, Darke SG (Royal Victoria Hosp, Bournemouth; Luton and Dunstable Hosp, England)
J Cardiovasc Surg 32:705–707, 1991   10–34

Introduction.—Digital soft-tissue ischemia and rest pain are the usual sequelae of atheroembolism. Two patients in whom typical muscular claudication symptoms developed in the presence of normal peripheral pulses from atherothromboembolism were examined.

Case Report.—Man, 54, suddenly had pain in both legs and buttocks, more marked on the left side, while walking briskly. The left foot was cyanosed, and both thighs and calves were tender. All peripheral pulses were palpable, and Doppler signals were normal. Exploration of the left calf revealed necrotic muscle tissue, and a below-knee amputation was necessary. Atheromatous debris was found within the small muscular vessels. Severe but transient pain occurred 4 years later in the buttocks, thighs, and right calf. Typical claudication occurred for 10 days, and angiography showed a small abdominal aortic aneurysm with adherent mural debris. A woven Dacron graft was placed. The right rectus muscle was atrophied, and histologic study showed atheromatous debris within arterioles.

▶ Both acute limb ischemia with absent pulses caused by macroembolization and sudden-onset digital ischemia with palpable peripheral pulses caused by microembolization of proximal atheromatous debris (the so-called blue-toe syndrome) are encountered with relative frequency and are readily recognized by experienced clinicians. This report makes us aware of a third, rare presentation of embolic disease: the sudden onset of claudication in a patient with normal pulses associated with extensive, selective atheromatous microembolization to skeletal muscles of the limb. To date, I have never recognized this, but I will be on the alert.—J. Mills, M.D.

11 Upper Extremity Vascular

Long-Term Follow-Up After Thoracic Outlet Decompression: An Analysis of Factors Determining Outcome

Green RM, McNamara J, Ouriel K (Univ of Rochester, Rochester, NY)

J Vasc Surg 14:739–746, 1991

11–1

Introduction.—Thoracic outlet syndrome resulting from neurologic causes remains a difficult therapeutic challenge. Because of the subjective nature of the symptoms, the lack of an objective test, and the risk of disastrous operative complications, some vascular surgeons avoid treating these patients. The results of first rib resection in 136 patients who underwent 147 rib resections during a 12-year period were reviewed.

Methods.—Surgery was offered to patients whose symptoms prevented work or normal activities, when symptoms occurred on abducting the shoulder to 90 degrees, or in whom physical therapy failed to improve function or lessen pain. Only 8 patients had classic findings caused by stretching of the distal C8/T1 roots or proximal lower trunk of the brachial plexus. Trauma occurred in 53 patients just before the onset of symptoms. Anatomical abnormalities were found in one third of patients; complete and incomplete cervical rib were most frequent.

Results.—During a mean follow-up of 5 years, 20 patients required secondary surgery in the neck. Fewer than half of the patients with a history of trauma returned to their pre-illness level of activity compared with nearly 80% of the others. Levels of patient satisfaction were high, regardless of a history of trauma. Coverage under worker's compensation negatively influenced the outcome (table), as did the presence of fixed joint abnormality or neurologic changes in the upper extremity.

Conclusion.—Many carefully selected patients who lack definite neurologic findings are able to return to their previous level of activity after a first rib resection. Trauma is an adverse prognostic factor, particularly in women who file a compensation claim. The value of any operation must be established in a long-term follow-up study in which patients are prospectively randomized to surgical or nonoperative treatment.

▶ I seriously doubt the very existence of neurogenic thoracic outlet syndrome in the absence of a distinct bony abnormality, primarily first rib anomaly or cervical rib. Between 5% and 10% of all workers in the West have

Impact of Type of Trauma and Gender on Return to Preillness Function

Status	Noncomp injury	Comp injury	Men noncomp/comp	Women noncomp/comp
Returned	16 (57%)	9 (36%)	6/7 vs 2/4 (86% vs 50%)	14/26 vs 3/16 (54% vs 19%)
Not returned	12 (43%)	16 (72%)	1/7 vs 2/4 (14% vs 50%)	7/26 vs 13/16 (27% vs 81%)
Total	28 (100%)	25 (100%)	11 (100%)	42 (100%)

Note: Comparisons: compensation vs. noncompensation injury: $P < .02$; men, compensation vs. noncompensation injuries: P not significant; women, compensation vs. noncompensation injuries: $P < .05$.
(Courtesy of Green RM, McMamara J, Ouriel K: J Vasc Surg 14:739–746, 1991.)

chronic complaints of neck, shoulder, and arm pain. The United States is the only country to ever attempt to address this chronic medical problem surgically. Beware of any condition for which there are no objective diagnostic criteria. The surgery is performed exclusively for the relief of symptoms, and the person judging the outcome of surgery is invariably the operating surgeon, who is hardly a disinterested observer.—J.M. Porter, M.D.

Severe Injuries Resulting From Operations for Thoracic Outlet Syndrome: Can They Be Avoided?

Mellière D, Becquemin J-P, Etienne G, Le Cheviller B (Paris-Val de Marne Univ)

J Cardiovasc Surg 32:599–603, 1991   11–2

Background.—Recent referral of 2 patients with critical ischemia of the upper limb after thoracic outlet syndrome (TOS) surgery prompted a national survey concerning severe complications caused by TOS operations.

Methods.—A survey was sent to all French vascular surgeons in private or public practice, asking about their experiences with complications of TOS surgery. The surgeons were asked to include patients referred to them and cases about which they had testified as an expert witness. Responses were received from 66 surgeons or surgical teams.

Findings.—Some of the respondents had performed TOS operations on hundreds of patients with no severe complications. However, others had seen rare but dramatic complications. Severing of the subclavian artery occurred in 4 patients, and the artery was injured in 4 others. All of these injuries occurred during the transaxillary approach. There were 4 cases of upper limb ischemia, 2 occurring after aneurysm repair through a supraclavicular approach. In 4 cases, the subclavian vein was injured, 3 during the supraclavicular route; repair was found to be difficult in each case. There were several cases of transient or definitive paralysis of the

Severe Complications After Operations for Thoracic Outlet Syndrome (French Inquiry, 1988)		
Complications	Transaxillary route	Supraclavicular route
Arterial injury	10	2
Arterial thrombosis	2	—
Phlebitis	1	—
Injury to subclavian vein	1	3
Hematoma, hemothorax	4	1
Severance of brachial plexus	2	—
Contusion of brachial plexus	14	3
Scapula alata	9	—
Phrenic nerve paralysis	1	4

(Courtesy of Mellière D, Becquemin J-P, Etienne G, et al: *J Cardiovasc Surg* 32:599-603, 1991.)

brachial plexus, long thoracic or phrenic nerve injury, and chylothorax (table).

Conclusion.—Complications of TOS surgery may occur with either approach and with experienced surgeons. Such an operation should be considered only when the diagnosis is sure and when the only option is decompression. The surgeon must choose an adequate approach, ensure good vision during surgery, and use meticulous technique. These complications are often very serious and may be more common than has been thought.

▶ The impressive injuries occurring during the performance of TOS surgery are sobering. The highly unpredictable likelihood of success, the significant incidence of injuries, and the significant likelihood of litigation all combine to make neurogenic TOS surgery generally unattractive.—J.M. Porter, M.D.

Late Upper Extremity Embolic Complications of Occluded Axillofemoral Grafts

Khalil IM, Hoballah JJ (New York Univ)
Ann Vasc Surg 5:375–380, 1991   11–3

Introduction.—Axillofemoral grafting has been used in lower limb revascularization with low morbidity and satisfactory patency rates. Axillary artery thrombosis and recurrent upper extremity emboli are infrequent complications of the bypass grafts, which tend to develop immediately or shortly after graft thrombosis. However, ischemic complications in the donor upper extremity can occur over an indefinite period after graft occlusion.

Methods.—Data were reviewed on 3 patients in whom emboli to the ipsilateral upper extremity developed at 9, 15, and 34 months after occlusion of their axillary femoral graft.

Results.—In all 3 patients, the anastomosis was located on the anterior surface of the artery. When the graft is tunneled superficial to the plane of the artery, there can be increased mechanical pull, which may further promote the "Y" elongation. If any of the axillary artery's branches are ligated at the time of surgery, limb ischemia may be aggravated if the artery occludes.

Conclusion.—The potential for upper extremity ischemia developing after occlusion of an axillofemoral graft is present for an indefinite period after surgery. The presence of a blind pouch in the graft stump or "Y" elongation of the artery with proliferative changes may contribute to this problem. Surgical techniques have been modified to alter mechanical factors that may contribute to occlusion. It is preferable to perform the anastomosis in the first portion of the axillary artery, medial to the pectoralis minor tendon and closer to the chest wall. This leaves the rich collateral network arising from the distal artery intact. Graft tunneling is recommended in the anatomical plane between the pectoralis muscles and along the midaxillary line.

▶ Not surprisingly, thrombosed grafts attached to the axillary artery are prone to late backwashed thrombosis and arm embolization. This can occur from a failed axillary-axillary bypass just as readily as from a failed axillofemoral bypass. We are seeing increasing numbers of these patients in our own practice, and they are clearly a cause for concern. From our preliminary experience, there is no amount of time with a failed graft beyond which the patient is "safe."—J.M. Porter, M.D.

Subclavian Artery Stenosis: Hemodynamic Aspects and Surgical Outcome
Branchereau A, Magnan PE, Espinoza H, Bartoli JM (Hôpital St Marguerite Université Aix-Marseille II, Marseille)
J Cardiovasc Surg 32:604–612, 1991   11–4

Background.—Obstructive lesions of the subclavian artery may produce the vertebrosubclavian steal syndrome. Ninety-seven patients with subclavian artery lesions were reviewed to define the relationship among symptoms, angiographic findings, and hemodynamic disorder detected by Doppler monitoring.

Clinical and Doppler Findings.—Ninety of the 97 patients, whose mean age was 58 years, had vertebrobasilar insufficiency (table). Fourteen of them had hemispheric transient ischemic attacks, whereas 7 had chronic upper limb ischemia. The total of 105 subclavian lesions in-

Frequency and Association of Vertebrobasilar Insufficiency Symptoms		
	Number of patients	Percent
Problems with balance	77	85.6
Visual disorders	58	64.4
Dizziness	35	38.9
Motor or sensory deficit	14	15.6
Vertigo	11	12.2
Dysarthria	1	1.1
Patients presenting with 1 symptom	21	
Patients presenting with 2 symptoms	38	
Patients presenting with 3 symptoms	20	
Patients presenting with 4 symptoms	13	
Total VBI	90	

(Courtesy of Branchereau A, Magnan PE, Espinoza H, et al: *J Cardiovasc Surg* 32:604-612, 1991.)

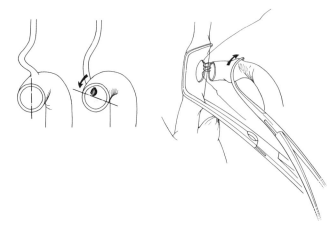

Fig 11–1.—A 90-degree backward rotation lowers the vertebral artery origin and avoids an excess of length and kinking of the vertebral artery. (Courtesy of Brancherau A, Magnan PE, Espinoza H, et al: *J Cardiovasc Surg* 32:604–612, 1991.)

cluded 29 occlusions and 76 stenoses greater than 50% of the vessel diameter.

Doppler examination of the vertebral artery, including a test for upper limb hyperemia, classified the patients into 3 groups. Thirty-five stage I patients had "pre-subclavian steal," with a sudden decrease in systolic vertebral blood flow and complete interruption of flow during hyperemia. Two thirds of these patients had severe vertebrobasilar insufficiency, and the same proportion had a 50% to 70% stenosis of the subclavian artery. Eighteen patients had findings of "intermittent" subclavian steal, with transient inversion of vertebral flow in systole and inversion lasting 1–2 minutes after hyperemia. A majority of these stage II patients had severe insufficiency, and nearly 80% had a 75% to 95% stenosis. Thirty-three stage III patients had permanent subclavian steal, a complete inversion of vertebral flow without diastolic flow and an increase in flow during hyperemia. Nearly three fourths of this group had severe vertebrobasilar insufficiency and either subtotal or complete subclavian occlusion. Hemodynamic stage correlated closely with the anatomical findings, but not with the severity of vertebrobasilar insufficiency. The severity of insufficiency related to the number of stenosed or occluded cerebral arterial trunks.

Results.—A total of 105 revascularization operations (Fig 11–1) were done. One patient died postoperatively, and 3 patients had a stroke, all after combined carotid surgery. There was one transient ischemic attack. Angiography demonstrated a patent reconstruction in 96 of 100 studies. Eight-two of 90 patients who were followed up for a mean of 54 months had a good neurologic outcome, whereas 8 patients had poor results.

Conclusion. Transposition of the subclavian artery into the common carotid appears to be a useful reconstructive procedure.

▶ The surgeons in Marseille have had an extraordinarily large experience with the surgical treatment of subclavian artery stenosis, most of which was undertaken for the treatment of vertebrobasilar symptoms. This is totally different from our own practice, in which we see less than 1 patient per year who we believe needs surgery for the treatment of symptomatic vetebrobasilar insufficiency.—J.M. Porter, M.D.

Surgery for Effort Thrombosis of the Subclavian Vein
Molina JE (Univ of Minnesota Hosp and Clinic, Minneapolis)
J Thorac Cardiovasc Surg 103:341–346, 1992   11–5

Background.—Primary thrombosis of the subclavian vein may occur primarily after a sudden effort using the arms. Physicians may be unaware of the need for urgent care before irreversible changes take place.

Patients.—Between February 1988 and March 1991, a total of 28 patients were seen with effort thrombosis. Six patients were seen within 5 days of having acute stage effort thrombosis of the subclavian vein. Seven others were seen subacutely 6 days to 2 weeks after the event, and 15 were seen in the chronic stage. Eight of the latter patients had an obstructed segment extending from 1 to 6 inches.

Treatment.—During venography, a catheter was placed with its tip within the thrombus, and urokinase, 3,000 U/kg/hr, was infused for 12–24 hours. After complete clot lysis, the first rib was resected by using a subclavicular approach (Fig 11–2). Fifteen patients had vein patch angi-

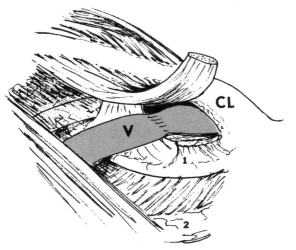

Fig 11–2.—Subclavian tendon muscle is transected from its insertion in first the rib and reflected upward to uncover the subclavian vein (V). A groove can be seen on the vein showing the site of pinching between the subclavius muscle (reflected) and the tendon of the anterior scalene muscle behind. *Abbreviations:* CL, clavicle; 1, first rib; 2, second rib. (Courtesy of Molina JE: *J Thorac Cardiovasc Surg* 103:341–346, 1992.)

oplasty as well. Bypass of a long-obstructed vein segment was attempted in 4 of the chronic patients with a length-obstructed segment.

Results.—Decompression was achieved and a normal vein caliber was restored in all patients who were seen in the acute or subacute stage, and in 86% of those with chronic thrombosis. In only 1 case did a saphenous vein bypass remain open.

Conclusion.—Emergency treatment of subclavian venous effort thrombosis can improve the outcome and prevent permanent disability.

▶ This author is almost correct. In my experience, the actual site of compression is about 1 inch medial to where it is shown in Figure 11–2, adjacent to the head of the clavicle bounded by the medial edge of the scalenus anticus laterally, and by the cephalad edge of the first rib interiorly. I do believe that thrombolytic therapy is optimal in the early patients, but I am unconvinced of the value of rib surgery as a routine procedure for all patients.—J.M. Porter, M.D.

Cervical Rib Variant: Report of a Case
Kosenak LM, Knorr EJ, DeRojas JJ, Katlic MR (Nesbitt Mem Hosp, Kingston, Pa)
Ann Vasc Surg 6:292–293, 1992   11–6

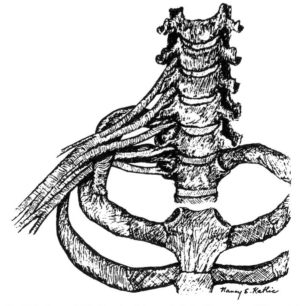

Fig 11–3.—Brachial plexus divided by the right cervical rib. (Courtesy of Kosenak LM, Knorr EJ, DeRojas JJ, et al: *Ann Vasc Surg* 6:292-293, 1992.)

Background.—Cervical ribs occur in 1% or less of the population. Although they occur most often in the lower cervical region, they may be seen as high as C-5. Only 5% to 10% of cervical ribs are symptomatic. It is assumed that the subclavian vessels arch over the cervical rib and that the brachial plexus is craniad to the structure. The plexus may, however, be split by the cervical rib.

Case Report.—Boy, 17 years, an athlete, had pain in the right shoulder, a weak right arm, and numbness in the arm and hand with the arm elevated. A right supraclavicular mass was noted, and clinical tests were consistent with a cervical rib. Bilateral cervical ribs were found on chest radiography. Conduction was slowed across the lower trunk of the right brachial plexus as it crossed the thoracic outlet. When exercises proved ineffective, the first and cervical ribs were resected via an axillary approach. The cervical rib was fused to the first rib and it split the trunks of the brachial plexus, with the lower trunk nerve passing dorsal to the extra rib (Fig 11–3). The symptoms resolved and the patient returned to full sports activities 2 months after operation.

Conclusion.—The brachial plexus is not always at a cranial-ventral site relative to a cervical rib. It is important to accurately identify all structures before resecting the cervical and first ribs.

▶ Most of us periodically have to operate on the cervical ribs. We have all been trained that the cervical rib elevates the neurovascular structures that are located exclusively on its cephalad surface. This fascinating article points out that the occasional patient with a cervical rib may have portions of the plexus posterior, or caudad, to the rib. I was not previously familiar with this anatomical variation.—J.M. Porter, M.D.

Critical Ischaemia of the Upper Limb
Quraishy MS, Cawthorn SJ, Giddings AEB (Royal Surrey County Hosp, Guildford, England)
J R Soc Med 85:269–273, 1992   11–7

Introduction.—Data were reviewed on 57 patients seen in 1980–1989 with critical ischemia in an upper extremity. The 43 female and 14 male patients were aged 17 to 85 years.

Causes.—Thirteen patients had emboli originating from the heart. Twenty-three others had arteritis, which affected large vessels in 7 cases and digital vessels in 16. The subclavian vessels were most often involved in the former cases. The diagnosis often was delayed, with the condition being mistaken for musculoskeletal pain. Nine patients had traumatic arteritis caused by either direct arterial injury or traction on a vessel. Six patients had acute-on-chronic atherosclerotic ischemia, and 4 had thoracic outlet compression that caused chronic ischemia. There were single cases of ischemia secondary to radiation fibrosis and disseminated intra-vascular coagulation.

Conclusion.—Critical ischemia in an upper extremity is an infrequent but challenging problem. Total extremity arteriography is indicated, except in those patients who are seen with classic embolic ischemia or direct arterial injury.

▶ These authors present a remarkable group of 57 patients with critical upper extremity ischemia encountered over a course of only 10 years. Ischemia resulted from a bewildering variety of different disease processes, which are well characterized herein. The authors appropriately emphasize the important role of arteriography in the evaluation of these patients.—J.M. Porter, M.D.

12 Carotid and Cerebrovascular Disease

Beneficial Effect of Carotid Endarterectomy in Symptomatic Patients With High-Grade Carotid Stenosis
North American Symptomatic Carotid Endarterectomy Trial Collaborators
N Engl J Med 325:445–453, 1991   12-1

Background.—Until the mid-1980s, the use of carotid endarterectomy increased dramatically, although there was no strong evidence of benefit. Use of this procedure has decreased in recent years. A United States and Canadian prospective randomized trial was performed to determine whether carotid endarterectomy reduces the risk of stroke in patients with a recent adverse cerebrovascular event and ipsilateral carotid stenosis.

Methods.—Fifty North American centers participated in the study. All study patients had had a hemispheric or retinal transient ischemic attack or nondisabling stroke within 120 days of entry to the study. Severity of carotid stenosis, as measured by angiogram, was used to stratify the patients into 2 groups: high-grade stenosis, defined as stenosis of 70% to 99%; and medium-grade stenosis, defined as stenosis of 30% to 69%. There were 659 patients in the high-grade stenosis group. All patients received medical care, including antiplatelet therapy, and 328 were randomized to receive carotid endarterectomy. Each case in which an endpoint was reached was studied in blinded, independent fashion. Follow-up was complete.

Results.—By 24 months after randomization, life-table estimates of the cumulative risk of ipsilateral stroke were 26% in the medically treated group and 9% in the surgically treated group. This reflected an absolute risk reduction of 17% and a relative risk reduction of 65%. For major or fatal ipsilateral stroke, the cumulative risk was 13.1% in the medically treated group and 2.5% in the surgically treated group. This corresponded to an absolute risk reduction of 10.6% and a relative risk reduction of 81%. Even when all strokes and deaths were included, surgical treatment still carried a 10.1% reduction in absolute risk. Evidence for the efficacy of surgery for patients with high-grade stenosis was so strong that randomization of this group was halted. The study of medium-grade stenosis was continued.

Conclusion.—For patients who have ipsilateral high-grade stenosis after hemispheric and retinal transient ischemic attacks or nondisabling strokes, carotid endarterectomy appears to be a highly beneficial treatment.

▶ This is probably the most important paper published to date on carotid endarterectomy. Vascular surgeons will do well to become extremely familiar with every part of this pivotal publication.—J.M. Porter, M.D.

Vascular Risks of Asymptomatic Carotid Stenosis
Norris JW, Zhu CZ, Bornstein NM, Chambers BR (Univ of Toronto; Repatriation Gen Hosp, Melbourne)
Stroke 22:1485–1490, 1991   12–2

Background.—Considerable evidence suggests that the asymptomatic neck bruit is a risk factor for later stroke, myocardial infarction, and death. Nevertheless, the risk of stroke is low. However, because most patients with bruit do not have significant carotid stenosis, an evaluation of the outcome of patients with proven carotid stenosis appears to be more important.

Methods.—A total of 696 patients with vascular laboratory-determined asymptomatic carotid stenosis seen over a mean period of 41 months were followed. The mean patient age was 64 years. Patients were followed clinically and by carotid Doppler ultrasound examinations.

Findings.—Seventy-five patients had transient ischemic attacks, and 29 had a stroke. A total of 132 patients had ischemic cardiac events during follow-up. Five patients died of stroke, and 59 died of cardiac causes. The annual rate of stroke was 1.3% in patients with 75% or less carotid stenosis and 3.3% in those with more marked stenosis. Patients with severe stenosis had an 8.3% annual rate of cardiac events, and an annual morbidity of 6.5%.

Conclusion.—Even moderate carotid stenosis increases the risk of cardiac ischemia and vascular death. The risk of stroke is increased in the presence of more than 75% stenosis, even in the absence of symptoms.

▶ This report by neurologists indicates that patients with diameter reduction of carotid stenosis greater than 75% have a combined transient ischemic attack and stroke rate of 10.5% per year, for a cardiac event rate of 8.3% per year and a death rate of 6.5% per year. It is crystal clear that symptomatic peripheral arterial disease, be it lower extremity or carotid, defines a patient population that is at extreme risk for morbid cardiovascular events, indeed a patient population approaching the end of life.—J.M. Porter, M.D.

Silent Stroke and Carotid Stenosis

Norris JW, Zhu CZ (Univ of Toronto)
Stroke 23:483–485, 1992

12–3

Background.—Silent cerebral infarction is a frequent finding on CT scans of patients with asymptomatic carotid stenosis, but its relationship to the stenosis is not clear.

Methods.—The CT findings and results of carotid Doppler examinations were compared for 115 patients with asymptomatic carotid stenosis, 203 with carotid transient ischemic attacks and stenosis, and 63 with transient ischemic attacks only.

Results.—At CT, lesions were seen in 47% of patients with carotid stenosis and transient ischemic attacks, 30% of those with ischemia alone, and 19% of those with asymptomatic carotid stenosis. Both central and peripheral infarcts were most frequent in the group with symptomatic stenosis. The scan findings correlated with the severity of carotid stenosis (table). In patients with symptomatic stenosis, 86% of the infarcts were on the same side as the stenosis.

Conclusion.—Ipsilateral cerebral infarction becomes more frequent as the severity of carotid stenosis increases. The presence of a silent cere-

Frequency of Central and Peripheral Infarctions According to Degree of Carotid Stenosis

Stenosis	*n*	Peripheral infarcts	Central infarcts	Positive CT scan (%)
Mild (35–50%)				
Symptomatic	41	7	3	24
Asymptomatic	193	7	7	7
Total	234	14	10	10
Moderate (50–75%)				
Symptomatic	34	6	6	35
Asymptomatic	84	2	6	9.5
Total	118	8	12	17
Severe (>75%)				
Symptomatic	128	40	17	52
Asymptomatic	156	18	10	10
Total	284	58	27	30

Abbreviation: n, number of stenosed carotid arteries.
(Courtesy of Norris JW, Zhu CZ: *Stroke* 23:483–485, 1992.)

bral infarct may indicate the need for endarterectomy in an asymptomatic patient.

▶ A remarkable number of patients with transient ischemic attacks only, as well as a remarkable number of asymptomatic patients with carotid stenosis, have cerebral infarction by CT scan. I do not know whether this represents a cause-and-effect relationship or a coincidental occurrence of simultaneous arterial disease at different locations.—J.M. Porter, M.D.

Which Asymptomatic Patients Should Undergo Routine Screening Carotid Duplex Scan?
Ahn SS, Baker JD, Walden K, Moore WS (Univ of California, Los Angeles)
Am J Surg 162:180–184, 1991   12–4

Introduction.—The usefulness of routine carotid duplex screening in patients without signs or symptoms of carotid disease, but with other symptomatic peripheral vascular disease has never been analyzed. To determine whether patients in this category will benefit from routine carotid duplex screening, 4,000 scans were reviewed retrospectively.

Between 1985 and 1989, 91 scans were performed for screening in 78 patients as part of their initial evaluation for peripheral artery disease. The patients' average age was 70 years; 69% were men and 31% were women. All had risk factors for atherosclerosis. An attempt was made to find a correlation between carotid disease and atherosclerotic risk factors and to determine which of these risk factors were predictive of significant carotid artery disease.

Results.—Nearly half (47%) the patients showed some evidence of atherosclerotic carotid artery disease. The carotid stenoses were 16% to 49% in 26 patients, more than 50% in 11, and more than 75% in 4. Two patients with a stenosis greater than 90% were alive and well after prophylactic carotid endarterectomy. Although individual risk factors for atherosclerosis did not predict the detection of high-grade carotid stenosis, an age of 68 years or older, in combination with other risk factors, was associated with an increased incidence of significant stenosis.

Conclusion.—In this patient group, all hemodynamically significant carotid lesions would have been detected if scanning were limited to men aged 68 years and older. Selective carotid screening of patients with peripheral vascular symptoms but no carotid symptoms will cost far less than the treatment and rehabilitation of a single stroke victim.

▶ A number of studies indicate that neurologically asymptomatic patients with lower extremity or coronary arterial disease have almost a 5% prevalence of carotid artery stenosis greater than 80%. Are screening tests worthwhile in these patients? I believe so, and I believe that the optimal screening test includes both a carotid duplex ultrasound and an abdominal ultrasound to rule out an unsuspected abdominal aortic aneurysm.—J.M. Porter, M.D.

Preoperative Carotid Artery Screening in Elderly Patients Undergoing Cardiac Surgery
Berens ES, Kouchoukos NT, Murphy SF, Wareing TH (Washington Univ, St Louis; Jewish Hosp of St Louis)
J Vasc Surg 15:313–323, 1992   12–5

Introduction.—The role of preoperative screening for carotid artery disease in older patients who have heart surgery remains uncertain. The prevalence of carotid artery disease in this group and the preoperative risk factors for carotid stenosis were identified in a prospective study.

Methods.—A total of 1,087 patients aged 65 years and older underwent carotid duplex ultrasonography before cardiac surgery. Ninety-one percent had coronary artery disease.

Results.—Carotid stenosis of at least 50% was found in 17% of the study group, and stenosis of 80% or greater was found in 6% (Table 1). Marked stenosis was associated with female gender, peripheral vascular disease, a history of transient ischemia or stroke, smoking, and the presence of left main coronary artery disease (Table 2). Carotid endarterectomy was performed in addition to heart surgery in 46 patients. Stroke occurred in 2% of all patients and in 6.5% of those who had carotid endarterectomy. The overall postoperative mortality was 5.2%.

Conclusion.—There are risk factors that allow subgroups of elderly patients scheduled for heart surgery to undergo screening for carotid artery disease before operation.

TABLE 1.—Prevalence of Carotid Artery Disease in 1,087 Patients

			No. of patients	
Severity of carotid artery stenosis	*No. of patients*	*%*	*Preoperative TIA or stroke*	*Carotid endarterectomy*
<50%/<50%	901	82.9	100	0
50-79%/<50%	97	8.9	15	5
50-79%/50-79%	24	2.2	4	0
80-99%/<50%	16	1.5	5	9
80-99%/50-79%	19	1.7	6	16
80-99%/80-99%	11	1.0	3	11
100/<50%	10	0.9	3	0
100/50-79%	3	0.3	2	0
100/80-99%	6	0.6	0	5
Total	1087	100%	138	46

(Courtesy of Berens ES, Kouchoukos NT, Murphy SF, et al: *J Vasc Surg* 15:313-323, 1992.)

TABLE 2.—Predictors of 80% Stenosis or Greater of 1 or Both Carotid Arteries
by Univariate and Multivariate Analysis

Variable	Univariate p value	Risk ratio	95% Confidence limits	Multivariate p value
TIA or stroke	0.0001	3.27	1.85 - 5.78	0.0001
Peripheral vascular disease	0.002	2.76	1.47 - 5.19	0.011
Left main disease	0.01	1.97	1.15 - 3.40	0.007
Female sex	0.03	1.79	1.08 - 2.97	0.003
NYHA class	0.03	1.54	1.05 - 2.24	
Hypertension	0.05	1.77	0.99 - 3.17	
Smoking history	0.07	1.62	0.97 - 2.71	0.026

(Courtesy of Berens ES, Kouchoukos NT, Murphy SF, et al: *J Vasc Surg* 15:313–323, 1992.)

▶ See the comments after Abstract 12–4. I believe that the optimal treatment of patients such as those described in this abstract is carotid surgery followed by coronary surgery. Based on numerous published reports of adverse outcome with combined procedures, we strive mightily to minimize the number of patients in whom we recommend simultaneous coronary and carotid artery surgery.—J.M. Porter, M.D.

Clinical Follow-Up and Progression of Carotid Atherosclerosis Determined by Duplex Scanning in Patients Suffering From TIA

Visonà A, Lusiani L, Sumner DS, Bonanome A, Papesso B, Pagnan A (Univ of Padua, Italy; Southern Illinois Univ, Springfield)
J Cardiovasc Surg 32:420–425, 1991   12–6

Background.—Transient cerebral ischemic attacks (TIAs) have long been thought to be a risk factor for stroke. Recent research suggests that TIAs may also be an indicator of ischemic heart disease. The association of carotid artery disease to TIA has not been established. Patients with TIAs referred for assessment of extracranial carotid arteries were reviewed to determine clinical outcomes and to document subsequent progression of lesions.

Methods.—A total of 109 patients with hemispheric ischemic attacks or amaurosis fugax were studied. Ninety-two patients reported lateralizing symptoms; 17 reported amaurosis fugax. Forty-eight percent of the plaques on the asymptomatic carotid arteries were homogeneous, whereas 52% were heterogeneous. Twenty-five patients (23%) underwent carotid endarterectomy, with the decision for surgery largely influenced by the duplex data. Surgical and nonsurgical groups appeared similar.

Outcomes.—During a mean follow-up of 40 months, the cumulative frequency of TIAs was 14%. There was no relationship between new

TIAs and the presence of known cardiovascular risk factors or plaque characteristics on duplex scanning. One patient died. None had any permanent neurologic deficits develop. The cumulative death rate was 6.5%, with myocardial infarction being the most common cause of death. Duplex scanning was used to determine anatomical progression of plaques in 22% of the internal carotid arteries. Progression of these plaques was unrelated to the development of new TIAs.

Conclusion.—Transient ischemic attacks do not seem to lead inevitably to stroke, as is commonly believed. In this series, death was more often caused by cardiac events rather than cerebrovascular ones. The clinical outcome of the patients with TIAs was not predictable based on various risk factors or plaque characteristics. The lack of correlation between symptoms and carotid lesions may suggest that TIAs are caused by other pathogenetic mechanisms than those studied.

▶ As interesting as this paper may appear to be, it is seriously flawed by the observation that 25 patients (23%) underwent carotid endarterectomy independent of the follow-up study. Their outcome results could have been severely skewed by this surgery. On the other hand, I think it is quite true that a number of patients have one or several TIAs, have only moderate carotid disease, and never have any further difficulty.—J.M. Porter, M.D.

Carotid Artery Disease in Young Adults
Castle DJ, Silber MH, Handler LC (Univ of Cape Town, South Africa; Groote Schuur Hosp, Cape Town)
S Afr Med J 80:278–281, 1991   12–7

Background.—Atherosclerosis is a less frequent cause of stroke in young adults, but nonatheromatous arteriopathies are seen more often in this group. The range of carotid artery disorders was examined in 10 male and 7 female patients, aged 14 to 39 years, who had stenosis or occlusion, or both, of at least 1 common or internal carotid artery (ICA). All the patients had neurologic symptoms.

Findings.—Three patients had atherosclerotic disease underlying cerebral infarction. Each had risk factors for such disease. Four other patients had large-vessel vasculitis, and 6 had noninflammatory arteriopathies. Three of the latter patients had findings of fibromuscular dysplasia. One patient (Fig 12–1) had abused cannabis and Mandrax (methaqualone and diphenhydramine). One patient had leg weakness secondary to internal carotid compression by a temporal glioma. In 3 cases, no cause of symptoms was apparent.

Outcome.—Two patients died during a mean follow-up of 20 months. Four others had further cerebrovascular events.

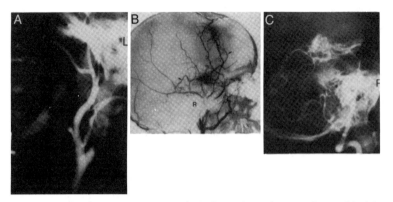

Fig 12–1.—Vasculopathy in patient who abused Mandrax and cannabis. **A,** occlusion of the left ICA 10 mm from its origin. **B,** occlusion of the distal right ICA and reconstitution of flow through anterior and middle cerebral artery branches (*filled arrows*) via rete mirabile from middle meningeal and superficial temporal arteries (*open arrows*). **C,** occlusion of distal basilar artery (*arrow*) with collateral filling of the superior cerebellar artery territory from posterior inferior cerebellar artery via leptomeningeal collaterals. (Courtesy of Castle DJ, Silber MH, Handler LC: *S Afr Med J* 80:278–281, 1991.)

Conclusion.—Carotid angiography can provide a definitive diagnosis in many young adults who have carotid artery disease and neurologic symptoms.

▶ This is a fascinating group of young patients with carotid artery disease producing neurologic symptoms. It provides a good, brief review of the arteritides, as well as the noninflammatory arteriopathies that may continue to this condition.—J.M. Porter, M.D.

High Frequency of Asymptomatic Visual Field Defects in Subjects With Transient Ischaemic Attacks or Minor Strokes
Falke P, Abela BM Jr, Krakau CET, Lilja B, Lindgärde F, Maly P, Stavenow L (Univ of Lund; Malmö, Sweden)
J Intern Med 229:521–525, 1991   12–8

Background.—Patients with TIAs or minor strokes were studied to determine the incidence of asymptomatic visual field defects by perimetric examination.

Methods.—Twenty-two consecutive male patients with TIA and 18 with minor stroke comprised the study sample. These patients underwent perimetry testing to evaluate cerebral visual field defects approximately 1 year after the event and again almost 6 months later. Regional cerebral blood flow was assessed within 1 month of the event using SPECT. Computed tomographic scanning was done the day after admission and 6 weeks afterward.

Results.—No patient had noticed any visual field symptoms, yet 29% of those with TIA and 57% of those with minor stroke had such defects.

Defects were located in the upper portion of the visual field in 85% of the cases. Computed tomography found new cerebral infarctions in 35% of the patients with TIA and in 61% of the patients with minor stroke. Defective blood flow was found in 85% of the TIA group and 76% in the minor stroke group.

Conclusion.—Patients with carotid TIA and/or stroke have a very high incidence of asymptomatic visual field defects, particularly in the upper half of the visual field. These findings do not correlate with CT and regional cerebral blood flow measurements.

▶ It is fascinating that such a remarkable percentage of patients with carotid TIAs and/or minor stroke have asymptomatic visual field defects. The obvious question is how does this compare with similar age-matched patients in the authors' clinic who do not have TIAs or minor strokes? Unfortunately, the lack of a case-control study and the absence of control data make the contained information far less valuable than it may otherwise have been.—J.M. Porter, M.D.

Carotid Endarterectomy and Prevention of Cerebral Ischemia in Symptomatic Carotid Stenosis

Mayberg MR, for the Veterans Affairs Cooperative Studies Program 309 Trialist Group (Univ of Washington, Seattle)
JAMA 266:3289–3294, 1991   12–9

Introduction.—Patients with symptoms of cerebral or retinal ischemia in the distribution of a hemodynamically significant internal carotid artery stenosis are believed to represent a distinct subgroup at increased risk for stroke.

Methods.—To determine whether carotid endarterectomy provides protection against subsequent cerebral ischemia in men with ischemic symptoms in the distribution of significant ipsilateral internal carotid artery stenosis, 16 university-affiliated Veterans Affairs medical centers participated in a prospective, randomized trial of men with TIAs or small strokes and > 50% stenosis of the ipsilateral carotid artery. Carotid endarterectomy plus best medical care was given to 91 patients, and best medical care alone was given to 98. The average follow-up was 11.9 months.

Results.—Stroke or crescendo transient ischemic attacks occurred in significantly fewer patients in the endarterectomy group (7.7%) than in the nonsurgical group (19.4%), for an absolute risk reduction of 11.7%. The benefit of surgery was more pronounced in patients with internal carotid artery stenosis of greater than 70% (table).

Conclusion.—Carotid endarterectomy can reduce the risk of subsequent ipsilateral cerebral ischemia in selected patients with symptoms of cerebral or retinal ischemia in the distribution of a high-grade internal

Secondary and Primary End Points

End Points	Surgical	Nonsurgical	Total
Secondary end points			
Crossover between groups	0	3	3
Withdrew from trial	4	5	9
Significant reaction to aspirin	2	1	3
Nonstroke death >30 d after randomization	4	2	6
Contralateral ischemia	0	1	1
Not available for follow-up	1	0	1
Total	**11**	**12**	**23**
Primary end points			
Events within 30 d of randomization			
Minor stroke	2	2	4
Major stroke	1*	0	1
Crescendo transient ischemic attack	0	4	4
Death	3†	0	3
Events >30 d after randomization			
Minor stroke	0	2	2
Major stroke	1	3	4
Crescendo transient ischemic attack	0	8	8
Total	**7**	**19**	**26**

* One Stroke occurred before surgery.
† Ruptured aortic aneurysm, pulmonary embolus, and cerebral hemorrhage occurred after discharge from the hospital.
(Courtesy of Mayberg MR, for the Veterans Affairs Cooperative Studies Program 309 Trialist Group: JAMA 266:3289–3294, 1991.)

carotid artery stenosis. In this subgroup, the risk of cerebral ischemia is much higher than once believed.

▶ This study shows a significant reduction in stroke or crescendo TIAs in patients with carotid disease and TIAs who are randomized to carotid endarterectomy, compared with those who are randomized to best medical care. However, the combined stroke and mortality rate of the operated patients was a disappointing 5.5%. This study again notes that patients with 50% to 70% carotid stenosis received less benefit then those with greater than 70% stenosis from carotid endarterectomy; this is currently a widely held position. See also the comments after Abstract 12–1.—J.M. Porter, M.D.

Spinal Accessory (11th) Nerve Palsy Following Carotid Endarterectomy
Sweeney PJ, Wilbourn AJ (Cleveland Clinic Found)
Neurology 42:674–675, 1992   12–10

Introduction.—Data were reviewed on 3 patients who sustained injury to only the 11th cranial nerve in the course of carotid endarterectomy. The 10th and 12th cranial nerves are injured in as many as 7% of pa-

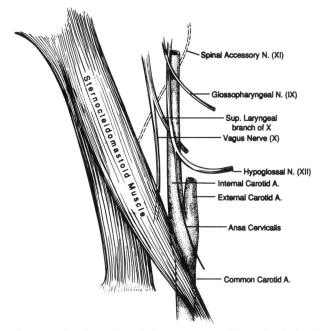

Fig 12–2.—Right neck, lateral view. The spinal accessory nerve is illustrated in *broken lines* coursing inferiorly deep to internal carotid artery and piercing the sternocleidomastoid muscle. (Courtesy of Sweeny PJ, Wilbourn AJ: *Neurology* 42:674–675, 1992.)

tients who have endarterectomy, but spinal accessory mononeuropathy is quite rare.

Causes and Effects.—Isolated partial palsy of the spinal accessory nerve is most often caused by surgery in the posterior triangle of the neck. Jugular venous cannulation is another possible cause. The nerve (Fig 12-2) provides motor innervation to the trapezius and sternocleidomastoid muscles, but sensory symptoms are prominent. Discomfort or pain is felt in the shoulder apex, lateral neck, and periauricular region. There may be a reduced range of ipsilateral shoulder motion, and patients may find it difficult to comb their hair or pull a sweater on or off. An altered clavicular alignment may produce a perception of asymmetry on the part of the patient.

▶ The vagus, recurrent laryngeal, superior laryngeal, hypoglossal, and glossopharyngeal nerves are widely regarded as being at risk for injury during carotid endarterectomy. To this list we must now also add nerve XI , the spinal accessory.—J.M. Porter, M.D.

Progression to Total Occlusion Is an Underrecognized Complication of the Medical Management of Carotid Disease

Perler BA, Burdick JF, Williams GM (Johns Hopkins Univ, Baltimore)
J Vasc Surg 14:821–828, 1991   12–11

Background.—Carotid artery disease may progress to total occlusion while the patient is under medical management. This may occur silently, or it may produce only mild neurologic symptoms.

Methods.—A group of 993 patients who had carotid angiography included 44 who had internal carotid artery occlusion caused by atherosclerotic disease. The 31 men and 13 women had a mean age of 65.9 years.

Findings.—The modes of clinical presentation ranged from stroke and retinal infarction to transient ischemic attacks and nonhemispheric symptoms. Ten of the 44 patients were asymptomatic. Hemispheric symptoms referable to the new occluded vessel had occurred in 5 of 9 patients seen with stroke, 5 of 8 with retinal infarction, 6 of 10 with transient ischemic attacks, and all 4 with amaurosis fugax. In all, 64% of the patients had ipsilateral symptoms a mean of 30 months before carotid artery occlusion was diagnosed.

Conclusion.—Total occlusion is a serious complication when symptomatic carotid artery disease is managed expectantly. More aggressive assessment and surgery for patients with symptomatic disease can prevent these occurrences.

▶ This study is flawed by its retrospective design, but it nevertheless reaches some important conclusions. The authors once again note that approximately 30% to 50% of patients with internal carotid artery occlusion have a stroke history appropriate to the lesion. A significant additional number of patients has neurologic symptoms. The important point is that this retrospective chart review indicated that 64% of all patients with internal carotid artery occlusion had experienced clear-cut ipsilateral symptoms of carotid stenosis before the occlusive event, and that only 28% of these patients had undergone any evaluation or had received any treatment. The authors advocate a more aggressive evaluation and surgical treatment of patients with symptomatic carotid disease, a position with which few of us can disagree.—J.M. Porter, M.D.

Delayed Postoperative Bleeding From Polytetrafluoroethylene Carotid Artery Patches

McCready RA, Siderys H, Pittman JN, Herod GT, Halbrook HG, Fehrenbacher JW, Beckman DJ, Hormuth DA (Methodist Hosp, Indianapolis)
J Vasc Surg 15:661–663, 1992   12–12

Introduction.—Routine patch angioplasty of the internal carotid artery after endarterectomy has been suggested as a way of reducing the risk of early postoperative thrombosis and recurrent carotid stenosis. However, patch angioplasty may be complicated by rupture of a saphenous vein patch, and rupture of polytetrafluoroethylene (PTFE) patches has also been reported.

Case 1.—Woman, 61, with asymptomatic 90% stenosis underwent left carotid endarterectomy with a PTFE patch. An expanding hematoma developed 36 hours postoperatively and produced respiratory distress. Two needle holes in the suture line were actively bleeding. Bleeding was controlled with Gelfoam and thrombin, and the patient recovered.

Case 2.—Woman, 70, underwent a carotid endarterectomy for preocclusive stenosis 6 weeks after a hemispheric stroke. The arteriotomy was closed with a PTFE patch. A large hematoma suddenly developed in the wound 4 days postoperatively, representing bleeding from a single needle hole in the suture line, which was readily controlled.

Case 3.—Man, 62, underwent a carotid endarterectomy with a PTFE patch. A rapidly expanding hematoma developed 36 hours later, which was caused by bleeding through 2 needle holes in the patch. The bleeding was controlled by Gelfoam and thrombin.

Conclusion.—These 3 patients were among 87 patients who underwent carotid endarterectomy during a 1-year period. Prosthetic PTFE patches, usually .4 mm in size, were used in 18 patients.

▶ Based on numerous impressive—if not conclusive—studies, the use of patches after carotid endarterectomy has become much more frequent in recent years. Patch material generally has consisted of saphenous vein, Dacron, or PTFE. Blow out of the saphenous vein patch has been well described. At least one report speaks to rupture of the PTFE patches. This report describes 3 patients who had significant delayed bleeding (through needle holes with a PTFE patch) that required return to the operating room between 1½ and 4 days after surgery. In each case, bleeding was controlled by the topical application of thrombin and oxidized cellulose. This occurred during the time interval when the same practice group used 18 PTFE carotid patches, 15 of which had no symptoms. I am unable to further evaluate this uncommon occurrence. Vascular surgeons should be familiar with this report (1).—J.M. Porter, M.D.

Reference

1. Rosenthal D, et al: *J Vasc Surg* 12:326, 1990.

Changes in Middle Cerebral Artery Flow Velocity and Pulsatility Index After Carotid Endarterectomy

Blohmé L, Pagani M, Parra-Hoyos H, Olofsson P, Takolander R, Swedenborg J (Karolinska Hosp, Stockholm)
Eur J Vasc Surg 5:659–663, 1991   12–13

Background.—Cerebral autoregulation partially compensates for the effect of carotid stenosis. After a hemodynamically significant stenosis is corrected, autoregulation must adjust to the new setting. Transcranial Doppler sonography was used to ascertain the hemodynamic changes after carotid endarterectomy in 32 patients undergoing 33 operations.

Methods.—The mean flow velocity (MV) and the pulsatility index (PI) were measured in the middle cerebral artery on multiple occasions after endarterectomy. A 2-MHz pulsed-wave monocrystal-focused transcranial Doppler transducer was used. Twenty-six patients were monitored for up to a year after endarterectomy.

Results.—Mean flow velocity peaked at 43% above baseline 6 hours after surgery (Fig 12–3). The PI also increased significantly after removal of the stenosis, and it remained increased 72 hours postoperatively (Fig 12–4). The increase in PI at 6 hours correlated with the degree of stenosis (Fig 12–5). The MV and PI remained increased at long-term follow-up. Only minimal changes occurred contralaterally in the 22 patients having readings made on both sides.

Conclusion.—The transcranial Doppler study may be a relatively simple and rapid means of assessing hemodynamics in patients undergoing carotid endarterectomy. An increase in cerebral blood flow, although less than early postoperatively, persists many months after surgery.

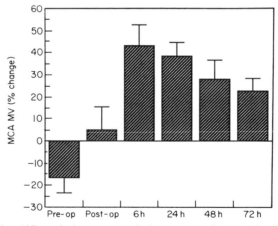

Fig 12–3.—The middle cerebral artery mean velocity percentage change on the operated side in 33 patients measured on 6 occasions before and after carotid endarterectomy. The values entitled *Pre-op* and *Post-op* are measured during anesthesia before and after the surgical procedure. (Courtesy of Blohmé L, Pagani M, Parra-Hoyos H, et al: *Eur J Vasc Surg* 5:659–663, 1991.)

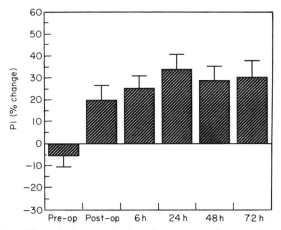

Fig 12–4.—The middle cerebral artery pulsatility index percentage change on the operated side in 33 patients measured on 6 occasions before and after carotid endarterectomy. The values entitled *Pre-op* and *Post-op* are measured during anesthesia before and after the surgical procedure. (Courtesy of Blohmé L, Pagani M, Parra-Hoyos H, et al: *Eur J Vasc Surg* 5:659–663, 1991.)

▶ Increasing information suggests that transcranial Doppler-detected cerebral flow velocity actually does correlate reasonably well with isotope measurements of cerebral blood flow. This study documents that transcranial Doppler findings after carotid endarterectomy indicate increased cerebral blood flow. The finding of increased flow in the middle cerebral artery on the operated side is hardly surprising, but it is gratifying. Perhaps this testing modality will be helpful in the objective diagnosis of the occasional patient with

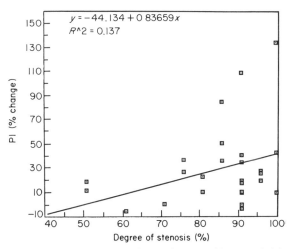

Fig 12–5.—Percentage change at 6 hours vs. degree of stenosis. (Courtesy of Blohmé L, Pagani M, Parra-Hoyos H, et al: *Eur J Vasc Surg* 5:659–663, 1991.)

cerebral hyperperfusion syndrome after carotid endarterectomy.—J.M. Porter, M.D.

Relation of Plasma Lipid and Apoprotein Levels to Progressive Intimal Hyperplasia After Arterial Endarterectomy

Colyvas N, Rapp JH, Phillips NR, Stoney R, Perez S, Kane JP, Havel RJ (Univ of California, San Francisco)
Circulation 85:1286–1292, 1992   12–14

Background.—An attempt was made to relate plasma lipoprotein levels to the proliferative response after arterial injury by estimating lipids, lipoproteins, and apoproteins in 20 patients who had recurrent stenosis shortly after carotid endarterectomy. Intimal hyperplasia was responsible for the stenoses. Twenty patients without recurrent stenosis also were studied.

Findings.—Reoperated patients had higher levels of plasma cholesterol total triglycerides and low-density lipoprotein (LDL) apoprotein B than did the control patients. The ratio of cholesterol level to LDL apoprotein B level was lower in the patients with restenosis. The high-density lipoprotein cholesterol level was lower in the patients with restenosis and, like the LDL apoprotein B level, was an independent predictor of the risk of restenosis.

Conclusion.—Increased lipid levels that are usually associated with an increased risk of atherosclerosis may predispose to intimal hyperplasia after carotid endarterectomy.

▶ These authors statistically relate recurrent stenosis occurring after carotid endarterectomy to an increased serum lipid level. Despite current analysis, the study is clearly retrospective in that the patients underwent surgery between 6 and 10 years ago.—J.M. Porter, M.D.

Selection of the Approach to the Distal Internal Carotid Artery From the Second Cervical Vertebra to the Base of the Skull

Mock CN, Lilly MP, McRae RG, Carney WI Jr (Brown Univ, Providence, RI)
J Vasc Surg 13:846–853, 1991   12–15

Objective.—A total of 12 cadavers were dissected bilaterally to define the limits of distal internal carotid artery exposure using several commonly recommended methods.

Results.—A standard anterior approach along the sternocleidomastoid muscle exposed the internal carotid artery to the level of the upper third of the second cervical vertebra (Fig 12–6). Dividing the posterior belly of the digastric muscle extended the upper limit of this exposure to the middle of the first cervical vertebra. Anterior subluxation of the mandi-

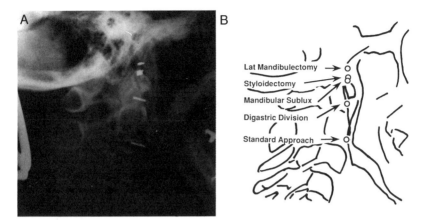

Fig 12–6.—**A,** a lateral cervical radiograph of a representative anatomical specimen. The metal clips were placed on the internal carotid artery (ICA) at the distal extent of the exposure obtained with each of the surgical techniques studied. From caudal to cephalad, the clips represent the distal exposure provided by (1) the standard approach, (2) the standard approach with division of the diagastric muscle, (3) the standard approach with division of the diagastric muscle and mandibular subluxation, (4) the standard approach with division of the diagastric muscle and mandibular subluxation and styloidectomy, and (5) all of the above plus lateral mandibulotomy. **B,** a schematic diagram of the radiograph in **A.** (Courtesy of Mock CN, Lilly MP, McRae RG, et al: *J Vasc Surg* 13:846:853, 1991.)

ble extended the distal exposure to the superior border of the first cervical vertebra. The addition of styloidectomy to the other maneuvers extended exposure by an additional .5 cm. Lateral mandibulotomy did not significantly improve exposure. Exposure of the internal carotid artery in the 1 cm just below the skull base requires a posterior approach with mastoidectomy.

▶ This interesting study, with data derived from cadaver dissection, defines the limits of distal internal carotid artery exposure that can be achieved using several frequently advocated methods. Division of the digastric muscle, anterior subluxation of the mandible, and styloidectomy are all helpful. Lateral mandibulotomy did not appear to add to the exposure.—J.M. Porter, M.D.

Direct Vein Graft Reconstruction of the Cavernous, Petrous, and Upper Cervical Internal Carotid Artery: Lessons Learned From 30 Cases
Sen C, Sekhar LN (Univ of Pittsburgh)
Neurosurgery 30:732–743, 1992   12–16

Introduction.—In 1985-1991, 30 patients underwent internal carotid artery reconstruction at the base of the skull, using saphenous vein, during surgical treatment of lesions at the cranial base. They constituted almost 9% of all patients in whom the cavernous or petrous part of the internal carotid was manipulated during treatment of a tumor.

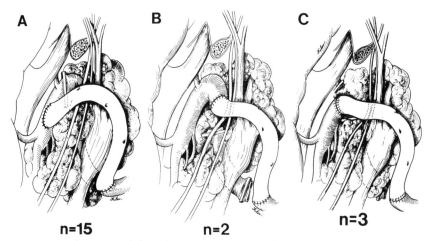

Fig 12–7.—Short vein graft from the petrous internal carotid artery (ICA). **A,** end-to-side supraclinoid ICA. **B,** end-to-end infraclinoid ICA with preservation of the ophthalmic artery. **C,** end-to-end supraclinoid ICA with obliteration of the ophthalmic artery. (Courtesy of Sen C, Sekhar LN: *Neurosurgery* 30:732–743, 1992.)

Methods.—Reconstruction is based on the results of balloon test occlusion of the internal carotid artery and the patient's age. The techniques included a petrous-to-supraclinoid/paraclinoid carotid anastomosis (Fig 12–7); a cervical-to-supraclinoid carotid vein graft (Fig 12–8); and a cervical-to-petrous carotid anastomosis. In 2 patients, a lacerated carotid artery was repaired with a saphenous vein patch graft.

Results.—The balloon test occlusion failed in 2 patients, and in 9 others, there was a decrease in cerebral blood flow to 15–30 mL/100 g/min. The patency rate after a mean follow-up of 18 months was 86%. Of 4 patients with an occluded graft, 3 were asymptomatic, and the fourth later died of massive cerebral infarction. Minor strokes occurred after graft surgery in 3 patients with inadequate collateral circulation, but all were leading independent lives. Revision was successful in 2 patients who had graft occlusion within 12 hours of surgery. Of the 19 benign tumors, 14 were totally removed. All 5 aneurysms were successfully eliminated.

Conclusion.—Direct vein graft reconstruction of the internal carotid artery has vastly improved the ability to treat neoplastic and vascular disorders at the cranial base.

▶ This is a fascinating report of what aggressive microvascular neurosurgeons are currently achieving with vein grafting to the internal carotid artery. It is impressive.—J.M. Porter, M.D.

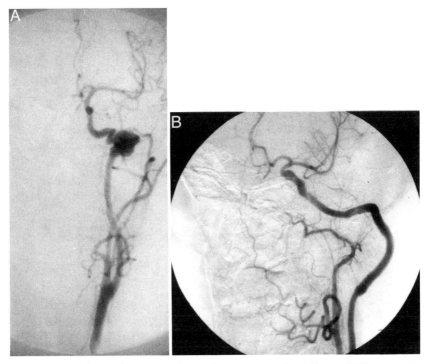

Fig 12–8.—A, left carotid arteriogram showing the petrous internal carotid artery (ICA) aneurysm. **B,** a long vein graft from the cervical to the supraclinoid ICA. (Courtesy of Sen C, Sekhar LN: *Neurosurgery* 30:732-743, 1992.)

Resolution of Petrous Internal Carotid Artery Stenosis After Transluminal Angioplasty: Case Report

Rostomily RC, Mayberg MR, Eskridge JM, Goodkin R, Winn HR (Univ of Washington, Seattle)
J Neurosurg 76:520–523, 1992   12–17

Introduction.—Percutaneous transluminal angioplasty—commonly used to treat peripheral vascular disease—recently has been applied to craniocervical lesions. A study patient who had progressive ischemic symptoms, despite maximum medical treatment for high-grade stenosis of the petrous part of the internal carotid artery, was effectively managed by percutaneous transluminal angioplasty.

Case Report.—Man, 68, had had progressive transient cerebral and retinal ischemic symptoms related to the left internal carotid artery circulation for 1 year. Flow through the left cervical internal carotid artery was reduced, but focal stenosis was not seen on duplex examination. Angiography showed focal 95% stenosis of the left intrapetrous internal carotid artery. A left thalamic infarct was seen on CT study. Angioplasty of the left petrous internal carotid artery was carried out in stages, reducing stenosis to less than 40%. Systemic heparin and then warfarin were administered. Symptoms have been absent for 2 years since angioplasty, with the patient receiving low-dose aspirin. A repeat angiogram showed 20% stenosis on the left side, with remodeling at the angioplasty site.

▶ The performance of percutaneous transluminal angioplasty of the intracranial carotid artery indicates the existence of a great deal of self-confidence among interventional radiologists. The dramatic clinical and radiologic improvement in a single patient after PTLA of the petrous internal carotid artery is described. I have no idea how widely applicable this technique may be, but it clearly may be of dramatic benefit in individual patients.—J.M. Porter, M.D.

Failure of Aspirin Plus Dipyridamole to Prevent Restenosis After Carotid Endarterectomy

Harker LA, Bernstein EF, Dilley RB, Scala TE, Sise MJ, Hye RJ, Otis SM, Roberts RS, Gent M (Scripps Clinic and Research Found, La Jolla, Calif; Emory Univ, Atlanta; Univ of California, San Diego; McMaster Univ, Hamilton, Ont)
Ann Intern Med 116:731–736, 1992   12–18

Background.—Previous reports have suggested that the combination of aspirin and dipyridamole may reduce the rate of progression of atherosclerotic disease in coronary and peripheral arteries, and it also may inhibit vascular lesions after mechanical injury. Aspirin/dipyridamole treatment was evaluated in 163 patients having 175 carotid endarterectomies.

Methods.—Eighty-three patients having 90 endarterectomies received 325 mg of aspirin plus 75 mg of dipyridamole, administered orally 12 hours preoperatively. A second dose was given within 8 hours after surgery and then 3 times daily for 1 year. The other 80 patients, having 85 operations, received placebo medication.

Results.—The incidence of restenosis exceeding 50% was 16% in treated patients and 14% in placebo recipients. Stenosis exceeding 20% also was more frequent in the actively treated patients. Intention-to-treat analysis revealed that stenosis greater than 50% developed in 26% of the operated arteries in treated patients and in 12% of those in the placebo group ($P = .18$).

Conclusion.—Aspirin plus dipyridamole probably confers no significant clinical benefit on patients having carotid endarterectomy.

▶ This well-designed and well-conducted prospective, randomized study of carotid endarterectomy indicates that the use of aspirin and dipyridamole not only fails to reduce the incidence of carotid stenosis, but actually may increase its frequency. There is overwhelming evidence that currently available antiplatelet drugs will not reduce the incidence of postoperative fibrointimal hyperplasia. They do, however, appear to be of clear benefit in both the primary and secondary prevention of myocardial infarction.—J.M. Porter, M.D.

Spontaneous Dissection of the Cervical Internal Carotid Artery: Presentation With Lower Cranial Nerve Palsies
Mokri B, Schievink WI, Olsen KD, Piepgras DG (Mayo Clinic and Found, Rochester, Minn)
Arch Otolaryngol Head Neck Surg 118:431–435, 1992   12–19

Background.—Spontaneous dissections of the internal carotid arteries are infrequent but not rare, and they are a fairly common cause of ischemic stroke in younger patients. Patients most often are seen with one-sided headaches followed by focal cerebral ischemic symptoms, or with unilateral headaches with an incomplete ipsilateral Horner's syndrome. A bruit may or may not occur.

Cranial Nerve Palsy.—Rarely, spontaneous internal carotid artery dissection produces a lower cranial nerve palsy with consequent dysphonia, dysarthria, dysphagia, and numbness of the throat. These patients may initially be seen by an otolaryngologist. The physicians studied 8 such patients, most of whom recovered to a substantial degree or completely. Cranial nerve XII was involved in all patients: nerves IX–XII in 4 of these, and nerves IX and X in one. Dissections have not recurred in the same vessels, and 90% of angiographic stenoses have resolved partially or completely. Rapid spontaneous neurologic improvement occurred in most patients.

Discussion.—Most physicians believe that these cases represent compression of the lower cranial nerves below the jugular foramen by the dissected vessel. The 8 study patients were among almost 120 patients seen with spontaneous dissection of the internal carotid artery.

▶ Spontaneous dissection of the internal carotid artery may be seen as a frank stroke, or with symptoms of headache, Horner's syndrome, or lower cranial nerve palsies. This interesting otolaryngology report details the findings in 8 patients with lower cranial nerve palsies accompanying carotid dissection.—J.M. Porter, M.D.

Familial Association of Intracranial Aneurysms and Cervical Artery Dissections
Schievink WI, Mokri B, Michels VV, Piepgras (Mayo Clinic and Found, Rochester, Minn)
Stroke 22:1426–1430, 1991   12–20

Introduction.—Saccular intracranial aneurysms of the circle of Willis are found in 2.5% to 5% of autopsies. Spontaneous cervical artery dissection is less frequent, but it is a cause of ischemic cerebrovascular disease in young and middle-aged individuals.

Methods.—Data were reviewed on 175 patients treated in 1970–1989 for spontaneous dissection of the cervical arteries.

Results.—In 3 families, siblings had both cervical artery dissection and intracranial aneurysm. They represented 1.7% of the patients reviewed.

Conclusion.—These data suggest an underlying arteriopathy common to both cervical artery dissection and intracranial aneurysm which, at least in some patents, may be inherited. Both lesions may involve an underlying anteriopathy combined with hemodynamic and degenerative factors. Both may be associated with such disorders as Ehlers-Danlos syndrome, Marfan's syndrome, collagen type III abnormality, and fibromuscular dysplasia. Similar risk factors, including hypertension, smoking, and oral contraceptive use, are related to both cervical artery dissection and subarachnoid aneurysmal bleeding. Co-existent saccular intracranial aneurysms are found in 5.5% of patients with cervical artery dissection compared with 1% in those without dissection. The occurrence of intracranial aneurysm and cervical arterial dissection in the same families provides support for the existence of a primary underlying arteriopathy in the pathogenesis of these disorders.

▶ The Mayo Clinic has recently reported the angiographic detection of saccular intracranial aneurysms in 5.5% of patients with cervical artery dissection, compared with 1% of patients without cervical artery dissection. This report describes the familial occurrence of intracranial aneurysms in cervical artery dissection, suggesting the occurrence of some type of underlying arteriopathy in the pathogenesis of these disorders. I am sure we will hear more about this in the future. In the meantime, I wonder whether the occasional patient we encounter with cervical internal carotid artery dissection should have detailed intracranial studies to detect aneurysm?—J.M. Porter, M.D.

Angiographic Frequency of Saccular Intracranial Aneurysms in Patients With Spontaneous Cervical Artery Dissection
Schievink WI, Mokri B, Piepgras DG (Mayo Clinic and Found, Rochester, Minn)
J Neurosurg 76:62–66, 1991   12–21

Background.—The pathogenesis of intracranial aneurysm and of spontaneous cervical artery dissection is not completely understood, but it is possible that a primary arteriopathy underlies both disorders.

Methods.—The association of intracranial aneurysm with spontaneous cervical artery dissection was studied by reviewing angiograms from 164 patients who had a diagnosis of spontaneous dissection of the extracranial carotid or vertebral artery.

Results.—A total of 13 intracranial aneurysms were found in 9 of the 164 patients, for an incidence of 5.5%. The incidence was 8.8% in females, whereas only 1 male (1.4%) was affected. The frequency of intracranial aneurysms in the general population in a recent angiographic series from the same institution was 1.1%.

Implication.—It is conceivable that an intracranial aneurysm distal to a narrowed cervical artery will increase in size after resolution of the dissecting process.

▶ This paper details the nonfamilial association of intracranial aneurysms in spontaneous cervical artery dissection described in the comment after Abstract 12–20.—J.M. Porter, M.D.

Combined Carotid Endarterectomy and Coronary Artery Revascularization: A Sobering Review
Bass A, Krupski WC, Dilley RB, Bernstein EF (Chaim Sheba Med Ctr, Tel-Hashomer, Israel; Univ of California, San Francisco; Scripps Clinic and Research Found, La Jolla, Calif)
Isr J Med Sci 28:27–32, 1992   12–22

Introduction.—Diffuse atherosclerotic disease involving multiple major vascular systems presents a difficult therapeutic challenge. These patients may be placed in considerable jeopardy if only 1 involved system is treated.

Methods.—During a 15-year period, 99 patients underwent combined single-stage carotid thromboendarterectomy and coronary bypass grafting at 3 centers. Coronary revascularization was urgent in 46 patients and emergent in 37. Nearly 80% of the patients had asymptomatic carotid stenosis of 80% or greater. Separate surgical teams performed carotid artery surgery and then myocardial revascularization. At least 3 coronary vessels were treated in 90% of the patients.

Results.—The mean patient age was 67 years. Almost half the patients had a previously myocardial infarct, and nearly 60% were hypertensive. Half the patients had smoked. Major neurologic complications occurred in 25% of patients, and stroke ipsilateral to the operated carotid vessel occurred in 11%. Multisystem failure and myocardial infarction each occurred in 8% of patients, and respiratory failure occurred in 5%. The overall mortality rate was 12%; 10 deaths were directly related to cardiac surgery, and 2 were a result of stroke.

Conclusion.—The frequent complications and deaths after combined surgery, even at centers with excellent records for each procedure when performed separately, suggest that the need for both procedures be assessed carefully. Prophylactic carotid endarterectomy has not been shown to reduce the neurologic risk of coronary bypass surgery significantly.

▶ This somber report by excellent clinical surgeons describes the outcome in 99 patients treated with combined carotid endarterectomy and coronary artery bypass at 3 different hospitals during a multi-year period. The overall major neurologic complication rate was 25%, with an 11% stroke rate ipsilateral to the operated carotid. These authors conclude, and I concur, that combined carotid and coronary operations frequently result in a high morbidity and mortality, even in institutions with excellent records for each operation performed separately. This reconfirms my belief that combined carotid-coronary surgery should be performed only on rare occasions.—J.M. Porter, M.D.

A Comparison of Two Doses of Aspirin (30 mg vs. 283 mg a Day) in Patients After a Transient Ischemic Attack or Minor Ischemic Stroke

Dutch TIA Trial Study Group
N Engl J Med 325:1261–1266, 1991   12–23

Background.—Aspirin appears to improve the outcome in patients who have transient cerebral ischemic attacks. However, the optimal dose remains uncertain.

Methods.—A total of 3,131 patients, who had either a transient ischemic attack or a minor stroke, participated in a double-blind randomized trial in which daily doses of aspirin (30 mg and 283 mg) were compared

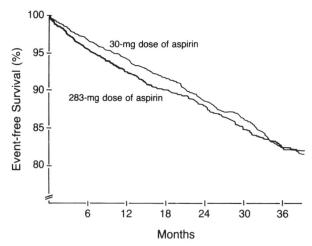

Fig 12–9.—Kaplan-Meier curves for the combined outcome event of death from vascular causes, nonfatal stroke, or nonfatal myocardial infarction, according to assigned treatment. (Courtesy of Dutch TIA Trial Study Group: N Engl J Med 325:1261-1266, 1991.)

to assess endpoints of death from all vascular causes, nonfatal stroke, or nonfatal myocardial infarction.

Results.—The overall incidence of death from vascular causes, nonfatal stroke, and nonfatal myocardial infarction was 14.7% in patients given 30 mg of aspirin daily and 15.2% in those given the higher dose (Fig 12–9). Major bleeding was slightly less frequent in the low-dose group, and minor bleeding was significantly less frequent. In addition, patients given the low dose had fewer gastrointestinal and other adverse effects.

Implications.—A 30-mg daily dose of aspirin is as effective as a 283-mg dose in preventing vascular events in patients seen after a transient ischemic attack or minor stroke, and it is safer. It may be best to begin treatment with a loading dose of at least 120 mg.

▶ The search continues to find an optimal dose of aspirin, in this case for treatment of patients with cerebral transient ischemic attacks. This study indicates that 30 mg of aspirin given daily is as effective in the prevention of vascular events as a 283-mg daily dose. As expected, the lower dose produces fewer drug-related complications. This appears to indicate that a daily "baby" aspirin is as effective as any other aspirin dose for this purpose.—J.M. Porter, M.D.

Swedish Aspirin Low-Dose Trial (SALT) of 75 mg Aspirin as Secondary Prophylaxis After Cerebrovascular Ischaemic Events
SALT Collaborative Group (Danderyd Hosp, Sweden)
Lancet 338:1345–1349, 1991   12–24

Background.—Antiplatelet treatment with aspirin is an established means of secondarily preventing arterial thrombotic disorders, but earlier trials often used high doses needed for analgesic and anti-inflammatory actions. Because lower doses are able to inhibit platelet function, the SALT examined the efficacy of daily administration of 75 mg of aspirin in preventing strokes and deaths after transient ischemic attacks or minor strokes.

Methods.—A total of 1,360 patients were entered into the study within 4 months of the qualifying event. Of these, 676 were assigned randomly to receive aspirin, whereas 684 received a placebo. The median follow-up was 32 months.

Results.—The risk of primary stroke or death was reduced by 18% in patients given aspirin. The risks of secondary outcome events such as stroke and 2 or more transient ischemic attacks within 1 week or myocardial infarction were reduced by 16% to 20%. Gastrointestinal side effects were only slightly more frequent in aspirin recipients than in patients given placebo. Bleeding, however, occurred significantly more often in patients given aspirin. All 5 fatal hemorrhagic strokes occurred in aspirin-treated patients.

Conclusion.—This is the first placebo-controlled trial showing that a daily dose of aspirin less than 300 mg can prevent stroke and death after an episode of cerebrovascular ischemia.

▶ In this study of about half as many patients as described in Abstract 12–23, patients who had had a TIA, minor stroke, or retinal artery occlusion within the previous 3 months were randomized to receive 75 mg of aspirin, given daily, or placebo. The aspirin group showed an 18% reduction in the risk of primary outcome events (stroke vs. death), compared with placebo. This study forms a nice companion to Abstract 12–23, which indicates that low-dose aspirin is as effective as high-dose aspirin.—J.M. Porter, M.D.

Neurologic Deficits Following Noncarotid Vascular Surgery
Harris EJ Jr, Moneta GL, Yeager RA, Taylor LM Jr, Porter JM (Oregon Health Sciences Univ and Portland VA Hosp)
Am J Surg 163:537–540, 1992   12–25

Objective.—All patients seen in a 3-year period with new postoperative focal neurologic events occurring within 2 weeks of a category I or II vascular procedure—excluding carotid artery surgery and arterial trauma—were reviewed. The objective was to determine the incidence and predictability of neurologic events after noncarotid vascular surgery.

Clinical Characteristics of Patients With Anterior
Circulation Neurologic Deficits (Group A) and Case
Controls (Group B) After Vascular Surgery

Variable	Group A (n = 12)	Group B (n = 12)	p
Mean Age (yr)	66.3 ± 4.4	61.7 ± 14.7	NS
Patients with previous neuro-logic events	42%	17%	NS
Intra-abdominal vascular oper-ations	75%	25%	<0.05
Emergent surgery	50%	8%	NS
>50% ipsilateral ICA stenosis	75%	0%	<0.001
Perioperative hypotension	42%	0%	<0.05

Abbreviations: NS, not significant: ICA, internal carotid artery.
Note: $P \geq .05$
(Courtesy of Harris EJ Jr, Moneta GL, Yeager RA, et al: *Am J Surg* 163:537–540, 1992.)

Findings.—Focal neurologic events followed 13 of 1,390 procedures (.9%). They included 10 anterior circulation strokes, 2 transient ischemic attacks, and a single posterior circulation stroke. One fourth of the strokes were fatal. Almost one third of the deficits occurred immediately after surgery, 54% between 4 and 72 hours, and 15% developed more than 3 days after surgery. New anterior circulation events after vascular surgery were statistically associated with intra-abdominal surgery, perioperative hypotension, and a 50% or greater internal carotid stenosis on the same side (table).

Conclusion.—Perioperative neurologic events are infrequent after noncarotid vascular surgery, but they occur more often than after other types of noncardiac, noncerebrovascular surgery.

▶ Stroke is distinctly uncommon after noncarotid vascular surgery, but it occurs at a rate considerably higher than that following other types of noncardiac nonvascular surgery. In many cases, these strokes appear to be associated with significant carotid artery stenosis.—J.M. Porter, M.D.

Urgent Therapy for Stroke: Part I. Pilot Study of Tissue Plasminogen Activator Administered Within 90 Minutes

Brott TG, Haley EC Jr, Levy DE, Barsan W, Broderick J, Sheppard GL, Spilker J, Kongable GL, Massey S, Reed R, Marler JR (Univ of Cincinnati; Univ of Virginia, Charlottesville; Cornell Univ Med College, New York; National Inst of Neurological Disorders and Stroke, Bethesda, Md)
Stroke 23:632–640, 1992   12–26

Background.—Acute thrombus formation and arterial occlusion are the critical pathologic events in at least 70% of strokes. Animal studies suggest that ischemic brain injury takes places when occlusion exceeds 2–3 hours. Recombinant tissue plasminogen activator (rt-PA) was assessed as urgent treatment for acute cerebral infarction in an open-label study.

Methods.—Seventy-four patients received .35 to 1.08 mg of rt-PA per kg, starting within 90 minutes of the onset of symptoms of acute ischemic stroke, using a dose-escalation design.

Results.—Three patients given higher doses of rt-PA had intracranial hematoma develop and then deteriorated neurologically. None of 58 patients given a maximum of .85 mg/kg had hematoma. Thirty percent of the patients had major neurologic improvement 2 hours after the start of treatment, and 46% at 24 hours. Significant improvement did not correlate with either increasing doses or the type of stroke.

Conclusion.—The potential clinical benefit from early administration of rt-PA warrants a randomized trial in patients with acute stroke.

▶ Thrombolytic therapy in the treatment of acute thrombotic stroke has the potential for great benefit, but it also has the potential for great harm. The obvious task is going to be the performance of a detailed and accurate risk benefit analysis. One also wonders how many new patients with stroke will be available for treatment within the short period required for optimal effect.—J.M. Porter, M.D.

Aneurysms of the Extracranial Internal Carotid Artery Due to Fibromuscular Dysplasia: Results of Surgical Management
Bour P, Taghavi I, Bracard S, Frisch N, Fiévé G (Hôpital Central, Nancy, France; Hôpital Saint Julien, Nancy)
Ann Vasc Surg 6:205–208, 1992   12–27

Patients.—Eight patients had surgical repair of aneurysms of the extracranial internal carotid artery, caused by fibromuscular dysplasia, in 1977 through 1990. The mean age of the 6 men and 2 women was 50 years. Five of the patients were seen with hemispheric symptoms. Most of the aneurysms were saccular (Fig 12–10) and were found at the C-2 or C-3 level.

Treatment.—A conventional cervicotomy was performed in all patients. Five patients underwent resection and graft repair, and 3 had resection with anastomosis. All specimens exhibited fibromuscular dysplasia of the arterial media.

Results.—No CNS-related morbidity or mortality occurred. One patient died of myocardial infarction 8 years after surgery. The other 7 were alive and free of new neurologic abnormalities after a mean follow-up of 13 years. Postoperative duplex studies or arteriograms showed that 7 patients had patent carotid vessels. One had occlusion at 18 months but was asymptomatic.

▶ Extracranial carotid aneurysms resulting from fibromuscular dysplasia are frequently diffuse and extend high in the cervical region. Excision and interposition saphenous vein grafting appears to be the procedure of choice for most of these.—J.M. Porter, M.D.

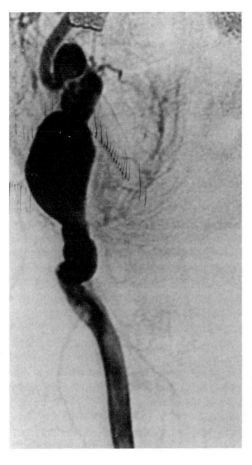

Fig 12–10.—Carotid arteriogram in a woman, 37, with fibromuscular dysplastic aneurysm of internal carotid artery extending from C-2 to C-4. (Courtesy of Bour P, Taghavi I, Bracard S, et al: *Ann Vasc Surg* 6:205–208, 1992.)

MRC European Carotid Surgery Trial: Interim Results for Symptomatic Patients With Severe (70–99%) or With Mild (0–29%) Cartoid Stenosis

European Carotid Surgery Trialists' Collaborative Group
Lancet 337:1235–1243, 1991   12–28

Background.—Patients who have had a nondisabling carotid territory ischemic stroke, transient ischemic attack (TIA), or retinal infarct, and are found to have stenosis at or near the bifurcation of the carotid artery on angiography, were randomized to surgery. Interim results are given of a multicenter, randomized trial designed to determine the operative and long-term risks of disabling stroke and the duration of nondisabled survival for patients with mild, moderate, or severe stenosis.

Methods.—During the past 10 years 2,518 patients at 80 centers were entered into the European Carotid Surgery Trial. All had a carotid territory nondisabling stroke or TIA, or a retinal infarct within the 6 months preceding randomization, and all had stenosis of the relevant carotid artery. Mild stenosis was defined as 0% to 29%; moderate stenosis was defined as 30% to 69%; and severe stenosis was defined as 70% to 99%. The patients were randomized to receive immediate surgery or no surgery. The mean follow-up to date is 3 years for 2,200 patients available for analysis of strokes lasting more than 7 days.

Results.—Moderate stenosis was seen in almost half the randomized patients. For this group, no conclusions could be drawn regarding the risk-benefit ratio of surgery, and full recruitment continues. Mild stenosis was seen in 374 patients. Even without surgery, these patients had little risk of ipsilateral stroke at 3 years; thus, the benefits of surgery were outweighed by the early risks. Severe stenosis was seen in 778 patients. In this group, the late benefits of surgery significantly outweighed its early risks. Overall, 7.5% of the patients with severe stenosis had a stroke or died within 30 days of surgery. During the next 3 years, however, patients who underwent immediate surgery had an extra 2.8% risk of ipsilateral stroke compared with 16.8% for controls. The surgery group also had a small reduction in the incidence of other strokes. The total risk of surgical death, ipsilateral stroke, or any stroke was 12.3% for the immediate surgery group compared with 21.9% for the control group. Disabling stroke or death occurred within 30 days of surgery in 3.7% of the patients. An extra 1.1% of surgery patients had a disabling stroke or died within 3 years compared with 8.4% of controls. The overall risk of any disabling or fatal stroke, including surgical death, was 6% in the surgery group compared with 11% in controls. In controls, however, the risks appeared to diminish after the first year, suggesting that delaying surgery by just a few months may make the overall difference nonsignificant.

Conclusion.—For patients with severe stenosis, carotid endarterectomy can avoid most ipsilateral ischemic strokes for the next few years. There is no apparent benefit of surgery in patients with mild stenosis, and recruitment continues in patients with moderate stenosis.

▶ This study stretches the definition of "randomized trial" to the limit. If the attending physician was "reasonably certain" after angiography that surgery was indicated, then the patient was declared ineligible for the trial. Thus, there is a major sampling error. In spite of this and other flaws in the study, it does corroborate the results of the NASCET trial, showing a clear advantage for carotid endarterectomy in symptomatic patients with 70% or greater internal carotid artery stenosis.—F.W. LoGerfo, M.D.

Regression of Carotid Plaques During Low Density Lipoprotein Cholesterol Elimination

Hennerici M, Kleophas W, Gries FA (Heinrich-Heine Univ, Düsseldorf, Germany)

Stroke 22:989–992, 1991 12–29

Introduction.—Studies in animals have shown that experimental atherosclerosis can be reversed. In humans, risk factor reduction and medical treatment can prevent the progression of atherosclerosis, but its reversal has not been demonstrated conclusively. High-resolution ultrasound duplex scanning was used to prospectively monitor the volume of carotid artery plaques in patients undergoing treatment for inherited hypercholesterolemia.

Patients.—Seven men with inherited heterogeneous low-density lipoprotein (LDL) receptor deficiency underwent heparin-induced extracorporeal LDL precipitation (HELP). This technique involves separating blood cells from whole blood, after which plasma is mixed with acetate buffer and heparin that precipitates LDL cholesterol and fibrinogen. Plasma is restored by filtration and bicarbonate dialysis. The technique can remove as much as 70% of LDL cholesterol per treatment. Low density lipoprotein cholesterol levels were measured before and after HELP, which was performed once a week. Plaque volume was measured with an ultrasound duplex prototype that combines high-resolution B-mode imaging with a specially designed 3-dimensional reconstruction facility. A 16-channel pulsed-Doppler flowmeter was used for the quantitative analysis of associated local blood flow disturbances. Ultrasound measurements were obtained at 3-month intervals.

Results.—During a mean follow-up period of 17 months, a total of 21 ultrasound studies of 4 flat and 17 soft carotid artery plaques were obtained. All patients had regression of carotid artery plaque. Regression occurred within 6 months in 6 patients and within 12 months in 1 patient. Thereafter, vessel wall changes persisted during continuous HELP treatment in 6 patients. Plaque progressed in 1 patient who still had intermittent increase of serum lipid levels despite HELP treatment. Doppler signal evaluations revealed no or only minor flow velocity pattern deterioration consistent with insignificant lumen obstruction at study entry.

Conclusion.—Heparin-induced extracorporeal LDL precipitation significantly reduced plaque volume in the carotid arteries of patients with inherited heterogeneous LDL receptor deficiency and markedly reduced their serum total cholesterol, LDL cholesterol, and fibrinogen levels.

▶ A reduction in the volume of carotid plaques was demonstrated after marked reduction in serum lipid levels in men with familial hypercholesterolemia. None of the carotid lesions were clinically significant, and none produced significant lumen obstruction. The lesions were likely to be foam cell lesions or fatty streaks, which are well known to regress with cholesterol reduction in experimental atherosclerosis. Whether fatty streaks evolve into or are precursors of clinically significant fibrocalcific plaques is unresolved. Thus, the observation that fatty streaks regress with cholesterol reduction may have little clinical relevance for carotid atherosclerosis. Most patients with clinically significant fibrocalcific plaques have normal or near normal serum cholesterol levels. The 1 carotid lesion in this study that was clinically significant (70% to 80% stenosis) developed during the time of cholesterol reduction, suggesting that mechanisms other than hypercholesterolemia are primarily responsible for carotid stenosis.—C. Zarins, M.D.

13 Grafts and Graft Complications

Improved Technique for Polytetrafluoroethylene Bypass Grafting: Long-Term Results Using Anastomotic Vein Patches
Taylor RS, Loh A, McFarland RJ, Cox M, Chester JF (St George's Hosp, London; Epsom District Hosp, Surrey, England; Taunton and Somerset Hosp, Taunton, England)
Br J Surg 79:348–354, 1992   13–1

Background.—The polytetrafluoroethylene (PTFE) graft is the best alternative for use in patients requiring infrainguinal arterial reconstruction who lack an adequate vein. Many optimistic reports on PTFE grafts have, however, proved to be premature, especially for anastomoses to the tibial and peroneal vessels. A modified operative technique based on incorporating a vein patch into the distal anastomosis was developed.

Methods.—The procedure is illustrated in Figures 13–1 through 13–5). The arteriotomy is 3–4 cm long, 4 to 5 times longer than the diameter of the 6-mm PTFE conduit. Distal anastomotic narrowing is largely avoided by trimming the graft appropriately and placing it so that the widest part overlies the distal limit of the anastomosis.

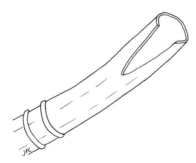

Fig 13–1.—The external support of the PTFE is removed over a length of 3–4 cm, and a short (1 cm) U-shaped slit is cut as shown. (Courtesy of Taylor RS, Loh A, McFarland RJ, et al: *Br J Surg* 79:348–354, 1992.)

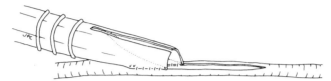

Fig 13–2.—The heel of the graft is sutured and slid down in parachute fashion. Suturing is completed along each side. Note the narrow angle between the graft and the artery. The PTFE is incised over a length of 3 cm. The proximal limit is fashioned in a U shape, the surplus graft being trimmed as shown by the *dotted lines*. (Courtesy of Taylor RS, Loh A, McFarland RJ, et al: *Br J Surg* 79:348–354, 1992.)

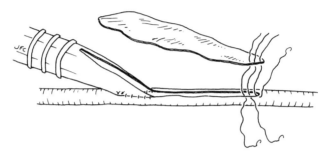

Fig 13–3.—The critical distal interrupted sutures between the vein patch and artery are all inserted under direct vision before any are tied. (Courtesy of Taylor RS, Loh A, McFarland RJ, et al: *Br J Surg* 79:348–354, 1992.)

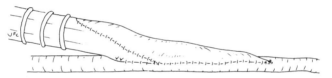

Fig 13–4.—Correct appearance of the completed vein patch that is tapered smoothly to enable a gradual reduction in diameter. (Courtesy of Taylor RS, Loh A, McFarland RJ, et al: *Br J Surg* 79:348–354, 1992.)

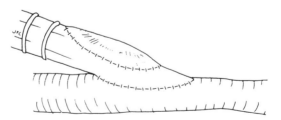

Fig 13–5.—In the proximal anastomosis, a 3-cm vein patch is inserted across the inlet of the PTFE graft. (Courtesy of Taylor RS, Loh A, McFarland RJ, et al: *Br J Surg* 79:348–354, 1992.)

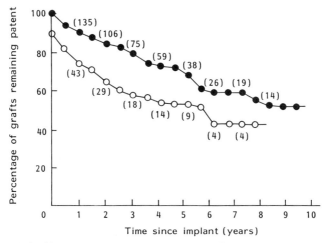

Fig 13–6.—Life-table curves comparing the primary patency of all popliteal grafts with infrapopliteal grafts. Above- and below-knee femoropopliteal grafts are designated by *closed circles*; femorotibial/peroneal grafts are designated by *open circles*. (Courtesy of Taylor RS, Loh A, McFarland RJ, et al: *Br J Surg* 79:348–354, 1992.)

Results.—In 256 patients operated on in 1982–1989, the 5-year patency rate was 71% for popliteal grafts and 54% for infrapopliteal grafts (Fig 13-6). All 6 immediate failures were bypasses to the ankle or foot level.

Conclusion.—An overall 5-year patency rate of 65% warrants the continued use of PTFE grafts if a suitable vein is not available.

▶ The first 3 abstracts in this section describe innovative technical methods for potentially improved prosthetic graft patency. For years, I have heard references to the Miller collar and the Taylor patch. This article describing the Taylor patch in detail is utterly remarkable. Using this technique in a large number of patients undergoing leg prosthetic grafting, the authors achieved the remarkable results of a 5-year primary patency of 71% with prosthetic grafting above and below the knee, and a 5-year primary patency of 54% with grafting to the infrapopliteal vessels. Postoperative anticoagulation was not used in these patients. These results are much superior to any previously reported with prosthetic grafting, and they are very close to those currently reported with vein grafting. This technique, if confirmed by other centers, may prove to be the most significant advance in lower extremity prosthetic bypass grafting to date.—J.M. Porter, M.D.

New Prosthetic Venous Collar Anastomotic Technique: Combining the Best of Other Procedures

Tyrrell MR, Wolfe JHN (St Mary's Hosp, London)
Br J Surg 78:1016–1017, 1991

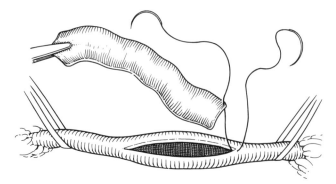

Fig 13–7.—A segment of vein has been split open longitudinally, and 1 corner is anastomosed to the apex of the arteriotomy. (Courtesy of Tyrrell MR, Wolfe JHN: *Br J Surg* 78:1016–1017, 1991.)

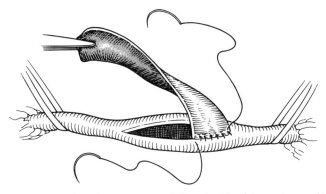

Fig 13–8.—The distal leading edge is anastomosed along the side of the arteriotomy. (Courtesy of Tyrrell MR, Wolfe JHN: *Br J Surg* 78:1016–1017, 1991.)

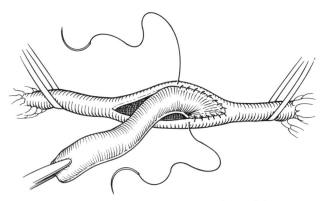

Fig 13–9.—The longitudinal length of vein is then anastomosed around the arteriotomy. (Courtesy of Tyrrell MR, Wolfe JHN: *Br J Surg* 78:1016–1017, 1991.)

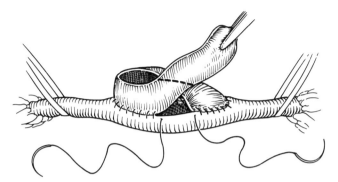

Fig 13–10.—A collar is formed and the redundant vein can be removed. The proximal edge of the vein collar is then anastomosed to the longitudinal edge. (Courtesy of Tyrrell MR, Wolfe JHN: *Br J Surg* 78:1016–1017, 1991.)

Introduction.—Reconstruction of single calf arteries using polytetra-fluoroethylene (PTFE) generally produces a poor outcome, with approximately one third of graft failures ascribed to progressive intimal hyperplasia at sites of anastomosis. Both a mismatch in anastomotic compliance and arterial distortion may contribute to this process.

Methods.—Miller and Taylor recently described modified distal PTFE-artery anastomotic techniques that have been associated with a significant improvement in intermediate-term PTFE-tibial bypass patency. However, the Miller collar produces turbulence because of its shape, whereas the Taylor patch requires direct PTFE-artery suturing, thereby increasing the likelihood of fibrointimal hyperplasia at this site. A new vein collar technique was developed to preserve the advantages of both while hopefully eliminating the disadvantages (Figs 13–7 through 13–12).

Conclusion.—This method provides a fully compliant venous collar while avoiding direct contact between the artery and graft. Greater graft longevity may result.

▶ This group at Saint Mary's Hospital in London describes an attractive modification of the Miller collar. They do not have clinical results with this

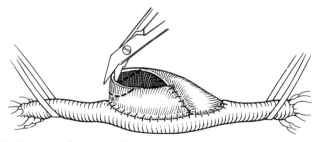

Fig 13–11.—A segment of posterior collar is incised to increase the size of the anastomosis between PTFE and the vein collar. (Courtesy of Tyrrell MR, Wolfe JHN: *Br J Surg* 78:1016–1017, 1991.)

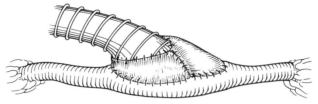

Fig 13–12.—The completed anastomosis. (Courtesy of Tyrrell MR, Wolfe JHN: *Br J Surg* 78:1016–1017, 1991.)

technique, so no patency figures can be quoted. When faced with the need to use a prosthetic leg bypass graft, I currently attempt to use the Taylor patch technique as described in Abstract 13–1.—J.M. Porter, M.D.

End-to-End Anastomosis Between a Prosthesis and a Vein of Different Diameters: A Technique That Maintains a Straight Vascular Axis
Merlini MP, Dusmet M (Hôpital Communal, La Chaux-de-Fonds and Centre Hospitalier Universitaire Vaudois, Lusanne, Switzerland)
Surgery 111:221–223, 1992   13–3

Introduction.—It may be difficult to make an end-to-end anastomosis between vessels of differing diameter—particularly when one vessel is a prosthesis. The resultant kinking can have adverse hemodynamic results.

Technique.—The anastomotic zone consists of a wide-mouthed flap from the small-diameter vessel and a decreasing flap from the large-diameter prosthesis (Fig 13–13). The length of the 2 flaps equals half the circumference of the prosthesis. The entire circumference of the vein equals the amount of tissue removed from the prosthetic circumference to make the base of its flap. At the base of the vein flap the circumference is cut along about two thirds of its length (Fig 13–14A and B). The flap length is determined by flattening the free end of the prosthesis and folding it back; the edge of the flattened segment is then cut; The free ends are then held side to side, and the vein is cut along two thirds of its circumference. The end of the vein is then flattened, and a segment is removed to leave a narrow-based, wide-ended flap. The end of the prosthesis is held against the cut vein edge to mark the width of the end of the flap on the prosthesis. The circumference at the flap base on the prosthesis is cut, using the free end of the vein's flap as a guide. The prosthesis flap is completed by joining the marking nicks and the end of the last cut. A running suture is then placed (Fig 13–15A–H).

Advantages.—This technique is especially helpful in composite femoropopliteal bypasses, in which there is a substantial difference in diameter between the vein and the prosthesis. It is not excessively demanding or time-consuming.

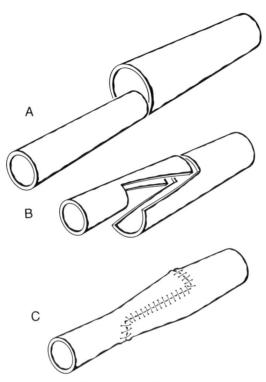

Fig 13–13.—**A,** 2 vessels of quite different diameter; **B,** after preparing flaps; **C,** completed anastomosis. (Courtesy of Merlini MP, Dusmet M: *Surgery* 111:221–223, 1992.)

▶ If one needs to perform an end-to-end anastomosis between conduits of significantly different diameters, this may be a superior way to achieve this. However, I suspect this technique will be infrequently useful. If one wishes to use a composite prosthetic venous graft, I believe the DeLaurentis technique mentioned in Abstract 10–24 is superior to an end-to-end anastomosis.—J.M. Porter, M.D.

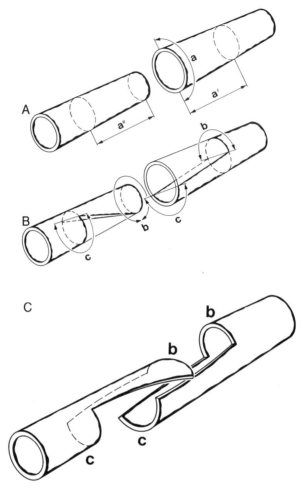

Fig 13–14.—A, *a* equals half of the circumference of the prosthesis. Each flap will be this long (*a* = *a'* = *a''*); **B,** *b* equals length of circumference of vein equals length of circumferential cut of prosthesis, and *c* equals two thirds of circumference of vein. This cut of vein will determine width of distal end of flap of prosthesis. **C,** completed flaps. (Courtesy of Merlini MP, Dusmet M: *Surgery* 111:221-223, 1992.)

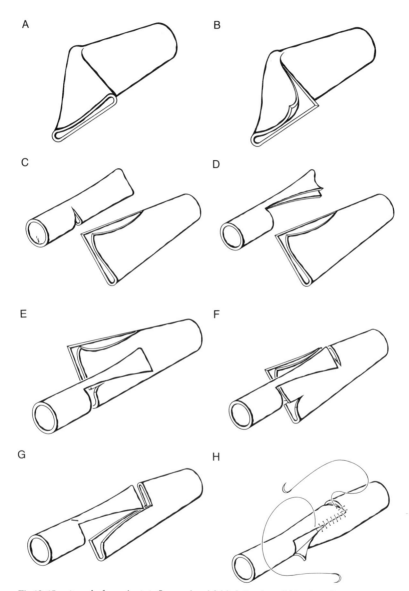

Fig 13–15.—**A,** end of prosthesis is flattened and folded. **B,** edge of this triangular segment is cut. **C,** end of 2 vessels are held side by side, and the circumference of vein is incised along two thirds of it. **D,** by cutting from the tip of the flattened end of the vein to transverse incision, flap is finished. **E,** holding vein against prosthesis, the end of the prosthesis flap is marked by 2 small nicks. **F,** similarly, the free end of the vein's flap is used as ruler to cut the circumference of the prosthesis. **G,** cutting from nicks to transverse cut on prosthesis, the second flap is finished. **H,** running suture between the complementary flaps. (Courtesy of Merlini MP, Dusmet M: *Surgery* 111:221-223, 1992.)

Intraabdominal Paraanastomotic Aneurysms After Aortic Bypass Grafting

Edwards JM, Teefey SA, Zierler RE, Kohler TR (Seattle VA Med Ctr)
J Vasc Surg 15:344–353, 1992

13–4

Life Table for Intra-Abdominal Para-Anastomotic Aneurysms

Time period (yr)	At risk	Developed aneurysms	Withdrawn	Interval aneurysm-free survival	Cumulative aneurysm-free survival	% Standard error
0	110	0	0	100	100	0.0
2	110	3	10	97	97	1.6
4	97	0	31	100	97	1.6
6	66	1	20	98	95	2.3
8	45	0	14	100	95	2.3
10	31	1	5	96	92	3.9
15	25	4	12	79	73	9.1
20	9	1	4	86	62	12.4
25	4	0	4	100	62	12.4

(Courtesy of Edwards JM, Teefey SA, Zierler RE, et al: J Vasc Surg 15:344–353, 1992.)

Introduction.—Femoral pseudoaneurysms occur in as many as 23% of patients given a prosthetic graft. Reported rates of intra-abdominal paraanastomotic aneurysms after bypass grafting of the abdominal aorta range from 1% to 15%.

Methods.—Abdominal sonography was performed annually to monitor 111 patients who underwent aortic graft surgery. A para-anastomotic aneurysm was defined as an aortic or iliac diameter exceeding 4 cm, or a focal outpouching of the lumen at or near a suture line.

Results.—In 11 (10%) patients, an intra-abdominal para-anastomotic aneurysm was found. The mean interval from surgery to detection of an aneurysm was 144 months; 3 lesions were found within 3 years of surgery, and 8 others were found after 7–28 years (table). There were 4 true aneurysms; all developed after repair of an abdominal aortic aneurysm. Pseudoaneurysms were more frequent after bypass for occlusive disease.

Conclusion.—At least 10% of patients may have a para-anastomotic aneurysm after elective aortic reconstruction for aneurysmal or occlusive disease. Abdominal sonography is the preferred screening measure and should be performed annually.

▶ It is sobering to note that, after a relatively short follow-up, 10% of 111 patients with abdominal aortic graft had para-anastomotic abdominal aneurysms. In 7 patients, these were believed to be pseudoaneurysms, and in 4 patients true aneurysms. The earliest aneurysm detected after surgery was found at 8 months. Based on this information, the authors advocate the use of yearly abdominal sonography for follow-up after aortic grafting. I believe this recommendation is reasonable, but I wonder whether it will pass muster with the funding agencies.—J.M. Porter, M.D.

Is Chronic Peritoneal Dialysis Safe in Patients With Intra-Abdominal Prosthetic Vascular Grafts?

Gulanikar AC, Jindal KK, Hirsch DJ (Dalhousie Univ, Halifax, NS, Canada)
Nephrol Dial Transplant 6:215–217, 1991   13–5

Introduction.—Long-term peritoneal dialysis is preferred to hemodialysis in patients who have extensive vascular disease or diabetes in addition to end stage renal disease. Patients in renal failure are at an increased risk of infection because of impaired cellular immunity. In patients with prosthetic vascular grafts, graft infection is a most serious complication.

Methods.—The risk of peritonitis was assessed in 6 patients older than 60 years of age with atherosclerotic vascular disease and renal failure. The patients had received an intra-abdominal prosthetic vascular graft 3–32 months before starting peritoneal dialysis. A Dacron velour graft was used in all patients, most often in the aortofemoral site.

Results.—Insertion of a peritoneal dialysis catheter was uneventful in all 6 patients. The mean duration of dialysis was 26 months. Peritonitis in 2 diabetic patients responded to standard treatment. No patient had clinical evidence of graft infection. The 4 surviving patients were continuing peritoneal dialysis.

Conclusion.—Prosthetic grafts become more resistant to infection the longer they remain in place. Patients with an intra-abdominal vascular prosthesis can safely undergo peritoneal dialysis. A dialysis catheter should be placed more than 6 weeks after surgery.

▶ We are all seeing an increased number of ESRD patients undergoing peritoneal dialysis, which is frequently required because of failure of peripheral hemodialysis access procedures. These authors ask the important question as to whether peritoneal dialysis is safe in patients who have prosthetic vascular grafts. They describe their experience with 6 patients with abdominal prosthetic vascular grafts who were undergoing peritoneal dialysis. The patients had undergone a mean of 26 months of dialysis, and 2 patients had had evidence of peritonitis that responded promptly to treatment. The authors conclude that patients with intra-abdominal prosthetic vascular grafts can be dialyzed safely intraperitoneally; they recommend delay of placement of the peritoneal dialysis catheter for 6 weeks after surgery.—J.M. Porter, M.D.

Axillo-Femoral (PTFE) and Infrainguinal Revascularization (PTFE and Umbilical Vein)

Johnson WC, Squires JW (New England Society for Vascular Surgery)
J Cardiovasc Surg 32:344–349, 1991   13–6

Background.—To evaluate the long-term performance of new vascular prostheses, The New England Society for Vascular Surgery (NESVS) began a vascular registry program in 1976. Long-term outcomes of axillo-femoral polytetrafluoroethylene (PTFE) grafts, infrainguinal PTFE grafts, and infrainguinal umbilical vein grafts placed between 1977 and 1983 were evaluated.

Methods.—Members of NESVS were asked to submit reports of their PTFE and umbilical vein bypass procedures voluntarily. New patient and follow-up data were requested every year thereafter. For the present report, 72 members reported 505 cases.

Results.—In 103 axillofemoral procedures, the 5-year primary patency rate was 55% for the bifemoral group, which was significantly greater than the 14% rate in the unifemoral group. There were 402 cases of infrainguinal reconstruction, including 55 patients with umbilical vein grafts. Five-year primary patency rates for femoropopliteal (F-P) above-knee PTFE grafts were 57% in patients with claudication, 46% in patients with rest pain, and 32% in patients with necrosis. Patency rates for

F-P below-knee grafts were 26% in patients with claudication, 17% in patients with rest pain, and 21% in patients with necrosis. The patency rates for umbilical vein grafts were 69% for F-P above-knee grafts and 45% for F-P below-knee grafts. No femoral tibial or peroneal prosthetic bypass graft was patent at 5 years. A routine duplex scan of 6 patent umbilical vein grafts 2–9 years after implantation reveal aneurysmal changes in 4.

Conclusion.—Compared with PTFE grafts at similar sites of anastomosis and indications for surgery, umbilical vein grafts may have increased patency rates, but aneurysm formation constitutes a significant problem. The PTFE grafts reported were not of the lightweight, thin-walled, or externally supported types in current use. A VA cooperative study to compare the efficacy of these types of grafts is currently under way.

▶ Voluntary vascular registries are always suspect, based on the possibility that only surgeons with the better results faithfully report, whereas surgeons with suboptimal results may choose not to participate. Nonetheless, the 5-year primary patency rate of 55% for axillobifemoral grafting is noteworthy, especially considering that these grafts were placed in the remote past, before the advent of the externally supported prostheses.—J.M. Porter, M.D.

Infrainguinal Polytetrafluoroethylene Grafts: Saved Limbs or Wasted Effort? A Report on Ten Years' Experience
Davies MG, Feeley TM, O'Malley MK, Colgan MP, Moore DJ, Shanik GD (St James'Hosp, Dublin)
Ann Vasc Surg 5:519–524, 1991   13–7

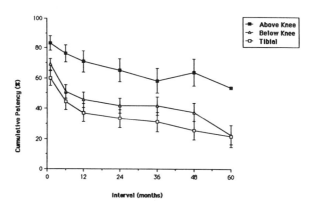

Fig 13–16.—Primary patency rates for above-knee popliteal (48), below-knee popliteal (113), and tibial vessels (63) groups. The values are mean ± SEM (Courtesy of Davies MG, Feeley TM, O'Malley MK, et al: *Ann Vasc Surg* 5:519–524, 1991.)

Introduction.—Since 1973, good short-term results have been achieved with polytetrafluorethylene (PTFE) for infrainguinal bypass. The results of PTFE grafts used for infrainguinal bypass over a 10-year period were reviewed.

Methods.—Of 224 infrainguinal (PTFE) reconstructions performed in patients with critical lower limb in 1978–1988, 48 were to the popliteal artery above the knee, 113 were to the popliteal artery below the knee, and 63 were to the tibial vessels.

Results.—The primary patency rate after reconstruction was 71% at 1 year and 54% at 5 years for above-knee popliteal reconstructions; 46% at 1 year and 23% at 5 years in the below-knee popliteal group; and 37% at 1 year and 22% at 5 years for reconstructions to the tibial vessels (Fig 13–16). The corresponding limb salvage rates were 81% and 73% (above-knee popliteal); 69% and 57% (below-knee popliteal); and 64% and 32% (tibial vessels). In 32 instances the graft became occluded but limb loss did not ensue. Forty-three percent of the patients were severely limited before reconstruction. At follow-up, 57% of the patients were independent, and only 17% remained severely restricted.

Conclusion.—The infrainguinal PTFE reconstruction provides good short-term limb salvage and improved mobility to patients with critical extremity ischemia who have a poor life expectancy.

▶ The question posed by the title is not answered by the subsequent data. Although there certainly exist some patients who do not have suitable vein for bypass, 224 PTFE bypasses in 10 years seem excessive. The authors do not state their definition of an unsuitable vein or which, if any, alternatives to ipsilateral saphenous vein were considered. No denominator for the total number of lower extremity bypass procedures is provided. The patency and limb salvage rates reported are substandard in every category (above- or below-knee or distal bypass), even considering the use of prosthetic graft material (1), and they are wholly inferior to those of autogenous vein bypass using alternative vein (2). I cannot help but compare these numbers with those listed in Abstract 13–1. I wonder whether the Taylor technique will make a real difference.—J.M. Porter, M.D.

References

1. Dalman RL, Taylor LM: *Ann Vasc Surg* 4:309, 1990.
2. Taylor LM, et al: *Am J Surg* 153:505, 1987.

PTFE or HUV for Femoro-Popliteal Bypass: A Multi-Centre Trial
McCollum C, Kenchington G, Alexander C, Franks PJ, Greenhalgh RM, The Femoro-Popliteal Bypass Trial Participants (Charing Cross Hosp, London; Queens Med Centre, Birmingham, England)
Eur J Vasc Surg 5:435–443, 1991   13–8

Objective.—The choice between human umblical vein (HUV) or poly-tetrafluoroethylene (PTFE) when the saphenous vein is inadequate for femoropopliteal bypass is not clear, despite extensive clinical experience. The results of 801 femoropopliteal bypasses were evaluated in a multi-center trial.

Study Design.—Prosthetic grafts were used in 252 femoropopliteal bypasses (31.5%) in which autogenous vein could not be used. Of these, 191 were randomized to either HUV or PTFE. Patients were given aspirin, 300 mg, plus dipyridamole, 150 mg, twice daily. Graft patency was expressed on an "intention to treat" basis by life table analysis. The mean follow-up period was 35 months.

Results.—Overall, 101 grafts failed, for a cumulative patency rate at 3 years of 53%. Patency was 60% in 549 saphenous vein bypasses. Prosthetic bypass patency above the knee was markedly better (65%) than that for below-knee bypasses (35%). This rate was comparable with the rate of 62% in 217 above-knee saphenous vein bypasses. Most failures occurred early, with failure rates of 52 per 1,000 patient-months in the first 3 months, 21 per 1,000 by 6 to 12 months, and nearly 10 per 1,000 in subsequent years. Graft failure was associated with poor compliance with platelet inhibitory therapy. Cumulative patency rates for the 87 HUV grafts were 68%, 63%, and 57% at 1, 2, and 3 years, respectively. Corresponding rates for the 104 PTFE grafts were 61%, 56%, and 48%. The difference of 9% at 3 years had a wide confidence interval and was not statitically significant. After thrombectomy in 19 grafts, however, the secondary patency rates at 3 years improved to 66% for HUV and only 49% for PTFE. The difference was statistically significant.

Conclusion.—In patients undergoing femoropopliteal bypass and receiving platelet inhibitory therapy, prosthetic grafts achieve patency rates similar to those with autologous vein above the knee. The difference in primary patency between HUV and PTFE was not statistically significant.

▶ This large study is somewhat curious in that the randomization of pros-thetics occurred only in patients who did not have acceptable vein, thus making an accurate comparison of these results to vein impossible. It is noteworthy that the 3-year patency with veins was only 60% in the femoropopliteal region, the same as that obtained by both prosthetics above the knee. The prosthetic bypasses to the below-knee popliteal fared much poorer. One of the major problems with this paper, in addition to the randomization problems, is the observation that above-knee vein graft patency at 3 years was only 60% not the stuff of which legends are made.—J.M. Porter, M.D.

Above-Knee Prosthetic Grafts Do Not Compromise the Ipsilateral Long Saphenous Vein

Budd JS, Langdon I, Brennan J, Bell PRF (Univ of Leicester, England)
Br J Surg 78:1379–1380, 1991   13–9

Background.—A number of surgeons prefer to use prosthetic graft materials for above-knee femoropopliteal bypass operations.

Methods.—The ipsilateral long saphenous vein was evaluated by B-mode ultrasonography in patients having had above-knee femoropopliteal bypass surgery utilizing prosthetic grafts. A total of 137 grafts were placed in a 10-year period, and 74 patients were available for assessment.

Results.—All but 3% of the veins examined were found to be suitable for use in future bypass surgery should this be necessary.

Conclusion.—An above-knee prosthetic bypass does not jeopardize the long saphenous vein.

▶ The authors conclude, and I am sure they are correct, that a well-placed above-knee prosthetic bypass does not jeopardize the greater saphenous vein. Although I am perfectly willing to accept this, I consider it to be monumentally irrelevant. Why would anybody use a prosthetic bypass anywhere in the leg if a perfectly acceptable greater saphenous vein is immediately available? A well-performed saphenous vein graft to an above-knee popliteal artery should have a primary patency approaching 90% at 5 years. This is much superior to the 50% to 55% reported by most above-knee prosthetic series. I continue to be unable to perceive any hint of logic in the argument that above-knee prosthetic grafts are preferable to a good vein.—J.M. Porter, M.D.

Biologic Fate of Cryopreserved Human Saphenous Allografts: Case Report and Hypothesis

Hoover WW, Kresowik TF, Cook RT (Univ of Iowa Hosp and Clinic, Iowa City)
J Cardiovasc Surg 32:708–710, 1991   13–10

Introduction.—Little is known about the early pathologic changes accompanying the use of cryopreserved venous allografts. The first report of the changes noted in such a graft recovered after 48 hours was reviewed.

Case Report.—Man 82, with critical ischemia in the left lower extremity underwent femoroperoneal bypass, with placement of a cryopreserved human saphenous vein allograft. He died of myocardial infarction 48 hours after operation. Examination of the graft showed karryorhexis and neutrophilic infiltration in the media, underlying a fibrin layer on the intimal surface (Fig 13–17). Im-

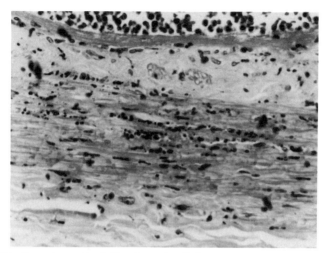

Fig 13–17.—Photomicrograph of allograft vessel wall demonstrating neutrophilic clustering and luminal fibrin deposition, and neutrophilic infiltrate in media with necrosis and karyorrhexis (Hematoxylin-eosin; original magnification, ×285). (Courtesy of Hoover WW, Kresowik TF, Cook RT: *J Cardiovasc Surg* 32:708–710, 1991.)

munoperoxidase studies confirmed luminal deposition of immunoglobulins and fibrinogen. There was no evidence of antemortem thrombosis.

Conclusion.—The changes seen in cryopreserved vein allografts may result from anoxia of the vascular wall, rather than immunologic mechanisms. Whether the changes represent the initial stage of intimal thickening and fibrosis remains to be determined.

▶ The dramatic microscopical changes observed in this cryopreserved human saphenous allograft removed 48 hours after surgery indicate that this cryopreserved tissue is by no means inert. I remain unconvinced that the current generation of cryopreserved allograft vascular tissue is superior to the previous cryopreserved allografts tried and abandoned a decade ago.—J.M. Porter, M.D.

Cryopreserved Saphenous Vein Allogenic Homografts: An Alternative Conduit in Lower Extremity Arterial Reconstruction in Infected Fields
Fujitani RM, Bassiouny HS, Gewertz BL, Glagov S, Zarins CK (Univ of Chicago)
J Vasc Surg 15:519–526, 1992   13–11

Objective.—Cryopreserved saphenous vein allogenic homografts were used for extremity salvage in 8 patients who underwent 10 lower extremity arterial reconstructions in the presence of infection.

Patients and Methods.—Six patients required complete or partial excision of 8 prosthetic grafts because of overt infection. All infected material was removed. One other patient had an infected femoral pseudoaneurysm, and 1 had extensive chemical burns. All the homografts were identical ABO/Rh matches with the recipients. No immunosuppression was administered. The mean follow-up was 9½ months.

Results.—One patient died shortly after surgery but had a patent graft. Two grafts became occluded, and 1 of these patients had patency restored by thrombectomy alone. The other 7 reconstructions remained patent, with eradication of the primary infection and no evidence of aneurysmal dilatation.

Conclusion.—In some cases when infection precludes the use of a prosthetic graft, a cryopreserved homograft saphenous vein can safely be placed when combined with aggressive antibiotic treatment.

▶ See the comments after Abstract 13–10. Perhaps these cryopreserved saphenous vein allografts do have increased resistance to infection. It is noted, however, that the mean follow-up in this series is only 9½ months, and that the maximum follow-up is 14 months. As the authors suggest, these cryopreserved grafts may be of value as interim conduits, and they may require replacement later.—J.M. Porter, M.D.

Mesh Tube-Constricted Varicose Veins Used as Bypass Grafts for Infrainguinal Arterial Reconstruction

Moritz A, Grabenwöger F, Raderer F, Ptakovsky H, Staudacher M, Magometschnigg H, Ullrich R, Wolner E (Univ of Vienna; Hosp of the Sisters of Mercy, Wels, Austria)
Arch Surg 127:416–420, 1992   13–12

Background.—Varicose veins generally are thought to be inadequate for use as graft material in arterial reconstruction because of their large and irregular caliber. Such veins may, however, be reduced in size by threading in a constricting tube, thereby creating bypass grafts of suitable caliber.

Methods.—Sixteen human varicose veins with a mean diameter of 13 mm, taken in stripping procedures, were placed in Dacron mesh tubes with an internal diameter of 6 mm (Fig 13–18). Paraffin casts showed that the veins were reduced by nearly 7 mm on average. Vein wall material formed folds in only 2 instances, in both of which the vein diameter was reduced by more than 10 mm. The folds did not lead to significant stenosis.

Clinical Cases.—Mesh-constricted varicose veins were used for bypass material in 11 patients having infrainguinal arterial reconstruction (table). One of the grafts occluded 2 months postoperatively, and 2 patients required reoperation; however, none of the complications were ascribed

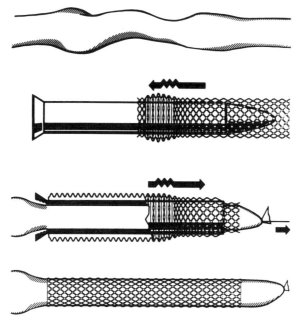

Fig 13–18.—The use of the mesh tube applicator. It consists of a metal tube with 1 funnel-shaped end and a removable bullet-shaped tip at the opposite end. The mesh tube segments are slipped over the tube and anastomosed to the length needed. The vein is threaded through the tube, and the mesh tube is slipped over the vein, resulting in a mesh tube-constricted vein. (Courtesy of Moritz A, Grabenwöger F, Raderer F, et al: *Arch Surg* 127:416–420, 1992.)

to vein constriction. The remaining grafts were functioning at a mean of 17 months after placement.

Conclusion.—Varicose veins may be substantially reduced in diameter and used as bypass grafts in arterial reconstruction without adverse effects resulting.

▶ I suspect that most of us have occasionally used a moderately varicose vein as a leg bypass. I certainly have, and I have been anecdotally impressed that they seem to work generally well as long as they are not sclerotic or phlebitic. These authors propose the interesting technique of simply enclosing varicose veins within size-reducing Dacron mesh tubes of 6-mm internal diameter, both to reduce the diameter of the varicose vein graft and to prevent future expansion. They present good results. Perhaps this will be a useful technique in an occasional patient.—J.M. Porter, M.D.

Patient Data

Patient No./ Sex/Age, y	Symp- toms	Wrap	Bypass	Remarks
1/M/65	IIb	Total	Fem-pop III	. . .
2/F /80	IV	Partial	Fem-crur sequential	Died 2 mo postoperatively
3/F /80	III	Partial	Popliteal- crural	Occluded 2 mo postoperatively
4/F /75	III	Partial	Fem-crur	Proximal stenosis after 16 mo
5/M/54	IIb	Partial	Fem-pop I	. . .
6/M/70	IV	Total	Fem-crur	. . .
7/M/61	III	Total	Fem-pop II	. . .
8/M/76	III	Total	Fem-pop III	. . .
9/F /56	IIb	Total	Fem-pop I	. . .
10/M/72	IV	Partial	Fem-pop III	Revision of end-to-end anastomosis
11/M/54	III	Total	Fem-pop III	. . .

Patients who received partially or totally mesh-reinforced and constricted varicose veins as infrainguinal bypass graft. The symptoms are listed in clinical stages. Femoropopliteal (*Fem-pop*) bypasses are differentiated by the popliteal segment (I, II, III) to which the distal anastomosis was made. *Fem-crur* indicates an infrapopliteal bypass.

(Courtesy of Moritz A, Grabenwöger F, Raderer F, et al: *Arch Surg* 127:416–420, 1992.)

Angiosarcoma at the Site of a Dacron Vascular Prosthesis: A Case Report and Literature Review
Weiss WM, Riles TS, Gouge TH, Mizrachi HH (New York Univ)
J Vasc Surg 14:87–91, 1991   13–13

Introduction.—The risk of cancer developing from a plastic foreign body is less in human beings than in murine species, but 5 sarcomas have been described in association with synthetic vascular prostheses.

Case Report.—Man, 56, underwent repair of an infrarenal aortic aneurysm with placement of a bifurcated woven double-velour Dacron graft. Pain developed in the left lower quadrant and lower back 35 years later, when CT showed a thickened distal aorta thought to represent thrombus interposed between the graft and the aortic wall wrap. Magnetic resonance imaging showed that blood flow was limited to the graft lumen. The mass was larger 2 months later, and left hydroureter and hydronephrosis were present. Exploration showed a vascularized tissue mass surrounding the graft. A high-grade angiosarcoma was diagnosed. The patient had liver metastases 11 months after en bloc resection of the mass with the graft. He is currently receiving chemotherapy.

Comment.—Of 32 sarcomas related to the aorta, 4 arose around a previously placed aortic prosthesis. Animal studies have implicated plastic polymers (including Dacron) as carcinogenic materials capable of inducing sarcoma.

Conclusion.—In the assessment of vascular masses, CT should be performed early. Angiography and MRI may help distinguish between a mass extrinsic to the graft, graft infection, and pseudoaneurysm. All emboli that are recovered should be examined pathologically.

▶ It is chilling to even consider that Dacron vascular grafts may induce angiosarcoma of the aorta. However, the implantation of hundreds of thousands of Dacron prostheses over the years, with only 32 reported aortic sarcomas indicates that any risk is well below the limits of statistical detection. The authors' admonition that this condition be considered in the differential diagnosis of any mass or thromboembolic event associated with a vascular prosthesis may be a bit overstated.—J.M. Porter, M.D.

Lack of Diameter Effect on Short-Term Patency of Size-Matched Dacron Aortobifemoral Grafts

Schneider JR, Zwolak RM, Walsh DB, McDaniel MD, Cronenwett JL (Dartmouth-Hitchcock Med Ctr, Hanover, NH)
J Vasc Surg 13:785–791, 1991   13–14

Introduction.—There appears to be a trend toward using smaller-diameter Dacron bifurcation grafts sized in proportion to the native arteries in patients with aortoiliac occlusive disease.

Methods.—The effect of graft diameter on both patency and function was investigated in 79 patients with an average age of 65 years who were given Dacron aortobifemoral bypass grafts for aortoiliac occlusive disease in 1985–1989. Of the patients, 65% were men, 25% were diabetic, and 94% were smokers. The mean follow-up period was 2 years.

Results.—Life-table survival was 92% at 3 years. All survivors were symptomatically improved, but there were 3 early and 5 late graft thromboses. When 48 patients given 12- or 14-mm diameter grafts were compared with 31 others given 16- or 18-mm grafts, graft diameter did not affect patency rates, which exceeded 80% in both groups at 3 years (Fig 13–19). Graft patency also was not influenced by age, diabetes, outflow status, the site of the distal anastomosis, or whether a knitted or woven graft was used.

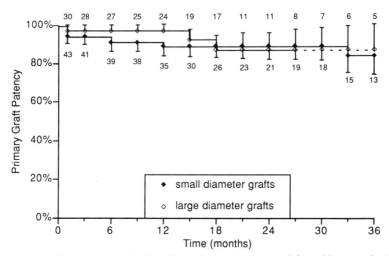

Fig 13–19.—Primary patency of small and large diameter Dacron aortobifemoral bypass grafts. The number of patients entering the next interval alive with a patent graft is indicated at each time point for both groups. *Error bars* indicate the standard error of the mean (*SEM*). The survival line is broken when the SEM exceeds 10%. (Courtesy of Schneider JR, Zwolak RM, Walsh DB, et al: *J Vasc Surg* 13:785–791, 1991.)

Conclusion.—When a Dacron aortobifemoral graft is matched with the native vessels, its patency is not a function of the actual graft diameter.

▶ Surgeons are creatures of strong habits, especially in areas unguided by appropriate data. Some surgeons tend to use large aortic bifurcation grafts, and some tend to use small grafts. It does not appear to make much difference. I, of course, intuitively know that the optimal size for most men is 16 × 8; for most women, it is 14 × 7.—J.M. Porter, M.D.

Sizing of Crimped Dacron Grafts
Reid JDS, Sladen JG (Univ of British Columbia; St Paul's Hosp, Vancouver, BC, Canada)
Am J Surg 163:541–543, 1992   13–15

Objective.—The stated size of Microvel Dacron grafts was compared with their actual internal diameter and also with ultrasound measurements made in the early postoperative period.

Methods.—Knitted, double-velour, collagen-impregnated Dacron grafts purported to be 7, 8, 9, and 10 mm in diameter were measured directly and with graded probes. Twenty randomly selected grafts were measured using a color flow duplex ultrasound unit within 3 months of implantation.

Calculated Diameter of Grafts

Graft	Circumference (mm) (±0.5 mm)	Calculated Diameter (mm)	Calculated Error
Dacron			
Microvel			
7 mm	26	8.3	(8.1–8.4)
8 mm	29	9.2	(9.1–9.4)
9 mm	33	10.5	(10.3–10.7)
10 mm	37	11.8	(11.6–11.9)
Vascutek			
8 mm	29	9.2	(9.1–9.4)
PTFE			
Gortex			
8 mm	25	8.0	(7.8–8.1)

Abbreviation: PTFE, polytetrafluoroethylene.
(Courtesy of Reid JDS, Sladen JG: Am J Surg 163:541–543, 1992.)

Results.—Graft circumference measurements yielded calculated diameters exceeding the stated graft size for Microvel and Vascutek Dacron grafts. The diameters of PTFE grafts, however, equaled the stated size (table). Unstretched grafts were 1.3–1.8 mm greater than their stated diameter. Ultrasound measurements showed the grafts to be 12% larger than stated.

Conclusion.—Microvel Dacron grafts are larger than their stated diameter, as are Vascutek Dacron grafts. Because flow velocity relates to graft diameter, this information is relevant when selecting a prosthetic vascular graft.

▶ I find it fascinating that certain Dacron grafts are larger than the manufacturer's stated diameter. I wonder why they cannot get it right.—J.M. Porter, M.D.

Axillobifemoral Bypass and Aortic Exclusion for Vascular Septic Lesions: A Multicenter Retrospective Study of 98 Cases
Bacourt F, Koskas F, French Univ Association for Research in Surgery (American Hosp, Neuilly, France; Group Hospitalier Pitié-Salpétrière; French Univ Assoc for Research in Surgery, Paris)
Ann Vasc Surg 6:119–126, 1992   13–16

Introduction.—Interruption of the aorta often is performed along with axillobifemoral bypass (ABFB) in patients with aortic infection or an aortoenteric fistula.

Methods.—Data were reviewed on 98 such patients who underwent ABFB and aortic exclusion, with 22 different surgical teams performing the operations.

Results.—The early mortality rate was 24%. The actuarial rate of primary patency was 82% at 2 years and 65% at 5 years, and the corresponding limb salvage rates were 90% and 82%. Within 8 months of surgery, 8 aortic stumps ruptured, and 2 of them were successfully repaired. Of 7 infections of the ABFB, 6 were treated effectively. All 8 axillary complications in the upper extremity were treated without sequelae. In 8 patients, the ABFB was replaced by a thoracic aortic bypass. Polytetrafluorethylene bypasses were infected less often than Dacron bypasses.

Conclusion.—Reinforcing the graft reduced the risk of occlusion appreciably. Occlusion occurred more often after grafting of occlusive lesions than after treatment of an aneurysm. Patients requiring emergency surgery had an early mortality of 30%.

▶ This report describes a mortality of 24% in patients with aortic infection or aortoenteric fistula treated by axillofemoral bypass and aortic exclusion. Graft patency at 2 and 5 years was 82% and 65%, respectively, with a limb-salvage rate of 90% and 82%. I see no reason to challenge fate by reimplanting a clean prosthesis in a contaminated field when results like this can be obtained with extra-anatomic bypass grafting.—J.M. Porter, M.D.

Total Excision and Extra-Anatomic Bypass for Aortic Graft Infection
Ricotta JJ, Faggioli GL, Stella A, Curl GR, Peer R, Upson J, D'Addato M, Anain J, Gutierrez I (Millard Fillmore Hosps, Buffalo, NY; Universita degli Studi di Bologna, Italy)
Am J Surg 162:145–149, 1991   13–17

Introduction.—Although aortic graft infection is an infrequent complication of aortic procedures, mortality rates range from 40% to 60%. Data on 32 patients with aortic graft infection were reviewed to establish current morbidity and mortality rates and to identify factors influencing surgical outcome.

Methods.—The patients came from 2 vascular centers and the private practice of 3 vascular surgeons. Records were reviewed, with special attention given to clinical presentation, diagnosis, and factors that might predispose to infection. The patients were divided according to operative management: partial removal with or without revascularization (12 patients) and total removal with or without revascularization (20 patients).

Results.—The mean patient age was 66 years; most (26) were men, and 8 had diabetes. Aortic graft infection occurred at a mean of 34 months after initial graft placement. Both surgical exposure of the groin (24 patients) and multiple vascular operations (16 patients) may have contributed to the subsequent development of graft infection. By far, the best results were obtained with total excision of the infected graft and remote bypass through a clean field. Their combination resulted in a mortality rate of 17% and an amputation rate of 11%. Late complications occurred only after partial removal.

Conclusion.—Total excision and extra-anatomical bypass should be the standard approach for aortic graft infection. No patient treated in this manner had late infection.

▶ The similarity of these numbers to those reported in Abstract 13–16 is striking. The best results in this report were obtained with total excision of the infected graft and remote bypass through a clean field, resulting in a mortality of 17% and an amputation rate of only 11%.—J.M. Porter, M.D.

Infected Femorodistal Bypass: Is Graft Removal Mandatory?
Cherry KJ Jr, Roland CF, Pairolero PC, Hallett JW Jr, Meland NB, Naessens JM, Gloviczki P, Bower TC (Mayo Clinic and Found, Rochester, Minn)
J Vasc Surg 15:295–305, 1992   13–18

Introduction.—Graft excision routinely performed for infected lower limb bypass grafts may not be necessary in all cases. The efficacy of aggressive local treatment was evaluated in 38 patients with 39 infected lower-limb bypasses.

Methods.—Prosthetic grafts were present in 33 limbs, vein grafts in 4, and composite grafts in 2; 27 (69.2%) of the infected grafts were made of polytetrafluoroethylene. The median time from graft placement to symptoms of infection was 48 days. *Staphylococcus aureus* was the most frequent pathogen. Nineteen infected femorodistal bypass grafts were partially or totally excised without reconstruction; 9 others were excised and femorodistal arterial reconstruction was performed, and 11 infected grafts were left in place.

Results.—In 5 patients, infection recurred, and 2 patients died of complications of graft infection. Of the 20 extremities at risk 10 were lost.

Summary of Results by Treatment Group

Treatment of graft infection	No. of grafts	Reinfection	Amputation	Deaths related to graft infection
Group 1				
Graft excision without reconstruction	19	1	7	1
Group 2				
Graft excision and femorodistal reconstruction	9	4	3	1
Group 3				
Local treatment without graft excision	11	0	1	1
Total	39	5	11	3

(Courtesy of Cherry KJ Jr, Roland CF, Pairolero PC, et al: *J Vasc Surg* 15:295–305, 1992.)

Limb salvage was significantly more likely when the graft was left in place (table).

Conclusion.—Aggressive local treatment of an infected lower extremity bypass graft (including drainage, débridement, and muscle transposition) may be effective in selected patients.

▶ These authors appropriately conclude that aggressive local treatment of arterial graft infection is occasionally successful. Despite this report and others of a similar nature, I continue to prefer total excision of the infected graft accompanied by remote bypass.—J.M. Porter, M.D.

Uptake of In-111 Labeled Leukocytes by Lymphocele: A Cause of False-Positive Vascular Graft Infection

Chung CJ, Wilson AA, Melton JW, Hartley WS, Allen DM (Med Univ of South Carolina, Charleston)
Clin Nucl Med 17:368–370, 1992   13–19

Introduction.—Although scintigraphy with ^{111}In-labeled leukocytes is a sensitive means of diagnosing infection of a prosthetic vascular graft, a number of factors may produce false positive findings.

Case Report.—Man, 59, had received an aortobifemoral bypass graft 3 years before, and he had had an enlarging right groin mass for 6 months, as well as progressive paresthesia in the lower extremities. Ultrasonography demonstrated fluid along both graft limbs in the left groin and increased uptake of ^{111}In activity (Fig 13–20). Angiography showed only small pseudoaneurysms. Computed tomography showed bilateral fluid collections that seemingly dissected along the graft. Surgery revealed a lymphocele with no evidence of graft infection. Similar findings were seen in the right groin 10 months later, and fluid aspiration was done.

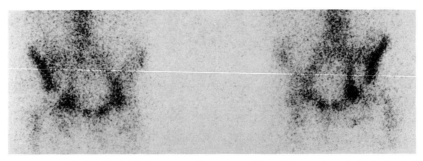

Fig 13–20.—In-111-labeled leukocyte scan demonstrates bilateral increased uptake in the inguinal areas along the graft. (Courtesy of Chung CJ, Wilson AA, Melton JW, et al: *Clin Nucl Med* 17:368–370, 1992.)

Conclusion—Lymphocele is a possible cause of falsely positive scintigraphic findings when a patient with a prosthetic vascular graft is examined with ¹¹¹In-labeled leukocytes for graft infection.

▶ In-111–labeled leukocyte scanning, is an important test for the detection of infected grafts. This interesting report of false positivity induced by lymphocele is noteworthy. Overall, the In-111 imaging has excellent sensitivity but, unfortunately, it has only fair specificity (too many false positive results).—J.M. Porter, M.D.

Clinical Usefulness of Tc-99m HMPAO Labeled White Blood Cell Imaging in Prosthetic Vascular Graft Infections
Mortelmans L, Verlooy H, Nevelsteen A, Wilms G, De Roo M (Univ Hosp Gasthuisberg, Leuven, Belgium)
Clin Nucl Med 17:11–13, 1992   13–20

Objective.—The use of leukocytes labeled with ⁹⁹ᵐTc-hexamethylopropyleneamineoxime (HMPAO) has been suggested as a relatively accurate means of detecting infection in a synthetic vascular graft. The value of this approach was confirmed in 2 patients.

Case 1.—Man, 67, with an aortobifemoral bypass graft in place for 7 years was seen with purulent drainage from the left groin, yielding *Staphylococcus aureus*. Ultrasound study showed a patent graft with an adjacent fluid collection, and contrast fistulography demonstrated a fistula extending along the left limb of the graft. The labeled leukocyte scan showed a collection of white blood cells in the left graft limb, as well as increased uptake in the right groin.

Case 2.—Man, 63, had hemipelvic pain a few years after iliacofemoral bypass grafting. A 7- × 3-cm abdominal mass was found. The white blood cell scan

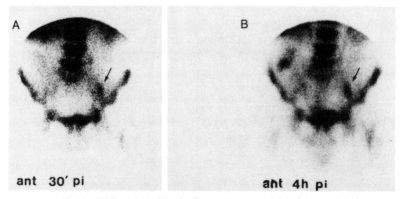

Fig 13–21.—Tc-99m HMPAO white blood cell scan 30 minutes (**A**) and 4 hours (**B**) after injection, anterior view. There is increased linear uptake in the iliacofemoral prosthesis (*arrow*). (Courtesy of Mortelmans L, Verlooy H, Nevelsteen A, et al: *Clin Nucl Med* 17:11–13, 1992.)

demonstrated linear uptake along the left part of the graft (Fig 13–21), which later was removed. Wound cultures yielded *Pseudomonas aeruginosa.*

Conclusion.—The ⁹⁹ᵐTc-HMPAO leukocyte scintigram is a relatively easy and accurate means of detecting infections of vascular grafts.

▶ These authors suggest that this radionuclide may be a better choice than In-111 for white cell labeling for detection of vascular graft infection.—J.M. Porter, M.D.

Evaluation of Muscle Flaps in the Treatment of Infected Aortic Grafts
Mehran RJ, Graham AM, Ricci MA, Symes JF (McGill Univ, Montreal)
J Vasc Surg 15:487–494, 1992   13–21

Background.—Standard management of an infected abdominal aortic graft by graft removal and extra-anatomical bypass carries significant morbidity and mortality. The value of using vascularized muscle flaps, with or without in situ replacement of the graft, was investigated.

Methods.—In 52 Landrace pigs, a segment of polytetrafluoroethylene graft was interposed in the infrarenal abdominal aorta and was infected by *Staphylococcus aureus.* A week later, groups of animals had retroperitoneal débridement only; débridement with graft replacement; wrapping of the graft with a rectus abdominis flap; wrapping with the seromuscularis of the jejunum; changing of the graft and wrapping with a rectus abdominis island flap; or a new graft with wrapping by a seromuscularis flap.

Results.—Graft infection was significantly less frequent when the graft was changed, regardless of the type of wrap used. Graft thrombosis also was much reduced in these groups, compared with that in control animals that had débridement only. Wrapping of the graft without replacing it controlled infection, but all grafts were thrombosed at re-exploration.

Conclusion.—Use of a vascularized tissue flap helps control infection of an aortic graft and may permit in situ replacement of an infected graft.

▶ On occasion, vascularized tissue flaps are certainly effective in dealing with occasional vascular infection problems in the extremities. I am not sure I am willing to consider using these flaps in the abdomen, despite the results of this innovative experimental study.—J.M. Porter, M.D.

Axillary Disruption of Axillobifemoral Graft
Wehmann TW, Rongaus VA (Cuyahoga Falls Gen Hosp, Cuyahoga Falls,

Ohio)
J Am Osteopath Assoc 91:813–815, 1991

13–22

Background.—Axillary disruption of axillofemoral grafts has not previously been described after appropriate graft placement medially on the axillary artery with proper subpectoral tunneling.

Case Report.—Man, 81, was found unconscious 6 weeks after technically proper surgery. The postoperative course had been relatively uneventful. Respiratory arrest ensued, and exploration showed that the polytetrafluoroethylene graft had separated from the axillary artery, despite an intact suture line on the artery itself. Cultures of the graft were negative.

Interpretation.—Anastomotic disruption in this patient was ascribed to trauma from cardiopulmonary resuscitation and external cardiac massage. An extra-anatomical bypass also bypasses normal protective mechanisms, creating a risk that is not ordinarily present when anatomical procedures are used.

▶ This article represents the second case report where it has been clearly documented that the sutures pulled through the wall of an 8-mm, thin-wall, ringed polytetrafluoroethylene (PTFE) used in the axillofemoral position (1). Most previous reports have focused on the lateral location of the anastomosis as a cause of disruption. However, in view of these recent case reports and the description of fractured fibrils in the PTFE material (see commentary for Abstract 13–23), increased attention should be directed toward the role of thin-walled PTFE used in this location.—F.W. LoGerfo, M.D.

Reference

1. Brophy CM, et al: *J Vasc Surg* 15:218, 1992.

Deterioration of PTFE-Prostheses Wall: A SEM Study
Geiger G (Univ Hosp Mannheim, Germany)
J Cardiovasc Surg 32:660–663, 1991

13–23

Background.—Aneurysms have been described in patients given single-layer prostheses of expanded polytetrafluoroethylene (ePTFE) prostheses, but not after placement of a 2-layer structure including an external PTFE wrap.

Methods.—A structural analysis of femoropopliteal ePTFE bypass grafts was done after amputation in 10 patients who had received such grafts previously, with implantation times varying from 5 to 94 months.

Results.—A homogeneous luminal structure was noted with fibrils interconnecting nodes of varying size (Fig 13–22). Irregularities appeared after 6 months, with PTFE nodes pressed together and the fibrils com-

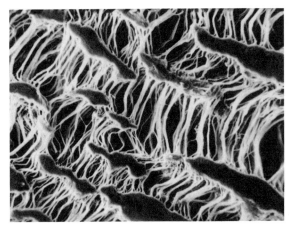

Fig 13–22.—Internal surface of an ePTFE prosthesis with uniform structure. Primary magnification, 1:1,000. (Courtesy of Geiger G: *J Cardiovasc Surg* 32:660–663, 1991.)

pressed or fractured (Fig 13–23). Structural changes were most evident in segments bridging the knee joint.

Conclusions.—The luminal surface of ePTFE prostheses becomes disrupted after one year in place. Less marked changes are found in an external PTFE wrap. In unwrapped prostheses, weakening of the wall can lead to aneurysm formation, especially at points of high mechanical stress. Hopefully, a PTFE-wrap combined with some means of external reinforcement will protect against complications such as aneurysm formation and lengthening of the graft, while at the same time extending the period of patency.

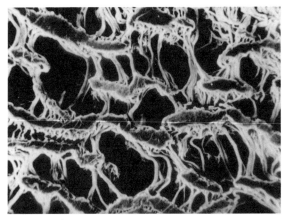

Fig 13–23.—Loss of uniform structure of the internal surface of the ePTFE prosthesis 12 months after implantation. Primary magnification, 1:1,000. (Courtesy of Geiger G: *J Cardiovasc Surg* 32:660–663, 1991.)

▶ Striking microscopic changes were noted in PTFE grafts after 12 months of implantation in patients. These authors hypothesize that such changes may underlie the formation of aneurysms and other examples of graft deterioration of PTFE. See also the comment for Abstract 13–22.—J.M. Porter, M.D.

14 Vascular Trauma

Utility of Arteriography in Penetrating Extremity Injuries
King TA, Perse JA, Marmen C, Darvin HI (Mt Sinai Med Ctr, Cleveland; Case Western Reserve Univ, Cleveland)
Am J Surg 162:163–165, 1991   14–1

Introduction.—There is considerable controversy regarding the use of routine arteriography in evaluating patients with penetrating injuries of the extremities. The clinical role for arteriography in extremity trauma was determined by examining arteriographic studies done on 82 consecutive patients with 98 extremity wounds between January 1984 and December 1988.

Patients.—The study group included 66 males and 16 females with a mean age of 27 years. None had symptoms of vascular disease before the injury. Sixty-five arteriograms were obtained, 57 because of the proximity of the wound or the trajectory of the injuring agent to a major neurovascular bundle, and 8 to localize a clinically apparent wound.

Results.—Eleven (19%) of the arteriograms obtained because of proximity identified a vascular injury, and 6 arteriograms obtained for clinical indications were positive (75%). Six wounds in each group required vascular repair, and all of these procedures were successful. Except for 1 patient who died of thoracic injuries, all were discharged in good condition. No amputations were necessary.

Conclusion.—Because not all vascular injuries are clinically obvious, arteriography plays an important role in diagnosing penetrating extremity wounds. The 11% rate of significant vascular injury justifies the use of proximity arteriography in extremity trauma, at least until better clinical criteria are defined or less invasive tests are developed.

▶ Arteriography, done only for the indication of proximity injury in penetrating extremity trauma, has taken a real bashing in recent years. This interesting study indicates that, in the experience of these authors, such arteriography was very productive. I think it is quite reasonable for high-volume trauma centers to selectively delete proximity arteriography if they are able to thoroughly evaluate the patient by other means. Those of us in other settings should continue the use of arteriography for this indication. (See also Abstracts 14–2, 14–3, and 14–4.)—J.M. Porter, M.D.

The Reliability of Physical Examination in the Evaluation of Penetrating Extremity Trauma for Vascular Injury: Results at One Year

Frykberg ER, Dennis JW, Bishop K, Laneve L, Alexander RH (Univ of Florida, Jacksonville)

J Trauma 31:502–511, 1991   14–2

Background.—Cases of penetrating extremity injury (PEI) that have any "hard" sign of vascular trauma (i.e., active hemorrhage, distal pulse deficit, distal ischemia, or bruit) are treated by prompt surgical exploration. For penetrating wounds that are in proximity to major extremity arteries that do not manifest any hard signs, exclusion arteriography is the standard method of evaluation. However, some believe that physical examination of occult cases of proximity PEI may be as reliable as arteriography and clearly safer and less costly. The use of physical examination in predicting the presence or absence of significant vascular injury after penetrating extremity injury was evaluated.

Methods.—Penetrating wounds between the inguinal ligament and midcalf in the lower extremity, and between the deltopectoral groove and midforearm in the upper extremity were studied. During the 1-year period, 273 male patients and 37 female patients were seen with 366 penetrating wounds to an extremity. Seventy-one percent of the wounds were in a lower extremity. In 78% of the wounds, the PEI was judged to be in proximity to major extremity vessels but produced either no signs or soft signs of vascular injury (a negative physical examination). Fifty-nine wounds (16%) were asymptomatic but were judged not to be in proximity to major extremity vessels, and 21 wounds had at least 1 hard sign of vascular injury (a positive physical examination). Most PEI resulted from gunshot wounds, but stabs and lacerations were most likely to result in major vascular injury to the extremity. Two missed vascular injuries were both in the asymptomatic proximity group.

Results.—Eleven arteriograms were performed during the initial evaluation of PEI. Twenty-three extremity vascular injuries required surgical intervention, and 21 produced at least 1 hard sign detectable by physical examination alone. Because all extremity wounds with hard signs had surgically significant vascular trauma, the positive predictive value of physical examination was 100% in this study population.

Conclusion.—The overall predictive value of physical examination of PEI for vascular injury approached 100% in this study. The 2 cases of delayed diagnosis in the asymptomatic proximity group were promptly treated and had no morbidity when they became clinically manifest, which suggests that the perceived dangers of delayed diagnosis of vascular injury may be overestimated. In light of costly diagnostic alternatives, physical examination is a reliable and safe method of evaluation for PEI.

▶ These authors conclude that physical examination alone is adequate to detect extremity arterial trauma, and that arteriography is not required for indication of proximity only. These results are interesting, but they are insufficiently persuasive to change my mind. Of course, once my mind is made up, almost no amount of data is sufficient to change it.—J.M. Porter, M.D.

Noninvasive Diagnosis of Vascular Trauma by Duplex Ultrasonography
Bynoe RP, Miles WS, Bell RM, Greenwold DR, Sessions G, Haynes JL, Rush DS (Univ of South Carolina School of Medicine, Columbia)
J Vasc Surg 14:346–352, 1991   14–3

Background.—Neither surgical exploration nor arteriography is a perfect approach to evaluating vascular injuries. On the other hand, observational management entails a risk of occult arterial injury without obvious signs. Duplex ultrasonography has been widely used to screen carotid plaques and deep venous thromboses.

Methods.—Duplex ultrasonography was carried out in a prospective series of 198 patients with 319 possible vascular injuries of the neck or an extremity. Only stable patients without obvious arterial injury were included in the study. Gunshot injuries were most frequent, followed by blunt trauma, stab wounds, and shotgun injuries.

Results.—Duplex ultrasonography correctly detected and localized vascular injuries in 23 patients. The injuries included arterial disruption,

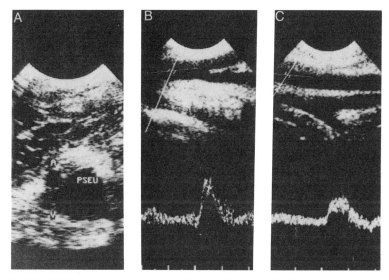

Fig 14–1.—Duplex ultrasonography of a gunshot wound to the thigh illustrating transversely (**A**) an acute traumatic extravasation (pseudoaneurysm) with a superficial femoral artery/superficial femoral vein arteriovenous fistula demonstrated longitudinally and proximally by disturbed superficial femoral artery flow (**B**) and arterialization of superficial femoral venous flow (**C**). (Courtesy of Bynoe RP, Miles WS, Bell RM, et al: *J Vasc Surg* 14:346–352, 1991.)

intimal flap, acute pseudoaneurysm (Fig 14–1), arteriovenous fistula, and arterial puncture by a shotgun pellet. Nineteen other patients were correctly found to have vasospasm or external arterial compression. Twenty patients had arterial repair, most on the basis of duplex ultrasonography alone. Two patients had minor pellet punctures that were missed, but neither required repair. One patient had a false positive duplex study. The technique was 95% sensitive and 99% specific, with an overall accuracy of 98%.

Conclusion.—Duplex ultrasonography appears to be as useful as exclusion arteriography in assessing vascular trauma. It poses no interventional risks and is a cost-effective approach.

▶ High-quality duplex ultrasonography may be a real plus in the evaluation of extremity and vascular trauma. I suspect that this may legitimately eliminate the need for arteriography in selected patients, but how many of us are able to perform high-quality duplex ultrasonography in the acute trauma setting? I suspect this will be a very difficult task to accomplish reliably.—J.M. Porter, M.D.

Can Doppler Pressure Measurement Replace "Exclusion" Arteriography in the Diagnosis of Occult Extremity Arterial Trauma?
Lynch K, Johansen K (Univ of Washington, Seattle)
Ann Surg 214:737–741, 1991   14–4

Background.—Contrast arteriography is an accurate way of ruling out occult arterial damage in an injured extremity, but it is costly, invasive, and time consuming. The value of Doppler-derived arterial pressure measurements in trauma victims was evaluated.

Methods.—The arterial pressure index (API) is the Doppler arterial pressure distal to the injury site divided by the pressure in the uninvolved arm. The API was determined in 100 consecutive injured extremities of 93 patients. Contrast arteriography then was performed.

Accuracy of Arterial Pressure Index < .90 Compared With
Arteriography and Clinical Outcome

Variable	Arteriography	Clinical Outcome
Sensitivity	0.87	0.95
Specificity	0.97	0.97
Positive predictive value	0.91	0.91
Negative predictive value	0.96	0.99
Overall accuracy	0.95	0.97

(Courtesy of Lynch K, Johansen K: *Ann Surg* 214:737–741, 1991.)

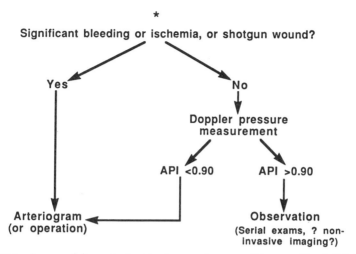

Fig 14–2.—A proposed diagnostic algorithm for extremity trauma. (Courtesy of Lynch K, Johansen K: *Ann Surg* 214:737-741, 1991.)

Results.—Twenty extremities had an API less than .9 and abnormal arteriographic findings. In 75 instances, both studies were normal. Compared with arteriography, an API less than .9 was 87% sensitive and 97% specific for arterial disruption (table). Both sensitivity and specificity improved when the API was compared with the clinical outcome.

Conclusion.—Estimation of the API may substitute for screening arteriography in patients with extremity injury, especially if close follow-up is assured (Fig 14–2).

▶ These authors in a major medical center conclude that simple ankle/brachial index determination can replace proximity indication arteriography with a very low likelihood of missing important injuries. They may be right, but I will still stick with arteriography.—J.M. Porter, M.D.

Successful Conservative Management of Iatrogenic Femoral Arterial Trauma
Rivers SP, Lee ES, Lyon RT, Monrad S, Hoffman T, Veith FJ (Albert Einstein College of Medicine/Montefiore Med Ctr, New York)
Ann Vasc Surg 6:45–49, 1992   14–5

Background.—In patients with femoral artery injury from diagnostic or interventional catheterization, emergency repair carries a significant rate of complications. A trial was begun of conservative management for patients with pseudoaneurysms or arteriovenous fistulas secondary to cardiac catheterization.

Conservative Management of Pseudoaneurysms

Series		Type of injury	Spontaneous resolution	Elective repair
Stein (1989)	n = 7	All penetrating trauma	5	2
Kotval (1990)	n = 3	Cardiac catheterization	3	0
Dennis (1990)	n = 5	All penetrating trauma	3	2
Kresowick (1991)	n = 9	PTCA	7	2
Present series n = 9		Cardiac catheterization and PTCA	8	1
Total n = 33			26 (79%)	7 (21%)

Abbreviation: PTCA, percutaneous transfemoral coronary angioplasty. (Courtesy of Rivers SP, Lee ES, Lyon RT, et al: *Ann Vasc Surg* 6:45–49, 1992.)

Patients and Methods.—Fifty-six of approximately 3,400 patients having transfemoral cardiac catheterization had femoral artery injuries. In 16 patients, it was possible to follow the natural course of the lesions. The patients, when hemodynamically stable, were placed on bed rest and had serial physical examination, duplex ultrasonography, and hematocrit estimates for at least 3 days.

Results.—Seven patients had a pseudoaneurysm, 6 had an arteriovenous fistula, and 3 had both complications. All but 1 of the pseudoaneurysms resolved spontaneously within 4 weeks. One patient given anticoagulant therapy required surgery for bleeding after 3 days of observation. Six of the 9 arteriovenous fistulas also resolved during the initial period of observation. The other 3 have remained asymptomatic during 4–20 months of follow-up.

Conclusion.—In this and other studies of conservative management for pseudoaneurysms after penetrating injury, nearly 80% of the lesions have resolved spontaneously (table). A period of observation is suggested for all hemodynamically stable patients, reserving surgery for those having hemorrhage, an expanding mass, or compromised cardiac output.

▶ Most pseudoaneursyms and arteriovenous fistulae arising incident to femoral artery catheterization resolve spontaneously without specific therapy. Others can be successfully thrombosed by duplex-guided external pressure. Considerably fewer of these lesions will require surgery in the future. See also Abstract 14–6.—J.M. Porter, M.D.

Postcatheterization Femoral Artery Injuries: Repair With Color Flow US Guidance and C-Clamp Assistance

Fellmeth BD, Buckner NK, Ferreira JA, Rooker KT, Parsons PM, Brown PR

(Mercy Gen Hosp, Sacramento Radiology Med Group, Sacramento, Calif)
Radiology 182:570–572, 1992   14–6

Background.—Compression repair of postcatheterization femoral artery injuries, guided by color flow ultrasonography, eliminates the need for surgery in most cases. Success has been achieved in more than 90% of cases using the method for as long as 2½ hours.

Methods.—Ultrasound-guided compression repair using a C-clamp device was attempted in 10 patients with clinical signs of femoral artery injury after a catheterization procedure. The upper arm of the clamp holds the ultrasound transducer, which can be moved to the best position for compression before being fixed in place. Lower compression pressure is tried after 20 minutes.

Results.—In 9 instances, the lesion was eliminated after a mean compression time of 59 minutes. The C-clamp effectively maintained the transducer in an effective position in 6 instances. Four patients required intervention to prevent slippage. The method was successful in all 4 patients receiving warfarin therapy.

▶ A spate of recent articles indicates that compression of postcatheterization arterial injuries (including both arteriovenous fistulas and pseudoaneurysms) using the duplex transducer head has been quite effective in inducing thrombosis of the lesion without further difficulty. These authors have devised an innovative clamp device, but I wonder whether having a human hold the probe might be preferable (1, 2). See also Abstract 14–5.—J.M. Porter, M.D.

References

1. Fellmeth BF, et al: *Radiology* 178:671, 1991.
2. Schwend R, et al: *J Vasc Tech* 15:83, 1991.

Spontaneous Thrombosis of Iatrogenic Femoral Artery Pseudoaneurysms: Documentation With Color Doppler and Two-Dimensional Ultrasonography
Johns JP, Pupa LE Jr, Bailey SR (Brooke Army Med Ctr, Fort Sam Houston, Tex)
J Vasc Surg 14:24–29, 1991   14–7

Background.—As many as 2% of femoral artery cannulations are complicated by pseudoaneurysm formation. A large-bore catheter or sheath and the cannulation of a poorly compressible vessel may contribute to pseudoaneurysm formation. Color Doppler imaging has recently been used instead of angiography for distinguishing between a pseudoaneurysm and hematoma. Prompt repair of these pseudoaneurysms has been proposed by some to avoid rupture or embolism.

Methods.—Both 2-dimensional ultrasonography and color Doppler imaging were used to diagnose and treat femoral artery pseudoaneurysms in 6 patients seen in an 18-month period with a pulsatile groin mass after catheterization. Pseudoaneurysm was diagnosed in these patients when the color Doppler study showed pulsatile systolic blood flow into an echolucent mass.

Results.—One patient underwent repair of a symptomatic pseudoaneurysm after the initial Doppler study. The other 5 patients underwent serial Doppler studies, which demonstrated resolution of the abnormality after a mean time of 18 days. One patient had surgical drainage of persistent hematoma, despite the absence of blood flow. Other complications did not occur during a mean follow-up of 233 days.

Conclusion.—Not all patients will small pseudoaneurysms after femoral artery cannulation require urgent surgical repair. Two-dimensional ultrasonography with Doppler color-flow imaging can distinguish those with an expanding mass and continued flow who require surgery from others who have stable or shrinking pseudoaneurysms.

▶ This conforms the information contained in Abstract 14–6.—J.M. Porter, M.D.

Acute Traumatic Aortic Aneurysm: The Duke Experience From 1970 to 1990

Duhaylongsod FG, Glower DD, Wolfe WG (Duke Univ, Durham, NC)
J Vasc Surg 15:331–343, 1992   14–8

Background.—Safe, expeditious repair of an acute traumatic aneurysm of the thoracic aorta is now possible, but significant numbers of patients still die of multisystem injuries.

Patients.—One hundred eight patients seen during decades with acute traumatic thoracic aortic aneurysms were studied. The mean patient age was 37 years, and the mean injury severity score (excluding aortic injury) was 17.5. Motor vehicle accidents accounted for three fourths of the patients.

Management.—Ninety-three patients lived long enough to come to surgery, which was done a median of 8 hours after injury. Shunts were used in 52.3% of the patients, bypass was used in 34.1%, and clamp/repair was used in 13.6%. In most patients, the aorta was repaired using a Dacron graft. The mean time of aortic occlusion was approximately 30 minutes in all groups.

Results.—There were 5 intraoperative deaths, 3 of them caused by aortic rupture and exsanguination. Twenty-two patients died postoperatively. Overall mortality was 39% of total admissions, but only 11 deaths were directly caused by thoracic aortic aneurysm. Associated injuries contributed to mortality in patients with late type transections (Fig

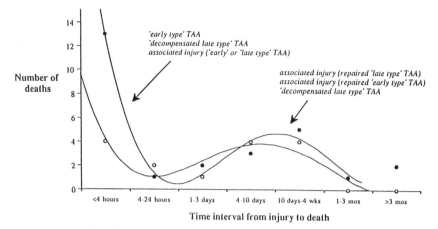

Fig 14–3.—Number of hospital deaths by time interval from injury to death. A bimodal distribution identifies 2 populations among patients with acute traumatic thoracic aortic aneurysm (TAA) (*open circle, 1970-1979; filled circle, 1980-1990*). (Courtesy of Duhaylongsod FG, Glower DD, Wolfe WG: *J Vasc Surg* 15:331-343, 1992.)

14-3). Five patients became paraplegic postoperatively; 4 had had shunt/bypass surgery and 1 had had clamp/repair.

Conclusion.—Patients with acute traumatic thoracic aortic aneurysms die chiefly of associated injuries, and these deaths have not declined substantially in the past 2 decades.

▶ The mortality rate among patients with traumatic thoracic aortic injury reaching the emergency room alive is almost 40%, and it has not improved in the past 20 years. An unknown, but doubtless very significant, percentage of these patients die immediately and never enter the trauma system. This paper provides an interesting discussion of the early type and late type injury patterns.—J.M. Porter, M.D.

Blunt Trauma to the Carotid Arteries
Martin RF, Eldrup-Jorgensen J, Clark DE, Bredenberg CE (Maine Med Ctr, Portland; State Univ of New York, Syracuse)
J Vasc Surg 14:789-795, 1991   14-9

Introduction.—Blunt injury of the carotid artery is infrequent but potentially dangerous. Eight patients with such injuries were examined in a 10-year period. Six of the patients had incurred a hyperextension injury and/or a cervical spine fracture.

Findings.—Arteriography demonstrated arterial dissection in 4 patients and thrombotic occlusion in 4. Two injuries were discovered while having CT of the head and neck. Two patients with asymptomatic common carotid artery occlusions and 1 with dissection causing transient ischemia successfully underwent arterial reconstruction. Three patients with internal carotid artery dissections were managed nonoperatively and had no more than minor neurologic deficit. Another patient had internal carotid artery thrombosis and a major fixed neurologic deficit that did not improve. One patient had asymptomatic thrombosis.

Conclusion.—Blunt injury of the carotid artery is a possibility in patient with hyperextension injury of the neck or cervical spine fracture, as well as those whose neurologic deficit not explained by intracranial trauma. Duplex scanning may be a helpful evaluative procedure. Surgery is indicated in selected patients who have an accessible lesion and a minor or no neurologic deficit. The asymptomatic patient with a small intimal flap or dissection may be adequately managed without surgery.

▶ The diagnosis of blunt carotid artery injury is frequently difficult and requires a high level of suspicion. This diagnosis should be suspected in patients with hyperextension injuries of the neck, cervical spine fractures and, especially, in patients with neurologic deficits not explained by intracranial trauma. Duplex scanning may be helpful. A typical clinical presentation is a lucid interval followed by the delayed development of a focal neurologic deficit.—J.M. Porter, M.D.

Peripheral Vascular Injuries in Children
Eren N, Özgen G, Ener BK, Solak H, Furtun K (Dicle Univ, Diyarbakir, Turkey)
J Pediatr Surg 26:1164–1168, 1991   14–10

Background.—Advances in vascular reconstruction have resulted in markedly lower rates of extremity amputation, even in difficult pediatric cases. An experience with the surgical treatment of 94 arteries and 39 veins in 91 children (mean age, 10.3 years) was reviewed.

Methods.—The children were treated at the study institution between 1978 and 1988. Most of the vascular injuries resulted from stab wounds,

Causes of Vascular Injuries		
Etiology	No.	%
Penetrating wound	37	40.7
Gunshot wound	31	34.1
Blunt trauma	21	23
Iatrogenic (surgical cutdown)	2	2.2
Total	91	100

(Courtesy of Eren N, Özgen G, Ener BK, et al: *J Pediatr Surg* 26:1164–1168, 1991.)

gunshot wounds, or traffic accidents; 2 cases occurred after surgical cut-down to establish venous access (table). Injured peripheral arteries were in the upper extremities in 43 patients and in the lower extremities in 51. Common clinical findings were no pulse distal to the area of injury (91.2%), open wounds (51%), coldness (51.6%), and pallor (42.8%). Twenty-one cases were associated with fractures.

Results.—Surgical methods of arterial repair consisted of end-to-end anastomosis in 61 children, autogenous saphenous vein graft replacement in 22, lateral suture in 8, and ligation in 3. Venous injuries were treated with end-to-end anastomosis in 19 patients, lateral suture in 6, saphenous vein graft replacement in 4, and ligation in 10. There were 8 cases of postoperative infection. Four patients required amputation. The patients who had amputation all had a delay of more than 18 hours from trauma to operation.

Conclusion.—Reconstruction of affected arteries is the most suitable surgical treatment of vascular injuries in children. Early treatment is essential for extremity preservation. Clinical findings are usually diagnostic, but arteriography is advised in the case of fractures and certain other situations.

▶ This sad report from Turkey documents the treatment of 94 arterial injuries in 91 children during a 10-year period. Stab wounds were the cause of the injury in 40% of the patients, and gunshot wounds were the cause in 23% of the patients. The age of these children ranges from 3 to 14 years, with a mean age of 10 years. The diagnostic and treatment methodology used is standard. To me, the noteworthy thing about this paper is the volume of severe trauma in such young children.—J.M. Porter, M.D.

Vertebrobasilar Ischemia After Neck Motion

Frisoni GB, Anzola GP (Università di Brescia, Spedali Civili, Brescia, Italy)
Stroke 22:1452–1460, 1991   14–11

Background.—Cerebral and brain stem ischemia after rotational head movements may result from chiropractic manipulation, simple falls, or spontaneous head turning. Of the 72 cases reported in the literature, 60 occurred after chiropractic manipulation. Vertebrobasilar distribution was involved in most cases. The possibility of identifying a population at risk is debated. Chiropractors claim that stroke after neck motion occurs in patients who have predisposing lesions, but physicians disagree. Three patients with vertebrobasilar ischemic stroke were studied. Two women and 1 man, aged 39–49 years, underwent chiropractic manipulation. In 2 patients, it was the first such procedure.

Case 1.—Man, 42, had mild hypertension but no other risk factors for stroke. Just after manipulation, this patient felt a sharp pain in the right side of his neck, followed by a brief syncope, paresthesias on the right side of his face, agitation, and an inability to stand. His symptoms did not progress over the next several hours. He was admitted, and a CT brain scan showed a small hypodense lesion in the right cerebellar hemisphere. A month later, brachial angiography showed a small right vertebral artery terminating into a normal posterior inferior cerebellar artery (PICA). Weeks later, MRI showed lesions in the lateral aspect of the right medulla and cerebellar hemisphere, both in the PICA distribution. This patient was discharged with good functional recovery, residual mild facial paresis, mild decreased pain, and temperature sensation in the right face and left limbs.

Case 2.—Woman, 39, had a sharp pain and severe vertigo and vomiting during chiropractic manipulation. Her symptoms did not progress in the hours after the procedure. This patient was also hypertensive and a moderate smoker. A brain CT scan done the next day showed a small hypodense cortical and subcortical cerebellar lesion in the right hemisphere within the PICA distribution. She had a good functional recovery with residual mild tendency to fall to the right when walking with closed eyes, miosis of the right eye, mild decreased pain and temperature sensation, and mild incoordination of the left lower limb.

Case 3.—Woman, 49, experienced vertigo, inability to stand, nausea, and repeated vomiting less than 1 hour after chiropractic manipulation. The symptoms did not progress. A brain CT scan showed a cerebellar hemorrhage involving the lower part of the upper vermis, mildly compressing the fourth ventricle. She was discharged without residual deficit, and later she underwent successful surgery for arteriovenous malformation ablation.

Conclusion.—Patients at risk cannot be identified beforehand. The presence of a vertebral artery terminating in PICA can be a contributing factor, although infrequently. However, its low frequency and the need for angiographic detection make it useless in daily practice. Vertebral ligament laxity is still speculation, but it may be prudent to avoid manipulating patients with known or suspected joint hypermobility. Development of neurologic symptoms during cervical manipulation always strongly contraindicates further chiropractic maneuvers. The cervical manipulation risk-benefit ratio always needs to be considered carefully, because possible complications are impossible to predict, can be very serious, and probably occur more often than believed.

▶ Many million chiropractic "neck adjustments" are performed annually in this country. A very small number of patients (only a few dozen have been reported to date) have had neurologic symptoms develop in close time proximity to the treatment associated with occlusion or obvious dissection of a vertebral artery. Thankfully, these symptoms usually improve and the patients return to near normal with the passage of time. Despite vascular surgeons' quick tendency to condemn chiropractic for this problem, it is noteworthy that a procedure that is performed more than 10 million times per year and is associated with a complication rate as trivial as that indicated by reports in the literature must be regarded overall as quite safe.—J.M. Porter, M.D.

Acute Foot Compartment Syndromes

Fakhouri AJ, Manoli A II (Wayne State Univ, Detroit)
J Orthop Trauma 6:223–228, 1992   14–12

Background.—Compartment syndrome is well recognized in the forearm and leg, but few reports of foot involvement have appeared. Data were reviewed on 12 such cases seen in 10 patients with a mean age of 33 years.

Findings.—All patients had incurred high-energy injuries: 6 in a fall from a height, 3 from crush injury, and 3 in a motor vehicle accident. There were 5 calcaneal fractures, 3 multiple metatarsal or phalangeal fractures (or both), and 2 Lisfranc fracture-dislocations with multiple metatarsal neck fractures. Tense swelling of the foot was the most consistent finding. The diagnosis was confirmed by pressure measurements in the medial, lateral, superficial, calcaneal, and interosseous compartments.

Treatment and Outcome.—Decompressive fasciotomy was carried out 3–13 hours after presentation, using a medial approach, combined medial and dorsal incisions, or combined medial, dorsal, and lateral incisions. All 4 patients with preoperative tingling and numbness gained at least partial relief. Most of those with severe pain had significant relief within 3 days of surgery. All the wounds healed well, and no infections occurred. Eight patients, however, had some degree of pain, discomfort, or stiffness after surgery, particularly when ambulating.

Discussion.—Classic signs of compartment syndrome are less reliable in the foot than they are elsewhere. Sensory deficit may reflect either nerve ischemia or direct nerve injury from the initial insult. The most consistent finding in all 12 cases was tense swelling of the foot. Tissue pressure measurements are necessary to reliably diagnose compartment syndrome in the foot.

▶ Compartment syndromes can, of course, occur in any fascial compartment in the body. Although they are most frequent in the calf, they certainly are not limited to this area. Foot compartment syndrome is an uncommon but potentially serious event. Surgeons caring for patients with extremity trauma must be familiar with this.—J.M. Porter, M.D.

Unstable Intertrochanteric Fracture Complicated by Pseudoaneurysm of the Deep Femoral Artery: Treatment by Transcatheter Embolisation

Edwards RD, Ingram S, McIntyre R (Western Infirmary, Glasgow, Scotland)
J Intervent Radiol 7:21–23, 1992   14–13

Background.—Pseudoaneurysm of the deep femoral artery is a recognized complication of orthopedic surgery of the femoral neck. In 1 case,

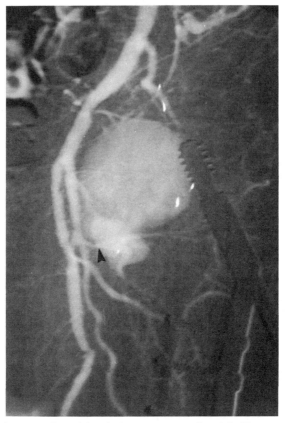

Fig 14–4.—Left common femoral digital subtraction angiography in left oblique anterior projection, showing a 7-cm pseudoaneurysm arising from the lateral circumflex branch of the deep femoral artery (*arrowhead*). (Courtesy of Edwards RD, Ingram S, McIntyre R: *J Interv Radiol* 7:21–23, 1992.)

a large pseudoaneurysm of the lateral circumflex branch of the deep femoral artery resulted from an unstable intertrochanteric fracture.

Case Report.—Woman, 82, incurred a 4-part intertrochanteric fracture of the left femur in a fall. She had a history of ischemic heart disease and parkinsonism. Considerable traction and mobilization of the femoral shaft were necessary to repair the fracture. Excellent anatomical reduction was achieved, but there was further femoral shortening and loss of reduction of the trochanteric fragments at clinic review. At 3 months, there was a tender 10-cm pulsatile mass on the anterior aspect of the thigh, which was shown by ultrasonography to be a pseudoaneurysm lined by thrombus. The 7-cm pseudoaneurysm arose from the lateral circumflex branch of the deep femoral artery (Fig 14–4). Placement of several coils was necessary to stop blood flow within the pseudoaneurysm. The patient was asymptomatic 6 months after the procedure.

Discussion.—Most pseudoaneurysms of the deep femoral artery complicating orthopedic surgery result from penetration of the arterial wall by a drill bit or screw. Laceration by sharp bone fragments also is a possibility. In this case, the artery may have been injured during surgical manipulation or later after loss of reduction. Transcatheter embolization is a useful alternative to surgical repair in elderly patients with co-existing medical disorders.

▶ It is amazing that orthopedists, with their drills, augers, reams, and various other medieval devices do not cause arterial damage more frequently.—J.M. Porter, M.D.

15 Venous Thrombosis and Pulmonary Embolism

Pattern and Distribution of Thrombi in Acute Venous Thrombosis
Markel A, Manzo RA, Bergelin RO, Strandness DE Jr (Univ of Washington, Seattle)
Arch Surg 127:305–309, 1992   15–1

Objective.—Duplex scanning was used to determine the site and extent of deep venous thrombosis in 833 patients examined in the past 3 years for suspected deep vein thrombosis. One fourth of the patients had positive studies.

TABLE 1.—Number of Limbs With Total or
Partial Obstruction

Vein Affected	R Leg		L Leg	
	Total	**Partial**	**Total**	**Partial**
CIV	4	2	12	6
EIV	18	6	30	9
CFV	33	24	46	33
SFV	51	26	67	33
PFV	26	5	30	8
Pop	48	29	63	31
PTV1	25	6	31	14
PTV2	24	11	31	15
GSV	13	7	15	8

Abbreviations: CIV, common iliac vein; *EIV*, external iliac vein; *CFV*, common femoral vein; *SFV*, superficial femoral vein (includes proximal, mid, and distal segments); *PFV*, deep femoral vein; *Pop*, popliteal vein; *PTV1* and *PTV2*, posterior tibial veins; *GSV*, greater saphenous vein. The values include bilateral cases.

(Courtesy of Markel A, Manzo RA, Bergelin RO, et al: *Arch Surg* 127:305–309, 1992.)

TABLE 2.—Isolated Deep Vein Thrombosis in
Different Veins of Both Legs

Vein Affected	R Leg	L Leg
IVC	0	0
CIV	1	0
EIV	0	0
CFV	3	4
SFV	6	7
PFV	0	0
Pop	11	13
PTV	7	4

Abbreviation: IVC, inferior vena cava; other abbreviations are as in Table 1. Both posterior tibial veins in each leg are considered together.
(Courtesy of Markel A, Manzo RA, Bergelin RO, et al: *Arch Surg* 127:305–309, 1992.)

Results.—Only 17% of the patients had both legs involved; in the others, the left leg was involved more often than the right. The superficial femoral, popliteal, and common femoral veins were most frequently affected (Table 1). Isolated occlusion of single veins was infrequent (Table 2). The above-knee region was involved in 95% of the patients with deep venous thrombosis, and the calf was involved in 40% (Table 3). Only partial obstruction occurred in 18% of the patients.

Conclusion.—Proximal venous thrombosis is a much more frequent cause for symptoms and referral for assessment than is isolated calf vein thrombosis.

▶ This careful publication contains an abundance of critical information. This excellent vascular laboratory found that, of the population referred to the vascular lab to rule out deep vein thrombosis, such thrombosis was actually present in 25% of the patients, and 95% of the patients had involvement of a major vein at or proximal to the popliteal vein. Isolated calf vein

TABLE 3.—Segment Involved by Deep Vein Thrombosis
in 209 Patients

Segment	Unilateral, No. (%)	Bilateral, No. (%)	Total, No. (%)
Proximal (above knee)	170 (81)	31 (141)	**200** (95)
Distal (below knee)	77 (37)	7 (3)	**84** (40)

(Courtesy of Markel A, Manzo RA, Bergelin RO, et al: *Arch Surg* 127:305–309, 1992.)

thrombosis was found in only 6% of the patients. This indicates that patients referred to the vascular lab to rule out deep vein thrombosis have a 25% likelihood of having venous thrombosis in their leg, and 95% of these venous thrombi are proximal and dangerous.—J.M. Porter, M.D.

Valvular Reflux After Deep Vein Thrombosis: Incidence and Time of Occurrence
Markel A, Manzo RA, Bergelin RO, Strandness DE Jr (Univ of Washington, Seattle)
J Vasc Surg 15:377–384, 1992   15–2

Objective.—Valve reflux was studied by duplex ultrasonography in 107 patients who had 123 legs involved by deep venous thrombosis and were under long-term follow-up. The studies were repeated after 1 week, 1 month, every 3 months for the first year, and then annually. The mean follow-up was 341 days. Reflux also was evaluated in 502 patients with negative results on duplex studies and no past history of thrombosis or chronic venous insufficiency.

Results.—Valve incompetence was present in 17 extremities (14%) in the group with acute deep venous thrombosis at the time of initial evaluation. Among those without initial reflux, the condition appeared in 17% of extremities within the first week (Table 1). More than two thirds of the extremities were affected within the first year of follow-up. At this time, the popliteal and superficial femoral veins were most frequently affected (Table 2). In subjects without initial thrombosis, reflux was found in the deep or superficial venous system in 6% of the extremities.

▶ Venous valvular reflux continues to develop for a long time after an identified venous thrombotic event. By 12 months, two thirds of patients with

TABLE 1.—Incidence of Reflux in Any Deep Vein
During Follow-up

Follow-up interval	Legs (n)	Reflux (%)	95%-CI
1 day	40	2 (5)	1-17
1 wk	54	9 (17)	8-30
1 mo	54	20 (37)	24-51
3 mo	61	32 (52)	39-65
6 mo	49	26 (53)	38-67
9 mo	36	20 (56)	38-72
1 yr	32	22 (69)	50-84
2 yr	24	15 (63)	41-81
3 yr	10	5 (50)	17-77

Abbreviation: CI, confidence interval.
(Courtesy of Markel A, Manzo RA, Bergelin RO, et al: *J Vasc Surg* 15:377–384, 1992.)

TABLE 2.—Incidence (Percent) of Reflux During
Follow-up Among Various Venous Segments

Follow-up interval	CFV	SFV	Pop	PTV	GSV
1 day	3	0	0	0	4
1 week	10	8	2	0	7
1 mo	13	20	10	9	20
3 mo	25	32	28	11	5
6 mo	26	31	34	6	20
9 mo	15	39	57	11	17
1 yr	33	37	58	18	25
2 yr	42	20	40	11	8
3 yr	46	29	50	0	33

Abbreviations: CFV, common femoral vein; SFV, superficial femoral vein; Pop, popliteal vein; PTV, posterior tibial vein; GSV, greater saphenous vein.
(Courtesy of Markel A, Manzo RA, Bergelin RO, et al: J Vasc Surg 15:377–384, 1992.)

deep vein thrombosis will have significant valvular insufficiency, primarily in the venous area involved in the thrombotic episode; however, it is not limited to these areas—not even to the same leg. I wonder how remote valvular insufficiency develops long after the thrombotic event.—J.M. Porter, M.D.

Frequency of Deep Venous Thrombosis in Asymptomatic Patients With Coronary Artery Bypass Grafts

Reis SE, Polak JF, Hirsch DR, Cohn LH, Creager MA, Donovan BC, Goldhaber SZ (Harvard Med School, Boston)
Am Heart J 122:478–482, 1991   15–3

Objective.—The frequency of clinically silent deep venous thrombosis (DVT) was determined by viewing the leg veins ultrasonographically in 29 asymptomatic patients who underwent coronary artery bypass graft surgery for myocardial revascularization.

Methods.—Both high-resolution B-mode ultrasonography and color Doppler imaging were done.

Findings.—Fourteen patients (48%) had a total of 20 documented leg vein thromboses. In all but 1 of the patients, DVT was restricted to the calf veins. One popliteal vein was involved. Half the thrombi were seen in the leg from which the saphenous vein was harvested (table). No patient had thrombosis suspected clinically, and there were no local signs resulting from vein harvest. Deep venous thrombosis was not associated with smoking or with the presence of varicose veins. No patient had clinically evident DVT or pulmonary embolism when followed for up to 11 months after coronary artery bypass graft surgery.

Results of Venous Ultrasound Examination ($n = 29$)

Results	N
No. of patients with DVT	14
No. of Patients with superficial vein thrombosis	2
Total number with DVT	20
Location of clots	
Popliteal vein (proximal)	1
Muscular veins (soleus, sural, gastrocnemius)	14
Peroneal vein	4
Posterior tibial vein	1
Leg with DVT (compared to SVG harvest site)	
Ipsilateral	10
Contralateral	10

Abbreviation: SVG, saphenous vein graft.
(Courtesy of Reis SE, Polak JF, Hirsch DR, et al: *Am Heart J* 122:478–482, 1991.)

Conclusion.—Asymptomatic DVT of the calf is surprisingly frequent; nearly half the study patients were affected after coronary artery bypass graft surgery.

▶ It has long been appreciated that DVT is infrequent in vascular patients, possibly because of heparin received during surgery. This study of patients undergoing bypass found that almost 50% had incidence of DVT, however, in all but 1 patient it was limited to the calf vein and appeared insignificant.—J.M. Porter, M.D.

Lower Extremity Calf Thrombosis: To Treat or Not to Treat?
Lohr JM, Kerr TM, Lutter KS, Cranley RD, Spirtoff K, Cranley JJ (Good Samaritan Hosp, Cincinnati)
J Vasc Surg 14:618–623, 1991   15–4

Single Vein Segment Involvement

	Segment involved	Patients
Propagators		$n = 13$
	PSOL	7 (54%)
	DSOL	4 (31%)
	PPTV	1 (8%)
	DPTV	1 (8%)
Nonpropagators		$n = 33$
	PSOL	15 (45%)
	DSOL	4 (15%)
	PPTV	6 (18%)
	DPTV	3 (9%)
	PPER	5 (15%)

Abbreviations: PSOL, proximal soleal vein; DSOL, distal soleal vein; PPTV, proximal posterior tibial vein; DPTV, distal posterior tibial vein; PPER, proximal peroneal vein.

(Courtesy of Lohr JM, Kerr TM, Lutter KS, et al: *J Vasc Surg* 14:618–623, 1991.)

Background.—Seventy-five patients with isolated calf vein thrombosis diagnosed by duplex ultrasonography were followed prospectively sequential duplex exams at 3-day to 4-day intervals.

Method.—A Biosound Phase II device with a 10-mHz phased linear-array probe was used to acquire duplex scans at 3- to 4-day intervals.

Results.—Twenty-four patients had propagation of thrombosis, in 11 instances into the popliteal vein or larger veins of the thigh, and in 13 to more proximal calf veins. Forty-nine patients had had surgery, but no particular procedures were significantly associated with propagation of thrombosis. The proximal soleal vein was the most commonly involved single vein segment, whether or not propagation occurred (table). Neither the extent of thrombosis nor the presence of bilateral involvement predicted propagation. In 4 instances, duplex scanning was done because of a highly probable ventilation-perfusion study.

Conclusion.—Deep venous thrombosis is not benign, even if it is initially limited to the calf. Long-term sequelae of deep venous insufficiency are as frequent as after more proximal deep venous thrombosis. Based on the likelihood of venous propagation and the high incidence of deep venous insufficiency in untreated patients, anticoagulation is recommended on a routine basis for patients with calf vein thrombosis, unless there is a high risk of complications from anticoagulation. Serial duplex scanning is an alternative approach to these patients.

▶ Fifteen percent of the patients with initially isolated calf vein thrombi (serially monitored with duplex scan) propagated thrombi into the popliteal or larger veins. There continues to be no consensus on the optimal treatment of truly isolated calf vein thrombus. Proponents of vigorous treatment cite the 15% to 20% incidence of major proximal vein propagation, as well as the long-term sequelae of valvular insufficiency, which may be reduced by anti-coagulation. Opponents cite the relatively infrequent complications of calf deep vein thrombosis and the high cost of routine treatment of all patients. Our current policy is not to treat with anticoagulation and to follow the patients with sequential duplex scans.—J.M. Porter, M.D.

Subcutaneous Low-Molecular-Weight Heparin Compared With Continuous Intravenous Heparin in the Treatment of Proximal-Vein Thrombosis

Hull RD, Raskob GE, Pineo GF, Green D, Trowbridge AA, Elliott CG, Lerner RG, Hall J, Sparling T, Brettell HR, Norton J, Carter CJ, George R, Merli G, Ward J, Mayo W, Rosenbloom D, Brant R (Univ of Calgary, Alta; Univ of British Columbia, Vancouver; Lions Gate Hosp, Vancouver; Northwestern Univ, Chicago; Texas A & M Univ, Scott and White Clinic, Temple; et al)
N Engl J Med 326:975–982, 1992   15–5

Background.—Compared with conventional unfractionated heparin, low-molecular-weight heparin has a high bioavailability and a prolonged half-life. However, there is little information on the relative efficacy of low-molecular-weight heparin in the treatment of deep vein thrombosis.

Methods.—Fixed-dose, subcutaneous, low-molecular-weight heparin given once a day was compared with adjusted-dose intravenous heparin given by continuous infusion in a multicenter, double-blind clinical trial as initial treatment for patients with proximal vein thrombosis. Objective documentation of clinical outcomes was used.

Findings.—Six of 213 patients given low-molecular-weight heparin and 15 of 219 given intravenous heparin had new episodes of venous thromboembolism. Major bleeding associated with initial treatment was noted in 1 patient in the low-molecular-weight heparin group and in 11 in the intravenous heparin group, representing a risk reduction of 91%. However, that apparent protection against major bleeding was lost during long-term treatment. Minor bleeding occurred infrequently. Mortality was 4.7% in the low-molecular-weight heparin group and 9.6% in the intravenous heparin group, for a risk reduction of 51%.

Conclusion.—Low-molecular-weight heparin is at least as safe and effective as intravenous heparin treatment. In addition, it is easier to give. Such treatment may enable patients with uncomplicated proximal deep vein thrombosis to be cared for on an outpatient basis.

▶ This and several subsequent articles document the intense interest in low-molecular-weight heparin. These authors conclude that low-molecular-weight heparin is at least as safe and effective as intravenous unfractionated heparin, and that it provides the opportunity for patients with uncomplicated deep vein thrombosis to be treated on an outpatient basis with subcutaneous drug administration, given only once daily.—J.M. Porter, M.D.

Comparison of Subcutaneous Low-Molecular-Weight Heparin With Intravenous Standard Heparin in Proximal Deep-Vein Thrombosis

Prandoni P, Lensing AWA, Büller HR, Carta M, Cogo A, Vigo M, Casara D, Ruol A, ten Cate JW (Univ of Padua, Italy; Academic Med Centre, Amsterdam)

Lancet 339:441–445, 1992   15–6

Introduction.—The efficacy of fixed-dose subcutaneous low-molecular-weight heparin (LMWH) therapy was compared with standard adjusted-dose intravenous heparin therapy in the treatment of deep vein thrombosis.

Methods.—Half of 170 consecutive symptomatic patients who had venographically confirmed proximal deep venous thrombosis received standard heparin therapy to prolong the activated partial thromboplastin time to 1.5–2 times the baseline value. The other patients received LMWH in doses adjusted for body weight for 10 days. Oral coumarin therapy was started after 1 week and continued for at least 3 months. Perfusion lung scanning was performed at baseline and on day 10, or earlier if clinically indicated.

Results.—Recurrent venous thromboembolism did not differ significantly in the 2 treatment groups, but venographic scores favored the LMWH group (table). Clinically significant bleeding was infrequent in both groups.

Conclusion.—Fixed-dose subcutaneous LMWH is at least as effective and safe as standard adjusted-dose intravenous treatment for symptomatic proximal vein thrombosis. Patients may be treated at home, because laboratory monitoring is not necessary.

▶ Abstract 15–5 from the prestigious *New England Journal of Medicine,* as well as this article from the *Lancet,* both conclude that subcutaneous LMWH is at least as effective and safe as standard unfractionated heparin treatment. These 2 important articles reach identical conclusions.—J.M. Porter, M.D.

Changes in Venographic Score

	No (%) of patients	
	Standard heparin (n = 85)	LMWH (n = 83)
Improvement ≥ 20%	20 (24%)	25 (30%)
Improvement < 20%	16 (19%)	25 (30%)
Unchanged	35 (41%)	28 (35%)
Worsening < 20%	6 (7%)	3 (3%)
Worsening ≥ 20%	8 (9%)	2 (2%)

(Courtesy of Prandoni P, Lensing AWA, Büller HR, et al: *Lancet* 339:441-445, 1992.)

Randomized Trial of Subcutaneous Low-Molecular-Weight Heparin CY 216 (Fraxiparine) Compared With Intravenous Unfractionated Heparin in the Curative Treatment of Submassive Pulmonary Embolism: A Dose-Ranging Study
Théry C, Simonneau G, Meyer G, Hélénon O, Bridey F, Armagnac C, d' Azemar P, Coquart JP (Hôpital Cardiologique, Lille, France; Hôpital A Béclère, Clamart, France; Hôpital Laënnec, Hôpital Necker, Paris; et al)
Circulation 85:1380–1389, 1992   15–7

Background.—Unfractionated heparin is generally used to treat minor and submassive pulmonary embolism, but it carries a significant risk of bleeding and its use requires hospital admission. Varying doses of Fraxiparine, a low-molecular-weight heparin, were evaluated in a series of 101 adult patients having angiographically proven pulmonary embolism with 15% to 55% pulmonary vascular obstruction.

Methods.—Patients received either standard heparin by continuous infusion, or Fraxiparine given subcutaneously in a dose of 400, 600, or 900 anti-Xa Institute Choay units per kilogram.

Results.—Inclusions ended when major bleeding developed in patients given the higher doses of Fraxiparine. The 400-unit dose proved to be as effective and as safe as unfractionated heparin. These groups had comparable angiographic improvement and similar rates of recurrence and bleeding.

Conclusion.—Fraxiparine is an effective alternative to unfractionated heparin for treating submassive pulmonary embolism.

▶ Low-molecular-weight heparin appears as effective as unfractionated heparin in the treatment of pulmonary embolism, as well as in the treatment of venous thrombosis. We will surely hear a great deal more about this substance in the future. See also Abstracts 15–5 and 15–6.—J.M. Porter, M.D.

The Significance of Venography in the Management of Patients With Clinically Suspected Pulmonary Embolism
Kruit WHJ, De Boer AC, Sing AK, Van Roon F (Bergweg Hosp, Rotterdam, The Netherlands)
J Intern Med 230:333–339, 1991   15–8

Background.—More than 90% of pulmonary emboli derive from deep venous thrombosis in the lower extremity. Lung scintigraphy is a very sensitive technique, but its specificity is quite variable. Pulmonary embolism is seen in perhaps 85% to 90% of the patients with substantial segmental perfusion defects and a ventilation mismatch, but 30% to 50% of the patients having proven embolism have such findings.

Methods.—Venography was evaluated prospectively in 169 patients clinically suspected of having pulmonary embolism. A ventilation-perfusion lung scan and impedance plethysmography were carried out, and patients with abnormal scan findings had bilateral venography of the lower legs.

Results.—Twenty-six percent of patients had normal scan findings and were not treated. Venography demonstrated thrombosis in 63 of the remaining 125 patients, and they received orally administered anticoagulants for 3 months. The remaining 62 patients with no leg thrombus received no treatment. New venous thrombosis developed during follow-up in 1 patient with a normal initial scan, 3 of those treated for thrombosis, and 1 with a negative venogram. One patient in the treated group had a pulmonary embolus. Thrombosis occurred in all but 7% of 41 patients whose scintigraphic findings were strongly suggestive of pulmonary embolism.

Conclusion.—Venography of the lower extremities can be helpful in patients clinically suspected of having pulmonary embolism if the lung scan does not provide adequate information.

▶ Between 50% and 75% of patients with pulmonary embolism have lower extremity deep vein thrombosis detectable by vascular lab or phlebogram at the time of pulmonary embolism diagnosis. I do not believe the presence or absence of lower extremity deep vein thrombosis is sufficient to enter into any decision-making algorithm concerning the treatment of patients with an abnormal ventilation perfusion lung scan consistent with pulmonary embolism. It seems to me that a pulmonary arteriogram would be a great deal more definitive than directing imaging attention to the legs.—J.M. Porter, M.D.

Autopsy-Verified Pulmonary Embolism in a Surgical Department: Analysis of the Period From 1951 to 1988
Lindblad B, Eriksson A, Bergqvist D (Univ of Lund, Sweden)
Br J Surg 78:849–852, 1991   15–9

Background.—Postoperative pulmonary embolism is an avoidable cause of death in many instances. Previous data have suggested a slight but significant reduction in pulmonary embolism in the 1970s.

Methods.—A review was undertaken of surgical patients in Malmö in 1951–1988 in whom pulmonary embolism was found at autopsy. Autopsies were done in 64% of 1,925 deaths occurring in 1981–1988. Nearly three fourths of the 811 patients dying within a month after surgery were autopsied.

Results.—Autopsy confirmed pulmonary embolism in 20.3% of all deaths and 31.7% of autopsies in 1981–1988. In 113 instances, pulmonary embolism was considered to be the cause of death, and it was a contributing factor in another 104 cases. Few patients had symptomatic deep venous thrombosis or pulmonary embolism before death. The overall rate of major pulmonary embolism remained constant at .3% during the review period. The reduction previously noted in the late 1970s continued into the 1980s. An increasing number of patients given prophylaxis against thrombosis had autopsy-proved pulmonary embolism.

Conclusion.—Pulmonary embolism is still an important cause of postoperative death, although it has decreased in frequency in the past 15 years. The incidence in the 1980s in an unselected surgical population is about the same as that reported in trials of thrombosis prevention.

▶ The remarkable Swedish Medical Record Department strikes again. Obviously, every part of every report of every autopsy ever conducted in Malmö is liable to form the basis for a major report in the medical literature. The authors conclude that pulmonary embolism has decreased in frequency during the past 15 years based on their autopsy study; however, I remain unconvinced that this type of retrospective review can really detect small changes.—J.M. Porter, M.D.

Postoperative Pulmonary Embolism After Hospital Discharge: An Underestimated Risk
Huber O, Bounameaux H, Borst F, Rohner A (Univ Hosp of Geneva)
Arch Surg 127:310–313, 1992   15–10

Series.—Pulmonary embolism (PE) is a rare but serious complication of surgery and immobilization. A total of 28,953 patients were admitted to a clinic of digestive surgery in 1980 through 1989, and two thirds of them underwent surgery.

Findings.—Symptomatic PE developed in 90 of these patients, .3% of the total series, during their hospital stay. Twenty-nine patients (.1%) were readmitted with PE within 30 days after discharge from hospital. In surgically treated patients, delayed PE occurred a median of 18 days after surgery and 6 days after discharge. Delayed PE was more frequent after ostensibly low-risk opeations such as herniotomy and appendectomy.

Conclusion.—The significant occurrence of PE after discharge of surgical patients provides the basis for prolonged prophylaxis. Inclusion of PEs within 30 days of discharge increases procedural PE rates by 30%.

▶ A significant number of pulmonary emboli occur many days after surgery and, frequently, many days after hospital discharge. When one makes a real effort to include all pulmonary emboli within 30 days of surgery, the incidence of apparent PE increases by as much as 30% over the incidence by the time of hospital discharge. This information also raises the issue as to whether prolonged prophylactic measures should be considered after hospital discharge.—J.M. Porter, M.D.

Rapid Anticoagulation Using Ancrod for Heparin-Induced Thrombocytopenia

Demers C, Ginsberg JS, Brill-Edwards P, Panju A, Warkentin TE, Anderson DR, Turner C, Kelton JG (McMaster Univ, Hamilton, Ont, Canada)
Blood 78:2194–2197, 1991   15–11

Introduction.—Approximately 1% to 5% of heparin-treated patients become thrombocytopenic. Thrombocytopenia itself rarely causes bleeding, but it may be complicated by venous or arterial thrombosis. Oral anticoagulant therapy can prevent recurrent venous thrombosis, but it requires time to become effective. Ancrod is a rapid-acting defibrinogenating agent that reportedly is an effective treatment for acute deep venous thrombosis.

Methods.—Ancrod was given to 11 consecutive patients who required anticoagulation for venous thromboembolism and who had acute heparin-related thrombocytopenia or a history of such thrombocytopenia. The diagnosis was based on a decrease in platelets of at least 50% or a platelet count less than $70 \times 10^9/L$ in temporal relation to heparin therapy. Ancrod was given as an intravenous infusion or subcutaneously in an initial dose of 1–2 U/kg, and the maintenance dose was adjusted to maintain a fibrinogen level of .5–1 g/L.

Results.—In all patients whose platelet count decreased during heparin therapy, ancrod therapy was followed by recovery of platelets a median of 6 days after discontinuing heparin. In 2 patients, venous thrombosis recurred during warfarin treatment after ancrod was withdrawn. No patient had arterial thrombosis while receiving ancrod.

Conclusion.—Ancrod is a reasonable choice for patients with heparin-induced thrombocytopenia who require anticoagulation. A targeted fibrinogen level of .5–1 g/L appears to be adequate.

▶ It is difficult to place ancrod in perspective. This is an interesting drug that appears to be effective, has been on the market for many years, and has been almost ignored. This drug is clearly effective in selective situations, and it probably is one that we should consider more often.—J.M. Porter, M.D.

Oral Contraceptive Estrogen Dose and the Risk of Deep Venous Thromboembolic Disease

Gerstman BB, Piper JM, Tomita DK, Ferguson WJ, Stadel BV, Lundin FE (Food and Drug Administration, Rockville, Md; Vanderbilt Univ, Nashville)
Am J Epidemiol 133:32–37, 1991   15–12

Background.—Little information is available about the thromboembolic disease risk associated with use of oral contraceptives containing less than 50 µg of estrogen. The rates of deep venous thrmobosis in patients using oral contraceptives containing varying rates of estrogen were estimated in a large cohort of Medicaid patients.

Methods.—A total of 2,739,400 prescriptions for oral contraceptives were analyzed in 234,218 patients between 15 and 44 years of age during nearly a 6-year period. The average follow-up was 33.2 days per prescription. Low-estrogen formulations were considered as those containing less than 50 μg of estrogen; intermediate-dose formulations contained 50 μg, and high-dose formulations more than 50 μg. Older patients, white patients, and those earlier in the study tended to receive the higher dose formulations. The low-estrogen cohort was used as the referent group, and relative risk of deep venous thrombosis was adjusted for age and calendar period.

Results.—The rates of thrombosis were 4.2 per 10,000 person-years for low-dose formulations, 7 for intermediate-dose formulations, and 10 for high-dose formulations. The adjusted relative risks were 1.5 for intermediate doses and 1.7 for high doses. When diagnostically confirmed cases were considered separately, relative risks were for intermediate doses and 3.2 for high doses.

Conclusions.—Oral contraceptives containing less than 50 μg of estrogen appear to reduce risk of deep venous thrombosis compared with formulations containing higher doses of estrogen. The design of this study overcomes some potential sources of bias but prevents estimation of relative risk of low-dose formulations. There appears to be a dose-response relationship between estrogen in oral contraceptives and venous thromboembolism across the dose range of products on the market.

▶ My interpretation of an abundance of literature is that anovulatory medications containing less than 50 μg of estrogen carry little or no measurable risk of increased venous thrombosis. An interesting question is whether women who have had 1 episode of deep venous thrombosis should continue to take oral contraceptives. If they are taking the modern version with very low-dose estrogen, I do not believe there is any significant increase in thrombotic risk.—J.M. Porter, M.D.

Intracardiac and Intrapulmonary Greenfield Filters: A Long-Term Follow-Up
Gelbfish GA, Ascer E (Maimonides Med Ctr, Brooklyn, NY)
J Vasc Surg 14:614–617, 1991   15–13

Background.—The best way of managing a misplaced or migrating Greenfield caval filter is uncertain. Attempts to remove the filter surgically from the heart or pulmonary artery may be too risky, but it is not clear that leaving a filter in place is safe over the long term.

Methods.—Three patients in whom a Greenfield filter was accidentally placed in the right side of the heart were treated. In 1 patient, the filter

Previous Reports of Intracardiac Intrapulmonary Filters

Author	Ref no.	Year	No. cases	Location	Intervention
Greenfield	1	1977	1	Heart	Operative removal
Greenfield	4	1980	1	Heart	Percutaneous reposition
Akins	5	1980	1	Heart	Operative removal
Scurr	6	1983	1	Heart	None
Castaneda	7	1983	1	Migrated to heart	None
Moore	8	1983	1	Migrated to heart	Operative removal
Friedell	9	1986	1	Migrated to PA	None
Hirsch	10	1987	2	Heart	Operative removal
Deutch	11	1988	1	Heart	Percutaneous removal

Abbreviations: PA, pulmonary artery.
(Courtesy of Gelbfish GA, Ascer E: *J Vasc Surg* 14: 614–617, 1991.)

migrated to the pulmonary artery. All patients were managed without attempting surgical removal.

Outcome.—In 2 cases, an attempt was made to remove the filter using a wire loop and sheath. Neither attempt succeeded and, in 1 case, the filter migrated to the right inferior pulmonary artery. None of the patients had complications when followed up for 2, 45, and 60 months, respectively.

Literature Review.—Ten cases of intracardiac or intrapulmonary filter were found on reviewing the English-language literature (table). Five ectopic filters were removed surgically, but clear indications were present in only 2. No patient had valvular incompetence or cardiac tamponade. Significant side effects did not occur when filters were left in place.

Conclusion.—Neither the authors' personal experience nor a review of the literature justifies the routine removal of ectopic caval filters. The potential morbidity from a filter must be weighed against the risk of attempted removal, whether operative or using a wire loop and sheath.

▶ Complications of intravascular foreign bodies continue to appear. It is interesting to note that simply leaving the filter in the right side of the heart or the pulmonary artery appears to be well tolerated.—J.M. Porter, M.D.

Floating Thrombi: Diagnosis and Follow-Up by Duplex Ultrasound
Voet D, Afschrift M (Univ Hosp, Gent, Belgium)
Br J Radiol 64:1010–1014, 1991   15–14

Introduction.—It is important to know whether certain thrombi pose an increased risk of embolization and, if so, how to identify them. Several reports in the past decade have suggested that floating iliofemoral thrombi carry a significant risk of pulmonary embolism.

Methods.—Floating thrombi (FT) were found on duplex scanning in 39 patients treated in 1987–1989 for above-knee deep venous thrombosis. In 30 patients, the evolution of the FT could be evaluated 2 weeks and/or 3 months after diagnosis. The criterion for FT was adherence of

Anatomical Distribution of Floating Thrombi (46 Veins)

	Veins with floating thrombus	
	Number	%
External iliac vein	7	15
Common femoral vein	18	39
Superficial femoral vein	5	11
Profunda vein	1	2
Popliteal vein	12	26
Long saphenous vein	3	7
Total	46	100

(Courtesy of Voet D, Afschrift M: *Br J Radiol* 64: 1010–1014, 1991.)

only the distal part of the thrombus to the vein wall, with the proximal segment moving freely in the blood stream when gentle calf pressure is applied.

Results.—The 44 FT in these patients were most prevalent in the common femoral vein, followed by the popliteal and then the external iliac veins (table). One third of the FT in the iliofemoral segment disappeared at follow-up, one third were unchanged, and almost one third were adherent to the vein wall. Only 13% of the floating segments remained visible after 3 months. In 13 patients, there were pulmonary embolisms before or after FT were diagnosed. More than one fourth of the FT were associated with malignant disease.

Conclusion.—Symptomatic pulmonary embolism occurred in 9% of 44 FT in these patients and in 14% of iliofemoral FT. All patients were undergoing therapeutic heparinization at the time of embolism.

▶ What is the real risk of the "floating thrombus" which we occasionally visualize in the ileofemoral venous system or even in the vena cava? These authors have found a lower incidence of pulmonary embolism than others have reported. This retrospective study does not definitively answer the question as to whether "floating" thrombi are more hazardous than adherent thrombi. I am not convinced that they are, and we continue to treat these patients in a standard fashion.—J.M. Porter, M .D.

Superior Vena Cava Occlusion in a Patient With Antiphospholipid Antibody Syndrome
Tomer Y, Kessler A, Eyal A, Many A, Shoenfeld Y (Chaim Sheba Med Ctr, Tel-Hashomer, Israel)
J Rheumatol 18:95–97, 1991   15–15

Introduction.—Many types of thromboembolic complications are known to occur in patients with antiphospholipid syndrome. Data were reviewed on a patient with an antiphospholipid syndrome associated with a lupus-like disease, which was complicated by a superior vena cava occlusion.

Case Report.—Woman, 55, had increasing facial edema. She had a lupus-like disease for 15 years and a history of 5 spontaneous abortions. The facial edema was attributed to steroid treatment, but it did not improve with a tapering of the dose. On admission to the hospital, congestion of the neck veins was noted, and the liver was palpable 3 cm below the costal margin. A CT scan of the chest revealed a thrombus in the superior vena cava that extended to the right jugular vein and was confirmed by Doppler ultrasonography. Treatment with heparin, 1,250 U/hour for 10 days, reduced the facial swelling. The patient was maintained on long-term warfarin therapy.

Conclusion.—The antiphospholipid syndrome is associated with a wide variety of conditions, including systemic lupus erythematosus. The thromboembolic complications associated with this syndrome are numerous, but this appears to be the first report of superior vena cava involvement. Physicians should be aware of this possibility when facial swelling appears in patients with antiphospholipid syndrome. Lifelong anticoagulant therapy may be necessary.

▶ Both arterial and venous thrombotic events can be caused by hypercoagulable abnormalities. One important abnormality is the antiphospholipid (or anticardiolipin) antibody. The other side of the coin, lupus anticoagulant, cross-reacts with anticardiolipin antibody in 80% to 90% of the patients; however, in a few patients they do not cross-react. When screening patients for hypercoagulable disorders, both of these should be checked.—J.M. Porter, M.D.

Duplex Scanning Versus Venography as a Screening Examination in Total Hip Arthroplasty Patients
Barnes CL, Nelson CL, Nix ML, McCowan TC, Lavender RC, Barnes RW (Univ of Arkansas for Med Sciences, Little Rock)
Clin Orthop 271:180–189, 1991   15–16

Background.—Improvements in pharmacologic and mechanical prophylaxis notwithstanding, deep vein thrombosis (DVT), and pulmonary embolism (PE) are still the leading causes of death and injury among hospitalized patients. Approximately 200,000 fatal pulmonary emboli occur annually in North America, more than half of which occur in hospitalized patients. Duplex scanning was studied to determine whether it is sensitive and specific enough to screen patients for popliteal and more proximal DVT before and after elective total hip arthroplasty (THA).

Results of Postoperative Duplex Scanning and
Venography (158 Patients)

		Duplex Scan	
Venogram	*No. Limbs*	*Normal*	*Abnormal*
Normal	289	283	6
Abnormal	19	4	15
Total	308	287	21

(Courtesy of Barnes CL, Nelson CL, Nix ML, et al: *Clin Orthop* 271:180–189, 1991.)

Methods.—A total of 158 patients were enrolled in the study. Combined B-mode/Doppler scanning was compared with venography in routine perioperative screening for DVT. Preoperative scans were done in the first 60 patients; the preoperative prevalence of 2% for proximal DVT was thought to not justify routine preoperative scanning.

Findings.—Duplex scanning had a postoperative sensitivity of 79%, specificity of 98%, and an accuracy of 79% when venographic findings were used as the gold standard. In this group of patients undergoing THA who were treated with mechanical and pharmacologic prophylaxis, the postoperative incidence of proximal DVT was 12%. When calf vein thrombosis was included, 30% had DVT after surgery (table).

Conclusion.—Duplex imaging is an attractive alternative to venography in the screening of patients undergoing THA. It is sensitive and specific enough to detect asymptomatic proximal DVT before and after surgery in patients undergoing this orthopedic procedure. Duplex scanning may now be considered the gold standard for detecting popliteal or more proximal DVT in this population.

▶ This is another clinical correlation of the performance of duplex scanning in comparison to phlebography in the detection of lower extremity venous thrombi. Duplex does very well. In my opinion it is that, with the availability of experienced vascular laboratory technologists, there is no longer any indication for using phlebography for the diagnosis of lower extremity DVT, including calf vein thrombi.—J.M. Porter, M.D.

Prevention of Thromboembolism After Spinal Cord Injury Using Low-Molecular-Weight Heparin

Green D, Lee MY, Lim AC, Chmiel JS, Vetter M, Pang T, Chen D, Fenton L, Yarkony GM, Meyer PR Jr (Northwestern Univ Med School; Rehabilitation Inst of Chicago; Mem Hosp, Chicago)
Ann Intern Med 113:571–574, 1990   15–17

Objective and Methods.—Many patients paralyzed by spinal cord injury have thromboembolism. The prophylactic value of low-molecular-weight heparin was examined in 41 patients who underwent daily clinical assessments and serial venous flow studies including duplex examinations. The patients received either 5,000 units of standard heparin 3 times daily, subcutaneously, or daily subcutaneous injections of 3,500 anti-Xa units of low-molecular-weight heparin. All the patients had a complete motor spinal cord injury within 72 hours before admission.

Results.—Five patients who were given standard heparin had thrombosis, including 2 who died of pulmonary embolism. Two other patients were withdrawn because of bleeding. None of the patients given low-molecular-weight heparin had either thrombotic events or bleeding. The difference between the 2 groups was significant (Fig 15–1).

Conclusions.—Low-molecular-weight heparin is an effective and safe way of preventing thromboembolism in cord-injured patients who are paralyzed. Whether multiply injured and brain-injured patients also will benefit remains to be determined.

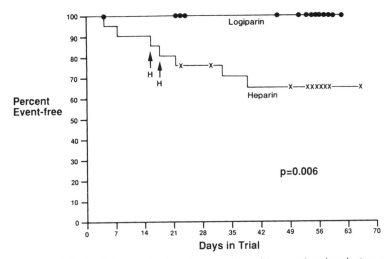

Fig 15–1.—A Kaplan-Meier plot showing when hemorrhagic (H, *arrows*) or thrombotic events occurred. The times at which patients left the trial are indicated by *filled circles* for low-molecular-weight heparin (*Logiparin*) and by *crosses* for standard heparin. The difference in event rates between the 2 groups was significant at P = .006 (log-rank test). (Courtesy of Green D, Lee MY, Lim AC, et al: *Ann Intern Med* 113:571–574, 1990.)

▶ It is sobering to realize that as much as 100% of all patients with complete motor paralysis after spinal cord injury have venous thrombosis. Apparently, almost the same number of patients with severe head trauma are also afflicted. Low-molecular-weight heparin appears to be effective in venous thrombosis prophylaxis in this very difficult patient group. In this study, the use of low-molecular-weight heparin was not associated with any complications of thrombosis or bleeding.—J.M. Porter, M.D.

Thromboembolism Following Multiple Trauma
Knudson MM, Collins JA, Goodman SB, McCrory DW (Univ of California, San Francisco; Stanford Univ Med Ctr, Stanford, Calif)
J Trauma 32:2-11, 1992   15–18

Background.—Deep venous thrombosis (DVT) and pulmonary embolism (PE) are potentially preventable causes of morbidity in trauma patients, but their true prevalence is uncertain. A Consensus Conference of the National Institutes of Health estimated that DVT occurs in approximately 20% of young patients with multisystem trauma. This study was an attempt to prospectively identify risk factors in 113 adults seen on a trauma service in a 1-year period.

Methods.—The patients were assigned to receive low-dose heparin (5,000 U given subcutaneously every 12 hours), or to wear sequential compression devices (SCDs). Duplex ultrasonography was used to detect thrombus in the common femoral through the popliteal veins, and ventilation-perfusion lung scanning was carried out when PE was suspected clinically.

Results.—Thromboembolism developed in 12% of the SCD group and in 8% of heparin-treated patients. Four patients had PE alone, and 3 had both DVT and PE. None of the patients with PE died, and no major complications resulted from prophylaxis. Compared with those without DVT/PE, patients with DVT/PE were older, required longer immobilization and more transfusions, and had PTT prolongation upon admission.

Conclusion.—A minority of adult trauma patients are at an increased risk of having DVT or PE develop. Both prophylaxis and close surveillance for DVT are warranted in these cases.

▶ This study emphasizes the seriousness of the problem of DVT in trauma patients, and it indicates that low-molecular-weight heparin is just as effective as the sequential pneumatic compression device, which is one of the most effective methods for DVT prophylaxis. I am convinced that low-molecular-weight heparin is going to be an important agent.—J.M. Porter, M.D.

Progression and Regression of Deep Vein Thrombosis After Total Knee Arthroplasty

Maynard MJ, Sculco TP, Ghelman B (Hosp for Special Surgery, New York)
Clin Orthop 273:125–130, 1991   15–19

Background.—Deep vein thrombosis (DVT) is a common finding in patients who have undergone total knee arthroplasty (TKA). There is considerable controversy regarding 2 aspects of the problem: the degree of danger posed by thromboses confined to the deep veins of the calf, and the choice and timing of prophylactic therapy for DVT.

Methods.—Patients selected for a prospective study were older than age 50 years and had indications for unilateral or bilateral primary TKA. Fifty-nine patients (76 knees) were evaluated with early (day of surgery or first postoperative day) and late (fourth to seventh day after surgery) postoperative venograms. Warfarin anticoagulation was started after the first postoperative venogram in those with positive studies.

Results.—Only 1 of the knees examined before surgery had a positive venogram. This patient, who had a history of pulmonary embolism (PE), had a thrombus formation in 1 deep calf vein. The overall positive rate for knees evaluated after operation was 47% for early and 54% for late venography. In the unilateral postoperative group, the rate of positive early venograms was 45%. Late venography yielded positive findings in 52%. Between the 2 evaluation times, 5 negative extremities had become positive and 2 positive extremities had become negative. In the bilateral group, there was a 50% positive rate at early venography and a 56% positive rate at late venography. Six extremities (18%) had additional clot formation between early and late venography. None of the patients showed symptoms of PE at any time during hospitalization. Twelve percent of the patients had deep vein clot proximal to the calf. Despite warfarin, 6% of patients with unilateral TKA showed clot propagation into the deep vein and to the calf between early and late venograms.

Conclusion.—Most thrombi related to TKA are formed in the intraoperative or immediate postoperative period. Thus, it is recommended that prophylaxis be targeted on these periods. Warfarin therapy at the time of the initial positive venogram did not entirely prevent propagation of thromboses into or above the popliteal vein.

▶ Deep vein thrombosis is a frequent complication of lower extremity joint replacement surgery. In these patients, DVT prophylaxis obviously is extremely important. In this study, between 40% and 50% of all patients had positive phlebograms, 12% of which had thrombus involvement in the large veins proximal to the calf.—J.M. Porter, M.D.

Prevention of Deep Vein Thrombosis After Total Knee Arthroplasty: Coumadin Versus Pneumatic Calf Compression

Hodge WA (Massachusetts Gen Hosp, Boston)
Clin Orthop 271:101–105, 1991   15–20

Background.—Deep vein thrombosis (DVT) has been reported in as many as 84% of patients having total knee arthroplasty without prophylaxis. Both warfarin and pneumatic calf compression (PCC) boots are thought to be effective in reducing the occurrence of DVT.

Methods.—Forty-eight consecutive patients undergoing knee arthroplasty received warfarin anticoagulation, and they were compared with 81 consecutive patients who were treated with sequential PCC boots. Lower limb phlebography was carried out 8–10 days postoperatively.

Results.—Deep vein thrombosis developed in 33% of the warfarin-treated patients, 6% of whom had thrombi in thigh veins. In the PCC group the incidence of DVT was 31%, with 6% having thigh thrombi. There were no treatment-related complications in either group. Warfarin treatment was almost 50% more expensive than the use of PCC boots.

Conclusion.—Both warfarin and PCC boots are safe and effective in limiting the occurrence of DVT after total knee arthroplasty, but economic factors suggest that PCC boots are the best option.

▶ See the comments after Abstract 15–19. Both warfarin and pneumatic compression devices appear effective in limiting the occurrence of DVT.—J.M. Porter, M.D.

Prevention of Deep Vein Thrombosis After Hip Replacement: Randomised Comparison Between Unfractionated Heparin and Low Molecular Weight Heparin

Leyvraz PF, Bachmann F, Hoek J, Büller HR, Postel M, Samama M, Vandenbroek MD (Vaudois Univ Hosp, Lausanne, Switzerland; Academic Med Ctr, Amsterdam; Hôpital Cochin, Paris; Hôtel-Dieu, Paris; Sanofi Research, Gentilly, France)
BMJ 303:543–548, 1991   15–21

Background.—There is controversy surrounding the best approach to preventing venous thromboembolic disease in patients undergoing total hip replacement. Low-molecular-weight heparin appears to be particularly effective. A prospective, open, randomized study was conducted to compare treatment with unfractionated vs. low-molecular-weight heparin.

Methods.—The study included 349 patients undergoing total hip replacement at 28 European orthopedic surgery departments during an 8-month period. The patients were randomized to receive either low-molecular-weight heparin with antifactor Xa activity or unfractionated

Frequency and Location of Deep Vein Thrombosis in 2
Study Groups. Figures Are Numbers (Percentages)
of Patients

Anatomical site	Patients receiving low molecular weight heparin (n=174)	Patients receiving unfractionated heparin (n=175)
Calf veins alone	17 (9·8)	5 (2·9)
Calf and proximal veins	3 (1·7)	12 (6·9)
Proximal veins alone	2 (1·1)	11 (6·3)
Total	22 (12·6)	28 (16)

Note: Bilateral phlebography was performed in all patients on days 9–11
after surgery.
(Courtesy of Leyvraz PF, Bachmann F, Hoek J, et al: BMJ 303:543–548,
1991.)

heparin. The former group received Fraxiparine, 41 IU/kg/day, for 3 days, then 62 IU/kg/day for 7 days, subcutaneously. The other group received subcutaneous unfractionated heparin every 8 hours, with the dose adjusted to maintain activated thromboplastin time at 2–5 seconds above control values. Ten days postoperatively, each patient underwent bilateral phlebography.

Results.—Deep vein thrombosis occurred in 16% of the unfractionated heparin group and in 12.65% of the low-molecular-weight heparin group (table). Thrombosis of the proximal vein occurred in 13.1% of the patients who received unfractionated heparin, and in 2.9% of those who received low-molecular-weight heparin. Pulmonary embolism occurred in 4 of the unfractionated heparin group vs. 1 of the low-molecular-weight heparin group. Both groups had a low incidence of bleeding complications.

Conclusion.—Low-molecular-weight heparin is at least as effective as unfractionated heparin in preventing deep vein thrombosis in patients undergoing total hip replacement. The low-molecular-weight regimen is more effective in preventing thrombosis of the proximal veins. This regimen is no more likely to result in bleeding complications and is easier to administer.

▶ Once again, low-molecular-weight heparin appears just as effctive as unfractionated heparin in preventing deep vein thrombosis, in this case after hip replacement. See also Abstract 15–18.—J.M. Porter, M.D.

Intermittent Pneumatic Compression Versus Coumadin: Prevention of Deep Vein Thrombosis in Lower-Extremity Total Joint Arthroplasty
Kaempffe FA, Lifeso RM, Meinking C (State Univ of New York, Buffalo; VA

Med Ctr, Buffalo)
Clin Orthop 269:89–97, 1991   15–22

Background.—Patients having joint arthroplasty in the lower extremity are at high risk of having venous thromboembolism develop, and the risk is compounded by older age.

Methods.—One hundred patients having total joint arthroplasty in the lower extremity were randomized to receive either warfarin therapy or intermittent pneumatic compression to prevent deep venous thrombosis (DVT). Ascending venography was used to diagnose DVT in most instances, but nuclear venography, Doppler examination, and impedance plethysmography also were used.

Results.—One fourth of the patients given warfarin and the same proportion of those treated by pneumatic compression had DVT develop. The latter method was more effective in patients having primary total hip arthroplasty, whereas warfarin was more effective in those undergoing primary total knee arthroplasty. More than one third of the patients having revision arthroplasty had DVT develop. Three fourths of all thrombi occurred proximally. Both treatments were safe. One of the 3 postoperative deaths might have resulted from pulmonary embolism.

Conclusion.—Pneumatic compression most effectively prevented DVT after hip arthroplasty, whereas warfarin was more effective in patients having knee arthroplasty.

▶ Pneumatic compression, warfarin, and low-molecular-weight heparin all appear effective in prevention of DVT with total joint arthroplasty.—J.M. Porter, M.D.

Prospective Randomized Trial of Sequential Compression Devices vs Low-Dose Warfarin for Deep Venous Thrombosis Prophylaxis in Total Hip Arthroplasty
Bailey JP, Kruger MP, Solano FX, Zajko AB, Rubash HE (Univ of Pittsburgh; Univ of Connecticut, Farmington)
J Arthroplasty 6:29S–35S, 1991   15–23

Objective.—In a prospective randomized study, the effectiveness of low-dose warfarin therapy and the use of sequential compression devices for deep venous prophylaxis were compared in patients aged 40 years and older who had elective primary or revision total hip arthroplasty. None had a history of venous disease or vein surgery.

Methods.—Fifty patients were assigned to receive thigh-length graded elastic compression stockings, which were applied immediately after surgery and were worn nearly continuously. Another 45 patients were assigned to receive low-dose warfarin therapy (10 mg the evening before surgery or 7.5 mg for older women). Thrombi were detected by lower extremity venography.

Results.—Venous thrombi developed in 27% of patients treated with warfarin and in 6% of those given elastic stockings, a significant difference. All thrombi in the former patients were in the calf, but 2 patients who were given elastic stockings had thrombosis in the thigh.

Conclusion.—Low-dose warfarin protected these patients against high thrombi more effectively than did elastic stockings, with no increase in the risk of bleeding. A sequential compression device for low-risk patients with no history of venous disease is now used in those who have total hip arthroplasty. All patients have postoperative venography or Duplex ultrasonography in the early postoperative period.

▶ In this study, the use of sequential compression devices significantly outperformed low-dose warfarin as a prophylactic agent.—J.M. Porter, M.D.

Comparison of Warfarin and External Pneumatic Compression in Prevention of Venous Thrombosis After Total Hip Replacement
Francis CW, Pellegrini VD Jr, Marder VJ, Totterman S, Harris CM, Gabriel KR, Azodo MV, Leibert KM (Univ of Rochester, NY)
JAMA 267:2911-2915, 1992   15–24

Background.—Treatment with the anticoagulants warfarin, dextran, or heparin is effective in reducing the incidence of postoperative thromboembolism after total hip replacement (THR). However, many surgeons do not routinely provide this prophylaxis because of concerns about bleeding complications occurring during surgery or in the postoperative period. External pneumatic compression (EPC) is one alternative for prophylaxis of postoperative deep venous thrombosis. By providing intermittent compression of the extremity, EPC decreases venous stasis and accelerates venous flow. The effectiveness and safety of warfarin and external pneumatic compression as prophylaxis for venous thrombosis after THR were compared.

Method.—In a prospective trial, 220 patients scheduled for elective primary THR were randomized to receive surgery and preoperative prophylaxis followed by venography; 201 underwent venography with no prophylaxis. Preoperative prophylaxis was either bilateral sequential EPC to both the calf and thigh, or warfarin in a low-intensity regimen beginning 10–14 days preoperatively. Outcome was measured by venography to detect venous thrombosis between postoperative days 6 and 8. Bleeding was assessed by surgical blood loss, transfusion requirements, changes in hematocrit level, and clinically identified bleeding complications.

Results.—The total incidence of venous thrombosis was 31% in the warfarin group compared with 27% in the EPC group, but the distribution of thrombi was strikingly different. Proximal thrombi were found in 3% of the warfarin-treated patients compared with 12% of those who received EPC. Calf vein thrombosis occurred in 21% of the warfarin-treated group and in only 12% of the EPC group. Most proximal thrombi in EPC-treated patients were located within 15 cm of the femoral head and were not continuous with thrombi in deep calf veins. Blood loss and bleeding complications were similar in the warfarin and EPC groups. The higher frequency of proximal clots in patients receiving EPC and their increased risk of pulmonary embolism or bleeding complications during treatment with heparin led to termination of the study.

Conclusion.—External pneumatic compression was significantly less effective than warfarin therapy in preventing proximal venous thrombosis after THR, and it was more effective in preventing calf vein thrombosis. This difference may be caused by the different causal mechanisms of the thrombi in these 2 locations. External pneumatic compression is judged to be superior to no prophylaxis in preventing proximal vein thrombosis, but it is significantly less effective than warfarin therapy.

▶ These authors conclude that low-intensity warfarin was more effective than EPC in preventing proximal venous thrombosis after THR, which obviously is an opposite point of view from that expressed in Abstract 15–23. I continue to believe that external pneumatic compression devices are quite effective in venous thrombosis prophylaxis if properly applied and used. Low-intensity warfarin anticoagulation also appears effective. I am unable to explain the discrepancy in these 2 reports.—J.M. Porter, M.D.

Aging and the Anticoagulant Response to Warfarin Therapy
Gurwitz JH, Avorn J, Ross-Degnan D, Choodnovskiy I, Ansell J (Beth Israel Hosp, Boston; Brigham and Women's Hosp, Boston; Hebrew Rehabilitation Ctr for Aged, Boston; Harvard Med School, Boston; Univ of Massachusetts, Worcester)
Ann Intern Med 116:901–904, 1992   15–25

Background.—Thromboembolic and vascular disorders that require long-term oral anticoagulant therapy with warfarin are relatively prevalent in the elderly, but there is particular concern about the risk of bleeding in these patients. An age-related increase in sensitivity has been proposed for oral anticoagulants. A cumulative 5% incidence of major bleeding has been reported during 1 year of treatment, with minor bleeding complications exceeding 20%.

Methods.—A total of 530 patients were monitored in an anticoagulation clinic during a 10 year period, 1980-1990. The series included 149 patients aged 60–69 years and 177 aged 70 years and older.

Results.—The older patients had more medical problems, took more medication, and weighed less than younger patients. The prothrombin time ratio adjusted for warfarin dose was significantly increased in older patients, even after controlling for relevant clinical and demographic variables. Women and patients using more medications were more sensitive to warfarin. Heavier patients and those using warfarin for more than 6 months were less sensitive.

Conclusion.—Older patients are more sensitive to warfarin and, therefore, require close monitoring, because the intensity of the anticoagulant effect is the chief predictor of bleeding in warfarin-treated patients. Age in itself appears to be an independent risk factor for bleeding complications from warfarin.

▶ The risk of warfarin anticoagulation in the older age groups outweighs its possible benefit, especially in patients with thromboembolic problems. I believe this paper correctly emphasizes that, although older patients are more sensitive to warfarin than younger patients, intense monitoring can certainly reduce the complication rate.—J.M. Porter, M.D.

Dermatan Sulphate: A Safe Approach to Prevention of Postoperative Deep Vein Thrombosis

Prandoni P, Meduri F, Cuppini S, Toniato A, Zangrandi F, Polistena P, Gianese F, Faccioli AM (Univ of Padua, Italy; Mediolanum Farmaceutici, Milan, Italy)
Br J Surg 79:505–509, 1992   15–26

Background.—Dermatan sulfate is a natural glycosaminoglycan that potentiates heparin co-factor II and, in animal studies, is an effective antithrombotic agent. It has proved to be less hemorrhagic than unfractionated calcium heparin (UFH) at equivalent antithrombotic doses.

Methods.—Dermatan sulfate (MF701) was compared with UFH in a randomized trial of 324 patients, aged 40 years and older, who were scheduled for elective major general surgery. Treatment with either 100 mg of MF701 given intramuscularly daily or 5,000 units of UFH given subcutaneously 3 times daily began before surgery and continued until discharge. The 316 evaluable patients had serial impedance plethysmographic studies. Sixty-two cases had testing with ^{125}I-labeled fibrinogen as well. A positive test of either type was confirmed by venography where possible.

Results.—Deep venous thrombosis occurred in 3.1% of the patients given MF701 and in 1.6% of heparin-treated patients, according to plethysmography alone. When both tests were carried out, the respective rates were 7.1% and 11.8%. Neither difference was significant. Clinical bleeding occurred in 6% of the patients treated with MF701 and in 18% of those given heparin. The need for transfusion or reoperation for bleeding was significantly less in the MF701 group.

Conclusion.—Dermatan sulfate is as effective as UFH in surgical patients, and it is less likely to cause significant bleeding.

▶ We are beset on all sides with many new agents reporting the superior modifiers of the coagulation process. This paper indicates that the dermatan sulphate is at least as effective as unfractionated heparin in venous thrombosis prophylaxis, and it appears to be associated with a lower rate of complication.—J.M. Porter, M.D.

Vena Caval Filter Use in Orthopaedic Trauma Patients With Recognized Preoperative Venous Thromboembolic Disease

Collins DN, Barnes CL, McCowan TC, Nelson CL, Carver DK, McAndrew MP, Ferris EJ (Univ of Arkansas, Little Rock)
J Orthop Trauma 6:135–138, 1992   15–27

Objective.—Because patients with surgically treated hip fractures are at risk for venous thromboembolism, the value of caval filters was examined in 35 patients who had pelvic or lower extremity fracutres requiring operative treatment. The patients also had documented acute deep venous thrombosis.

Methods.—A total of 36 caval filters of various makes were placed, and low-dose warfarin was given with the goal of maintaining the prothrombin time at 1.3–1.5 times the control value for as long as 3 months.

Results.—No patient died of pulmonary embolism. There were no significant complications from filter placement, but 8 patients had asymptomatic complications, including caval thrombosis and penetration. One patient with a tilted filter required replacement.

Conclusion.—A combination of a vena caval filter and low-dose warfarin is an effective and relatively safe means of managing patients with acute deep venous thrombosis who require operative treatment of a pelvic or lower extremity fracture.

▶ These authors advocate the prophylactic placement of a vena caval filter in patients with lower extremity deep vein thrombosis who are facing orthopedic surgery. I suppose this recommendation is reasonable, but I am unable to generate much enthusiasm for the prophylactic use of vena caval filters. In fact, we seem to have little use for vena caval filters in general.—J.M. Porter, M.D.

Clinical Trials With Low Molecular Weight Heparins in the Prevention of Postoperative Thromboembolic Complicatins: A Meta-Analysis

Lassen MR, Borris LC, Christiansen HM, Schøtt P, Olsen AD, Sørensen JV, Rahr H, Jensen HP (Aalborg Hosp, Aalborg, Denmark)
Semin Thromb Hemost [Suppl] 17:284–290, 1991   15–28

Introduction.—Theoretically low-molecular-weight heparin (LMWH) should prevent thrombosis more effectively than unfractionated heparin, and it should be less likely to induce bleeding. Animal studies have supported these possibilities. In addition, LMWH has a longer half-life and is more bioavailable.

Methods.—The availability of LMWH preparations from several manufacturers prompted an analysis of 42 published trials (all randomized controlled studies) of LMWH in general and orthopedic surgery. Meta-analysis was performed to yield odds ratios with 95% confidence intervals.

Results.—Two studies comparing LMWH and placebo in general surgery indicated considerable efficacy for LMWH. Analysis of 17 studies comparing LMWH with twice-daily, low-dose heparin (using the radioactive fibrinogen uptake test for diagnosis) demonstrated that LMWH was more effective prophylactically in some, but not all, of the studies. Thrice-daily low-dose heparin appeared to be less effective than LMWH, but the study designs were inconsistent. In elective hip surgery, LMWH appeared superior to placebo, dextran, and thrice-daily administered low-dose heparin. In addition, LMWH was better than placebo and low-dose heparin in acute hip surgery.

Conclusion.—These data indicate that LMWH is as effective and as safe as other pharmacologic methods of preventing thrombosis, but comparative clinical trials are needed to show which preparations are most effective.

▶ These authors have performed a meta-analysis of 42 published randomized, control studies in general and orthopedic surgery comparing LMWH with unfractionated heparin in the prevention of postoperative thromboembolic complications. They conclude that LMWH is both safe and effective in the prevention of postoperative thromboembolic complications. This will doubtless be an important agent.—J.M. Porter, M.D.

16 Chronic Venous and Lymphatic Disease

Epidemiology of Chronic Venous Ulcers
Baker SR, Stacey MC, Jopp-McKay AG, Hoskin SE, Thompson PJ (Fremantle Hosp, Fremantle, Australia)
Br J Surg 78:864–867, 1991   16–1

Background.—The prevalence and clinical characteristics of chronic venous ulceration were studied in a metropolitan population of 238,000 in Perth, Western Australia.

Methods.—Patient accrual was by referral from health professionals and institutions and by self-referral. Venous disease was identified with photoplethysmography.

Results.—Of the 242 patients with chronic leg ulcers, 138 (57%) had an abnormal venous filling time, yielding a prevalence of venous ulcers of .62 per 1,000 population. There were 49 men and 89 women, the median age being 75 years. The prevalence of chronic venous ulceration increased significantly with age, 90% of the patients being older than 60 years of age. This group comprised 16.7% of the study population, for a prevalence of 3.3 per 1,000 population. An abnormal venous filling time was the only abnormality in 64% of limbs with venous ulcers. The remaining 36% had additional etiologic factors, including arterial ischemia, rheumatoid arthritis, and diabetes mellitus. The most common site of ulceration was the gaiter area. The median duration of ulceration was 26 weeks, and the duration of ulceration was longer than 26 weeks in 46% of the limbs. Recurrent ulceration was present in 76%, and more than 10 episodes of ulceration had occurred in 28%. A history of deep venous thrombosis was present in only 17% of patients, but another 79% had other predisposing factors.

Conclusion.—The prevalence of chronic venous ulceration in this population is .62 per 1,000 population, and it increases with increasing age. The condition is most common in patients older than 60 years of age.

▶ This article addresses the interesting question of causation of leg ulcers in a defined population. In the authors' experience, 57% of all leg ulcers resulted from venous disease. In 36% of the patients with presumed venous ulcers, contributory factors were seen, including diabetes, rheumatoid arthritis, arterial ischemia, and thrombocythemia. This epidemiologic article is of interest but, undoubtedly, these authors underestimated the prevalence of ulcers, becuase there is no assurance whatsoever that they saw all leg ulcers in their metropolitan population.—J.M. Porter, M.D.

Influence of Phlebographic Abnormalities on the Natural History of Venous Ulceration
Stacey MC, Burnand KG, Thomas ML, Pattison M (St Thomas' Hosp, London)
Br J Surg 78:868–871, 1991   16–2

Introduction.—A number of methods are available to assess functional abnormality in limbs with venous ulceration. Whether abnormalities detected on ascending and descending phlebography correlated with the natural history of ulceration, with calf pump function as assessed by foot volume plethysmography, and with transcutaneous oxygen measurements was determined.

Patients.—Seventy-three patients with 85 affected limbs participated in the study. The median patient age was 63 years. Limbs with post-thrombotic changes were classified into 2 groups, those with changes limited to the calf and those with more extensive changes involving the superficial femoral vein.

Results.—All limbs had an abnormal half volume refilling time on foot volume plethysmography and a Doppler arterial ankle/brachial pressure index greater than .9. Post-thrombotic changes were seen in 44 limbs on ascending phlebography, 28% extending into the superficial femoral vein. In the limbs with normal deep veins on ascending phlebography (48%), 11 had evidence of localized incompetence of the calf communicating veins, and 14 had long saphenous vein incompetence, deep vein reflux to the level of the knee or below, or both. Sixteen limbs had no phlebographic abnormalities. The limbs with post-thrombotic changes extending into the femoral vein had a significantly longer history of ulceration and more ulcer recurrences than did the limbs with normal deep veins or those with calf vein damage.

Conclusion.—Limbs at risk of recurrent ulceration can be readily identified with phlebography. Although these limbs had extensive post-thrombotic changes, there was no associated delay in ulcer healing.

▶ This excellent group provides a detailed phlebographic report of a large number of patients with healed venous ulcers. As one may predict, more extensive phlebographic disease was associated with a longer history of venous ulceration and more episodes of venous ulcer recurrence. Although there is nothing particularly surprising in this paper, it does present important phlebographic confirmation of the diffuse venous abnormalities seen in patients with venous ulceration.—J.M. Porter, M.D.

A Prospective, Randomized Trial of Unna's Boot Versus Duoderm CGF Hydroactive Dressing Plus Compression in Management of Venous Leg Ulcers

Cordts PR, Hanrahan LM, Rodriguez AA, Woodson J, LaMorte WW, Menzoian JO (Boston Univ)
J Vasc Surg 15:480–486, 1992   16–3

Background.—As many as a half million Americans may have leg ulcers secondary to chronic venous insufficiency, but there has been little improvement in conservative treatment. Unna's boot still is a frequently used measure. Duoderm CGF dressing provides considerable comfort but a recent report indicated that, without compression, healing takes longer than with Unna's boot.

Methods.—Duoderm CGF plus compression with a Coban wrap was compared with Unna's boot in 30 patients with leg ulcers. The 2 groups were similar in age, gender, initial area and duration of ulceration, and duplex scan findings.

Results.—Half the ulcers treated with Duoderm and 43% of those treated with the Unna's boot healed completely. The rate of healing correlated most closely with the initial area of ulceration. Adjusting for this parameter, healing occurred more rapidly in patients treated with Duoderm (Fig 16–1).

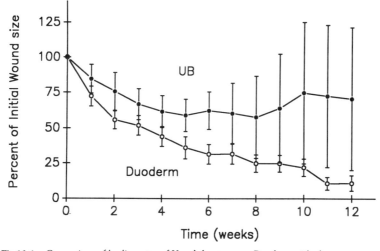

Fig 16–1.—Comparison of healing rates of Unna's boots versus Duoderm with ulcer areas expressed as a percent of initial ulcer area. Because 2 patients on Unna's boot markedly deteriorated and 1 patient showed minimal improvement, standard errors for Unna's boot become quite large when approaching 12 weeks. Analysis of variance reveals no significant difference in healing rates between the 2 groups. (Courtesy of Cordts PR, Hanrahan LM, Rodriquez AA, et al: *J Vasc Surg* 15:480–486, 1992.)

Conclusion.—Venous stasis ulcers may heal more rapidly when treated with Duoderm CGF dressing and compression than when Unna's boot is used.

▶ These authors struggle mightily to prove that Duoderm is superior to Unna's boot. I am unconvinced. There are many things wrong with this study, including a number of patients' refusal to be randomized to the Unna boot group. However, this paper does present an interesting discussion of the difficulties in assessing ulcer healing, pointing out that the use of square centimeters and percentage healing may give quite different results. I do not use either Duoderm or Unna's boot for the healing of venous ulcers. A simple gauze pad covering placed under a nylon stocking covered by a 30–40 mm below-knee elastic stocking, permitting the patient to ambulate, seems to work extremely well in our experience. I do not recall using a Unna's boot in the past 25 years, and I do not think Duoderm is any better.—J.M. Porter, M.D.

Color Doppler Ultrasound of the Post-Phlebitic Limb: Sounding a Cautionary Note

Baxter GM, Duffy P, MacKechnie S (Southern Gen Hosp, Glasgow, Scotland)
Clin Radiol 43:301–304, 1991   16–4

Background.—Color Doppler ultrasonography is an accurate means of diagnosing acute venous thrombosis in the lower extremity. A variable number of patients will present again with an episode of recurrent leg swelling frequently leading to repeat leg duplex ultrasonography. This study was designed to define the duplex natural history of deep venous thrombosis.

Methods.—Twenty patients with deep venous thrombosis, diagnosed by both ultrasonography and venography, were followed up prospectively. The 16 patients with femoropopliteal thrombosis were rescanned at 1, 3, and 6 months, and the 4 with calf vein thrombosis only were restudied at 1 week and at 1 and 3 months.

Results.—Only half the patients with above-knee thrombosis exhibited complete recanalization by 6 months. The others could not be distinguished from patients with acute nonocclusive thrombus. Three patients with calf vein thrombosis had complete recanalization, and 1 had popliteal extension of thrombus.

Conclusion.—All patients with above-knee venous thrombosis should have repeat ultrasound study at 6 months to provide a baseline against which to compare future duplex exams in case the patient is seen again with a new episode of leg swelling. Such a policy should assist with the difficult task of determining whether such a new episode means a new episode of DVT, which may require retreatment.

▶ This paper brings up the very interesting question of just how good color duplex ultrasound is in assessing patients with a known post-phlebitic limb and recurrent episode of swelling who also may have a recurrent episode of DVT. In a small number of patients with acute deep venous thrombosis, these authors note that, by 6 months, only about half the patients had complete recanalization; the other half had partial recanalization. When a patient with partial recanalization is seen, one cannot reliably differentiate the partially recanalized thrombotic abnormalities from fresh subocclusive thrombus, which should be treated with heparin. These authors suggest that all patients with deep venous thrombosis should have a 6-month duplex ultrasound test to establish a baseline against which to assess future abnormalities. I agree.—J.M. Porter, M.D.

Ambulatory Stab Evulsion Phlebectomy for Truncal Varicose Veins
Goren G, Yellin AE (Vein Disorders Ctr, Encino, Calif; Univ of Southern California, Los Angeles)
Am J Surg 162:166–174, 1991   16–5

Background.—Primary varicose veins are traditionally treated by routine ligation of the saphenofemoral junctional valve and ankle-to-groin stripping of the entire greater saphenous vein. However, this approach is based on hemodynamic assumptions that are no longer valid. Stab evulsion phlebectomy is a new surgical technique for treating trunk and tributary varicosities. The procedure is safe and effective, can be done in an ambulatory setting, and is based on hemodynamically accurate principles.

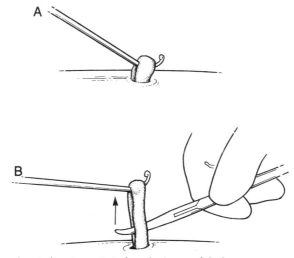

Fig 16–2.—A, the vein loop is exteriorized. **B,** the 2 arms of the loop are separated. (Courtesy of Goren G, Yellin AE: *Am J Surg* 162:166–174, 1991.)

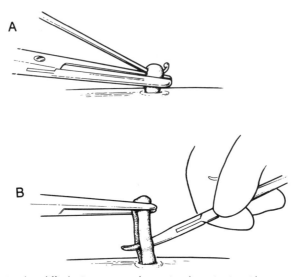

Fig 16–3.—A, when difficulty is encountered, grasping the varicosity with a mosquito or Kocher forceps will facilitate the delivery of the vein. **B,** the 2 arms of the loop are separated. (Courtesy of Goren G, Yellin AE: *Am J Surg* 162:166–174, 1991.)

Surgical Procedure.—Stab evulsion phlebectomy is performed using locoregional anesthesia. The procedure causes minimal tissue trauma and provides maximal cosmesis. After high ligation, small stab wounds 1.5–3 mm long are made along the border of the premarked varicosities. Specially designed hooks, or phlebextractors, are used to remove trunk and tributary varicosities through these minute incisions (Figs 16–2, 16–3, and 16–4). It is possible to remove vein segments of up to 5–6 cm through each incision. Incisions are closed with adhesive strips, and bleeding is usually minimal.

Patients.—During a 9-month period, 56 patients underwent stab evulsion phlebectomy on 69 varicose limbs. Thirteen patients had bilateral involvement. Fifty-seven limbs had primary varicose veins and 12 had recurrent varicosities. Fifty-two limbs had long saphenous vein varicosities, and 31 had an incompetent saphenofemoral junctional valve. Only 22 of the 69 limbs had associated main saphenous truncal incompetence. Twenty-nine limbs (42%) have been followed for at least 6 months.

Results.—Three patients had transient nerve palsies caused by the locoregional anesthesia, but the symptoms resolved within 24 hours. Three patients had bleeding from stab sites when they got up from the operating table, but the bleeding was promptly controlled by pressure reinforcement of the dressing. None of the patients had late hemorrhage. Two patients had localized phlebitis 2 weeks after operation, presumably from a clotted vein segment left in situ. The phlebitis resolved within 5–7 days with ibuprofen, compression, and continued ambulation. There were no wound infections. Prophylactic antibiotics were not

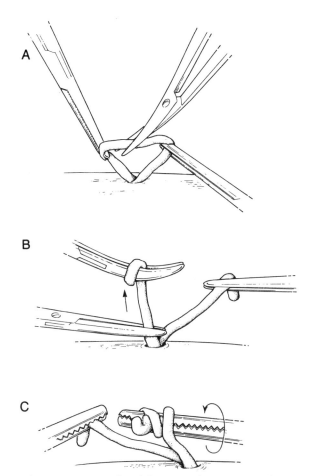

Fig 16–4.—A, the 2 arms are grasped, and the varicose loop is transected. Segments of vein are evulsed by **(B)** direct traction on each arm; **(C)** by twisting the vein on the forceps. (Courtesy of Goren G, Yellin AE: *Am J Surg* 162:166–174, 1991.)

used. No recurrent varicose veins were identified after a follow-up period of 3–9 months.

Conclusion.—Ambulatory stab evulsion phlebectomy effectively removes all trunk and tributary varicosities while leaving undamaged trunk veins in situ for future vein grafting, if needed.

▶ Stab evulsion phlebectomy for varicose veins has clearly been one of the major advances in varicose vein surgery of this or any other decade. Traditional 1- to 2-inch incisions, which produce unsightly scars, are no longer state-of-the-art for varicose vein surgery. The tiny incisions (2–3 mm in length) that are used with stab evulsion phlebectomy give just as good results and produce virtually no visible scarring (1).—J.M. Porter, M.D.

Reference

1. Rivlin S: *Br J Surg* 62:913, 1975.

Venous Wall Function in the Pathogenesis of Varicose Veins

Clarke GH, Vasdekis SN, Hobbs JT, Nicolaides AN (St Mary's Hosp, London)
Surgery 111:402–408, 1992   16–6

Background.—Three theories have been proposed to explain varicose veins: valve incompetence, weakness of the vein wall, and increased arterial inflow associated with multiple arteriovenous communications.

Methods.—Thirty-six extremities with superficial venous incompetence and 51 control limbs were assessed by duplex Doppler scanning and ambulatory venous pressure measurements. Elasticity of the venous system was studied by strain-gauge plethysmography. Changes in venous pressure and volume were monitored as a cuff was inflated to occlude venous outflow to calculate the elastic modulus.

Findings.—Vein wall elasticity was significantly reduced in high-risk extremities (as identified on occupational, family history, symptomatic, and physical grounds), and arterial inflow was increased in comparison with normal extremities. Valve incompetence was not, however, more prevalent in high-risk limbs.

Conclusion.—The role of venous valves in the development of varicose veins is subsidiary to both the altered elastic properties of the veins and the rate of arterial inflow.

▶ The calculation of elastic modulus from pressure/volume relationships strikes me as a bit too contrived to be convincing. Many, many assumptions underlie the measurement of this complex relationship. These authors purport to demonstrate a significant reduction in vein wall elasticity in the pathogenesis of varicose veins. I am unconvinced.—J.M. Porter, M.D.

Venous Valvular Insufficiency: Influence of a Single Venous Valve (Native and Experimental)

Dalsing MC, Lalka SG, Unthank JL, Grieshop RJ, Nixon C, Davis T (Indiana Univ Med Ctr, Indianapolis)
J Vasc Surg 14:576–587, 1991   16–7

Background.—Incompetent venous valves are responsible for chronic venous insufficiency in the lower extremity in more than 90% of the cases. The immediate and long-term venous hemodynamic effects of a single competent venous valve in the proximal superficial vein (SFV valve) were examined.

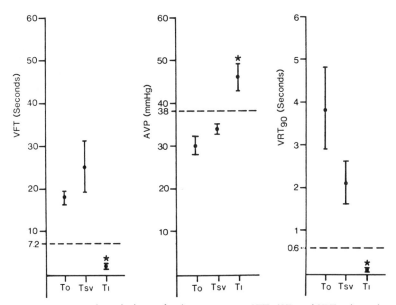

Fig 16–5.—Mean and standard error for the measurement VFT, AVP, and VRT_{90} obtained in the normal canine lower limb (T_0), when a single competent proximal SFV valve remained (T_{sv}), and after all valves have been rendered incompetent (T_1) in the short-term study-single SFV valve. The *asterisk* signifies a difference from the normal valve condition of $P \leq .05$. (Courtesy of Dalsing MC, Lalka SG, Unthank JL, et al: *J Vasc Surg* 14:576–587, 1991.)

Methods.—The time to maximal ankle venous pressure after standing (VFT), and to 90% of that time after exercise (VRT_{90}), were measured along with the minimal postexercise pressure (AVP) in greyhound dogs before intervention, after leaving only the SFV valve in place, and again after complete venous valvulotomy. After 3 weeks, some dogs underwent SFV native valve or autogenous venous valve transplantation, and

TABLE 1.—Numeric Data Gathered From the Long-Term Study-Single SFV Valve as Expressed by the Mean and Standard Error of the Mean

Valve condition	Valve type	VFT (sec)	AVP (mm Hg)	VRT90 (sec)
			Hemodynamic parameter	
TO	NVT	15.2 ± 1.95	30.75 ± 2.14	1.9 ± 0.17
	EVT	17.6 ± 2.12	21.3 ± 2.56	3.22 ± 1.21
TCVI	NVT	2.9 ± 0.26	39.75 ± 2.32	0.26 ± 0.07
	EVT	4.5 ± 1.75	38.9 ± 4.56	0.25 ± 0.07
TSV	NVT	17.0 ± 2.2	41.0 ± 2.08	0.75 ± 0.06
	EVT	7.06 ± 1.54	44.7 ± 3.36	0.83 ± 0.19

(Courtesy of Dalsing MC, Lalka SG, Unthank JL, et al: *J Vasc Surg* 14:576–587, 1991.)

TABLE 2.—The Comparison of Native and Experimental
Venous Valve Transplants as Analyzed by Venous
Pressure Measurements

	VFT		Hemodynamic parameter	
Comparison	*NVT*	*EVT*	*AVP*	*VRT$_{90}$*
T$_O$ vs T$_{CVI}$	0.009	0.001	0.0017	0.0001
T$_O$ vs T$_{SV}$	NS	0.006	0.0002	0.0003
T$_{CVI}$ vs T$_{SV}$	0.0002	NS	NS	0.0418

Note: Only for VFT did the 2 valves differ in their basic pattern of response ($P = .0095$) and necessitate separate comparison for each valve condition (T_0, T_{cvi}, T_{sv}). *Abbreviations:* T_0, control; T_{cvi}, chronic venous insufficiency; T_{sv}, single valve condition; NVT, native valve transplant; EVT, experimental valve transplant.

(Courtesy of Dalsing MC, Lalka SG, Unthank JL, et al: *J Vasc Surg* 14:576–587, 1991.)

venous pressure measurements were repeated 3 weeks after valve transplantation. The autogenous valves were taken from the opposite extremities. All animals received aspirin.

Results.—All venous hemodynamic parameters were significantly altered by complete venous valvulotomy (Fig 16–5). One remaining valve, however, preserved normal venous hemodynamics in the short-term study. Only the VFT differed significantly with the native valve transplant and experimental valves in place (Tables 1 and 2). Venous pressure after

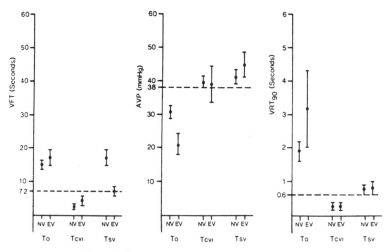

Fig 16–6.—Mean and standard error graphically presented for the measurements of VFT, AVP, and VRT$_{90}$ obtained in the normal canine lower limb (T_0), after all valves have been rendered incompetent (T_{cvi}), and 3 weeks after transplantation of a native (NV) or experimental (EV) valve into the incompetent limb (T_{sv}). (Courtesy of Dalsing MC, Lalka SG, Unthank JL, et al: *J Vasc Surg* 14:576–587, 1991.)

standing improved significantly only after native valve transplantation (Fig 16–6). Ambulatory venous pressure remained significantly higher than normal after transplantation of either valve type. The VRT_{90} improved by valve transplantation, but it did not become normal.

Conclusion.—A single competent valve in the proximal SFV is critically important in terms of venous hemodynamics. Transplanting a venous valve, however, does not markedly improve venous hemodynamics over the insufficiency state in the long term. Popliteal vein valve repair or repair of multiple valves may prove more effective.

▶ There is a simply stated problem facing those who wish to reconstruct or transplant a single competent valve into the lower extremity deep-vein circuit either at or proximal to the popliteal artery: Just how important is a single valve? These authors present a remarkably detailed study examining this question in animals. This is a remarkably well-performed and well-analyzed study, and it is commended to anyone interested in lower extremity venous valve reconstruction.—J.M. Porter, M.D.

The Valvular Anatomy of the Iliac Venous System and Its Clinical Implications

LePage PA, Villavicencio JL, Gomez ER, Sheridan MN, Rich NM (Uniformed Services Univ of the Health Sciences, Bethesda, Md; Walter Reed Army Med Ctr, Washington, DC)
J Vasc Surg 14:678–683, 1991   16–8

Background.—The role and the importance of the valves in the hemodynamics of the venous circulation and in the pathophysiology of varicose veins has long been recognized and thoroughly described. However, literature on the valvular system of the internal iliac vein and its tributaries is scarce. Vulvar and gluteal varices were observed, and retrograde venograms performed on patients with vulvar varices and symptoms of pelvic congestion syndrome were analyzed. The presence of varices of the vulva, posterior thigh, and the pelvic congestion syndrome are correlated with insufficiency of the internal iliac venous system. The anatomy and valve distribution of the pelvic veins in human cadavers were examined to determine the physiology and pathophysiology of the venous circulation in the pelvis.

Methods.—Dissection of 42 human cadavers yielded 82 common and external venous systems and 79 internal iliac vein specimens. Each specimen consisted of common, external, and internal iliac veins and tributaries of the latter. On dissection, the anatomical variations of the internal iliac vein trunk and the location of valves in the complete iliac venous system were recorded.

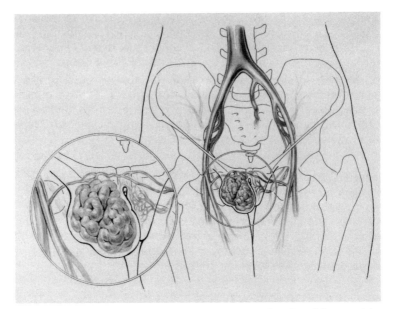

Fig 16–7.—Artist's conception of the iliac venous system and the branches of the internal iliac vein that more often contribute to the formation of vulvar varices. The internal iliac vein receives blood from parietal and visceral tributaries. The parietal tributaries are the superior and inferior gluteal, sciatic, ascending lumbar, internal pudendal, and obturator veins. The visceral branches drain the venous plexuses of the pelvic organs: hemorrhoidal and vesicoprostatic plexuses in men, and uterine, gonadal, and vaginal in women. A large cluster of vulvar varices is illustrated in the insert connecting the saphenous system (through the external pudendal veins) with the internal iliac incompetent obturator and internal pudendal veins. (Courtesy of LePage PA, Villavicencio JL, Gomez ER, et al: *J Vasc Surg* 14:678–683, 1991.)

Findings.—The internal iliac vein consisted of a single trunk in 73% of the specimens and 2 separated venous trunks in 27% of the specimens. The internal iliac trunk had valves in the main trunk in 10.1% of the specimens and in the tributaries in 9.1% of the specimens. The external iliac vein had one valve in 26.2% of the specimens. The right external iliac vein had almost 3 times as many valves on the left.

Conclusion.—Well-developed valves of the internal iliac vein were demonstrated for the first time in a series of cadaver dissections. The scarcity of valves in the pelvic veins suggests that varicose veins in the vulva or elsewhere develop not only because of valvular incompetence, but also because of genetic anomalies and hormonal and hemodynamic factors present during pregnancy (Fig 16–7).

▶ This group has had a long interest in the clinically important, but much ignored problems of posterior thigh and vulvar varicose veins, and the pelvic congestion syndrome in women. They have performed detailed anatomical dissection in cadavers to further define the normal venous anatomy of the internal iliac venous system. Very few valves were found in these veins, and this anatomical peculiarity doubtless plays a significant role in this entire group of clinical problems.—J.M. Porter, M.D.

Klippel-Trenaunay Syndrome: The Risks and Benefits of Vascular Interventions

Gloviczki P, Stanson AW, Stickler GB, Johnson CM, Toomey BJ, Meland NB, Rooke TW, Cherry KJ Jr (Mayo Clinic, Rochester, Minn)
Surgery 110:469–479, 1991   16–9

Introduction.—Klippel-Trenaunay syndrome (KTS) is a rare congenital disorder characterized by varicose veins, hypertrophied soft tissues and bones, hemangioma (usually of the capillary port-wine type), and an absence of significant arteriovenous shunting.

Methods.—Data were reviewed on 144 patients in whom KTS was diagnosed. Hemangioma, the most consistent feature, was present in 95% of the patients and varicosities were seen in 76% (Fig 16–8). In more than two thirds of patients, the disease was limited to a lower extremity.

Results.—Most of the patients did well without any treatment or with elastic compression only. In the past decade, 9 patients had surgery for a vascular malformation of the lower extremity. In 7 of them, varicose

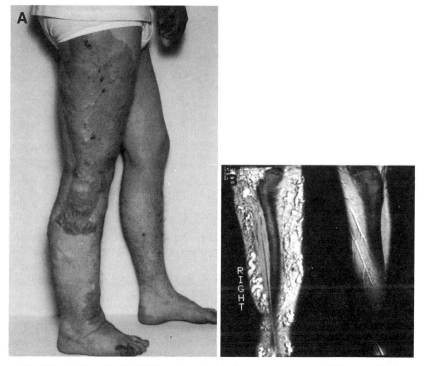

Fig 16–8.—**A,** Man, 18, with KTS involving the right lower extremity. **B,** an MRI scan of the lower extremities reveals large varicose veins in the superficial compartment of the calf. (Courtesy of Gloviczki P, Stanson AW, Stickler GB, et al: *Surgery* 110:469–479, 1991.)

veins or a hemangioma were removed. None of these patients were cured, but all 5 who had resection of varicose veins and 1 of the 2 patients who had a hemangioma resected improved; 2 other patients who had removal of varicose veins elsewhere deteriorated symptomatically. One patient was doing well after deep venous reconstruction for atresia of the superficial femoral vein using the contralateral saphenous vein.

Conclusion.—Presently, MRI and contrast venography are performed in all patients with KTS who are candidates for surgery. Excision of hemangiomas should be approached cautiously. Complete removal of either varicose veins or hemangiomatous tissue seldom is possible and will not halt bony hypertrophy.

▶ We continue to see 2 or 3 new patients with this syndrome every year, which leads me to conclude that there is a significant number of individuals in our population who are afflicted with this potentially disfiguring developmental disorder. This paper presents a nice overview of this problem and rightly stresses the importance of elastic compression therapy as the primary treatment modality. The authors appropriately emphasize that only a rare patient requires varicose vein or hemangioma excision, and that this should be approached very hesitantly by conservative surgeons. Some of these patients will have segmental deep vein hypoplasia or aplasia. The role of any deep vein reconstruction in these patients is undefined, but I am sure it will be very infrequently applicable. Magnetic resonance imaging is recommended to assist in any preoperative visualization of venous abnormalities.—J.M. Porter, M.D.

Magnetic Resonance of the Inferior Vena Cava

Colletti PM, Oide CT, Terk MR, Boswell WD Jr (Univ of Southern California, Los Angeles)
Magn Reson Imaging 10:177–185, 1992   16–10

Methods.—Magnetic resonance imaging was carried out in 54 patients, 30 men and 24 women with a mean age of 51 years, who had abnormalities of the inferior vena cava (IVC). Thirty-two patients had intrinsic IVC abnormalities, 16 had extrinsic compression, and 6 had a dilated IVC. Spin-echo imaging was performed in all cases, and MR angiography was done in 21 patients.

Results.—Magnetic resonance angiography demonstrated the IVC and the superior mesenteric vein in normal subjects (Fig 16–9). The most frequent intrinsic lesion of the IVC was renal-cell carcinoma (Fig 16–10). Presaturated spin-echo images demonstrated intrinsic lesions advantageously, but collateral vessels were best studied by MR angiography using the time-of-flight technique.

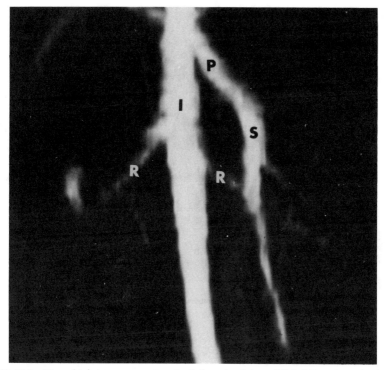

Fig 16–9.—Normal inferior vena cava. Anterior 2-dimensional time-of-flight MR angiography shows normal inferior venea cava (*I*), renal veins (*R*), portal vein (*P*), and superior mesenteric vein (*S*). (Courtesy of Colletti PM, Oide CT, Terk MR, et al: *Magn Reson Imaging* 10.177–185, 1992.)

▶ Magnetic resonance imaging is going to have an increasingly important effect on our future practice pattern. This study shows remarkable visualization of the venous abdominal system with current generation equipment. Imagine what the refinement of new generations of MR equipment is going to produce. I continue to believe that contrast arteriography and phlebography will be used less often as a diagnostic test in the future.—J.M. Porter, M.D.

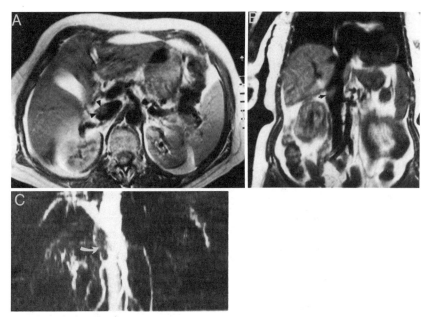

Fig 16–10.—Level I renal cell carcinoma with invasion of the inferior vena cava in a woman, 58. Axial TR 2,000, TE 20 view of abdomen (**A**) shows a small tumor in the inferior vena cava (*arrowheads*). Coronal TR 500, TR 20 sequence again shows small level I module in the inferior vena cava (**B**) (*arrows*). Anterior 2-dimensional TOF MR angiography (**C**) shows low-signal area within inferior vena cava (*arrow*). (Courtesy of Colletti PM, Oide CT, Terk MR, et al: *Magn Reson Imaging* 10:177–185, 1992.)

Leiomyosarcoma of the Inferior Vena Cava: Analysis and Search of World Literature on 141 Patients and Report of Three New Cases

Mingoli A, Feldhaus RJ, Cavallaro A, Stipa S (Creighton Univ, Omaha, Neb; Univ of Rome, Italy)
J Vasc Surg 14:688–699, 1991   16–11

Background.—Leiomyosarcoma of the inferior vena cava (IVC) is a rare and potentially curable malignancy. Too few long-term follow-up results have been reported to generalize about the results of treatment.

Methods.—Personal experience with 3 cases and also data on 141 previously reported patients with IVC leiomyosarcoma were reviewed.

Results.—Two of the authors' patients did well after surgical removal of the tumor, but 1 died of metastatic disease despite adjuvant chemotherapy and radiotherapy. The findings in 1 case are shown in Figures 16–11 and 16–12. In the reported series, 27.9% of 82 patients who underwent radical tumor resection lived 5 years, and 14.2% survived 10 years. Patients with tumors involving the middle segment of the IVC did better than those with lower-segment tumors. Both abdominal pain and

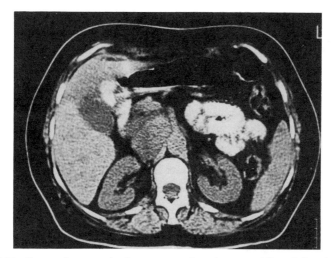

Fig 16–11.—Computed tomography shows a retroperitoneal mass partially occluding the IVC (*arrow*). (Courtesy of Mingoli A, Feldhaus RJ, Cavallaro A, et al: *J Vasc Surg* 14:688–699, 1991.)

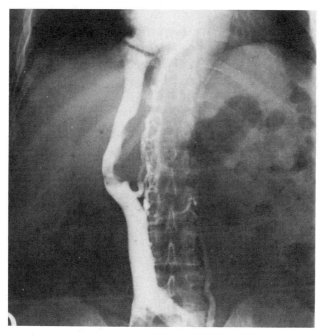

Fig 16–12.—Inferior vena cavagram shows partial occlusion of the IVC with tumor protrusion into the lumen. The IVC is deviated toward the right by the mass. (Courtesy of Mingoli A, Feldhaus RJ, Cavallaro A, et al: *J Vasc Surg* 14:688–699, 1991.)

the absence of a palpable abdominal mass were favorable prognostic factors. Forty-eight patients were inoperable.

Conclusion.—Early surgery remains the best approach to IVC leiomyosarcoma. Hopefully, modern noninvasive imaging methods will allow even earlier diagnosis and consequently improved survival.

▶ Primary sarcoma of veins and arteries appear to be both rare and devastatingly malignant in a majority of patients. These authors have produced a concise review of the world's literature on this topic.—J.M. Porter, M.D.

Indirect Lymphography With Isovist-300 in Various Forms of Lymphedema
Gan J-L, Chang T-S, Fu D-D, Liu W, Luo J-C, Cheng H (Shanghai No. 2 Med Univ; Plastic Hosp of Hangzhou, Hangzhou, China)
Eur J Plast Surg 14:109–113, 1991   16–12

Introduction.—Direct lymphography is a useful means of diagnosing extremity lymphedema by demonstrating large peripheral collectors and lymph nodes, but it is invasive, and the oily contrast material that is used may produce granulomatous adenitis or secondary lymphangitis. An alternative approach, indirect lymphography, is based on the new-generation contrast medium, Isovist.

Methods.—Indirect lymphography was performed using Isovist-300 in 20 patients with lymphedema of an extremity. Only 1 patient had primary lymphedema. Contrast medium normally appears roundish in the vertical projection 2–3 minutes after it is injected. Lymphatics fill centripetally from the intradermal deposit; 1–4 lymph collectors are seen arising from the deposit.

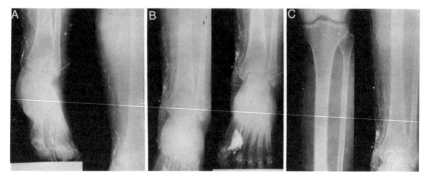

Fig 16–13.—Indirect lymphography in secondary lymphedema. **A,** demonstration of dilated lymph collectors with dermal backflow. **B,** dilatation and tortuosity of lymphatic vessels are evident. **C,** at 10 minutes after injection, the lymph collectors are increased in number. Demonstration of spread dermal flow and disappearance of valvular images. (Courtesy of Gan J-L, Chang T-S, Fu K-D, et al: *Eur J Plast Surg* 14:109–113, 1991.)

Results.—In secondary lymphedema, the lymph collectors appeared dilated and tortuous, and they sometimes were discontinuous. Widespread retrograde dermal flow was evident, and a reticular pattern of lymphatics was noted subcutaneously (Fig 16-13). The number of fine initial lymphatics without lymph collectors was increased. There were no systemic side effects.

Conclusion.—Indirect lymphography by intradermal infusion of Isovist can demonstrate abnormal dermal lymph vessels in patients with lymphedema of an extremity.

▶ Direct lymphography with injection of an oil-based contrast media has become a thing of the past, and it is no longer a relevant diagnostic test in modern medicine, except possibly in evaluation of lymphoma. Indirect lymphography is based on the injection of a water-soluble contrast media, known as Isovist-300, into the digital web space of the foot. The subsequent flow of contrast is followed with a fluoroscopic monitor with delayed filming. Remarkably good direct view of the distal lymphatics, so called "initial lymphatics," are obtained. It appears that the thigh views are much less impressive, but these authors theorize that virtually all obstructive or hypoplastic lymphatic diagnoses can be made from the initial view. This may actually be more valuable than the isotopic technique of lymphoscintigraphy, which has recently become rather widely used. See also Abstract 10–22.—J.M. Porter, M.D.

Mechanism of Action of External Compression on Venous Function
Sarin S, Scurr JH, Smith PDC (Middlesex Hosp, London)
Br J Surg 79:499–502, 1992   16–13

Background.—External compression is an age-old means of treating venous disease. Today the availability of graduated compression stockings has made this approach more acceptable to patients, but how compression works remains uncertain.

Methods.—Both lower extremities of 36 patients aged 45–65 years were examined by duplex ultrasonography. Popliteal venous reflux was identified in 17 extremities, long saphenous vein (LSV) reflux was found in 19, and short saphenous vein (SSV) reflux was present in 21. A water-filled adjustable pressure cuff was placed about the knee and was gradually inflated during ultrasound imaging.

Observations.—Reflux was abolished before the vein became occluded in 24% of the affected popliteal veins, 42% of the LSVs, and 14% of the SSVs. The cuff pressures needed to restore valve function were significantly lower than those required to occlude the veins.

Conclusion.—Compression may control venous disease by promoting the coaptation of valve cusps to restore competence.

▶ We have all struggled mightily to determine the beneficial effect of wearing elastic compression hosiery in patients with significant chronic venous disease, and we have all been unable to define convincing hemodynamic changes. These authors propose the innovative concept that external compression may restore competence to dilated valve.—J.M. Porter, M.D.

Prevalence of Venous Disease: A Community Study in West London
Franks PJ, Wright DDI, Moffatt CJ, Stirling J, Fletcher AE, Bulpitt CJ, McCollum CN (Charing Cross and Westminster Med School and Royal Postgraduate Med School, Hammersmith Hosp, London; University Hosp of South Manchester, Manchester, England)
Eur J Surg 158:143–147, 1992   16–14

Objective.—The prevalence of venous disease was determined using a self-administered questionnaire in a community sample of 2,103 individuals (aged 35–70 years) in west London, England.

Results.—Varicose veins were described by 25% of the 1,338 subjects completing the questionnaire (Fig 16–14). Deep venous thrombosis or pulmonary embolism was reported by 6% of the group (Fig 16–15), and phlebitis was reported by 5% (Fig 16–16). Seven percent of the patients had worn support stockings, and 6% had received anticoagulants at some time. In all, 31% of respondents reported having had some form

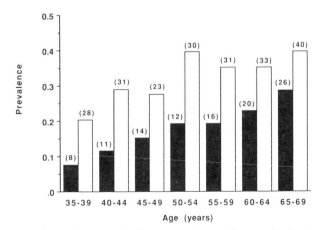

Fig 16–14.—Prevalence of varicose veins by age group in a random sample of patients registered with 3 general practices in west London. *Solid bars* indicate men; *open bars,* women. The numbers of patients are given in parentheses. (Courtesy of Franks PJ, Wright DDI, Moffatt CJ, et al: *Eur J Surg* 158:143–147, 1992.)

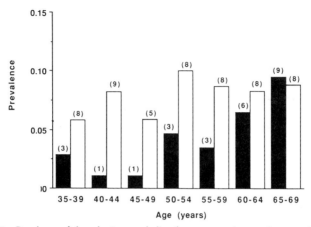

Fig 16–15.—Prevalance of thrombosis or embolism by age group in a random sample of patients registered with 3 general practices in west London. *Solid bars* indicate men; *open bars*, women. The numbers of patients are given in parentheses. (Courtesy of Franks PJ, Wright DDI, Moffatt CJ, et al: *Eur J Surg* 158:143–147; 1992.)

of venous disease. Selected clinical exam validation studies indicated that the survey response was nearly 90% accurate.

Conclusion.—Varicose veins and phlebitis were likelier to occur in older subjects and females in this population. Thrombosis and pulmonary embolism correlated with diabetes, female gender, and older age.

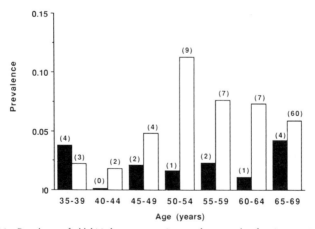

Fig 16–16.—Prevalence of phlebitis by age group in a random sample of patients registered with 3 general practices in west London. *Solid bars* indicate men; *open bars*, women. The numbers of patients are given in parentheses. (Courtesy of Franks PJ, Wright DDI, Moffatt CJ, et al: *Eur J Surg* 158:143–147 1992.)

Venous disease may constitute a larger health care burden than has been recognized.

▶ A written survey technique is, of course, suspect as a means of obtaining prevalence data. However, in this case, clinical exam validation indicated that the survey was approximately 90% accurate. Venous disease clearly affects some populations far greater than others. In my experience, the Northern European population has a far greater prevalence of both varicose veins and deep vein thrombosis than does the American population.—J.M. Porter, M.D.

Femoral Vein Valve Repair Under Direct Vision Without Venotomy: A Modified Technique With Use of Angioscopy
Gloviczki P, Merrell SW, Bower TC (Mayo Clinic and Found, Rochester, Minn)
J Vasc Surg 14:645–648, 1991   16–15

Introduction.—Kistner recently described a closed method of external suture repair of an incompetent femoral vein valve. Although venotomy is avoided and handling of the vein wall is minimized, visual control is lacking. A method is available to repair a valve without venotomy while using angioscopy to ensure accurate suture placement.

Technique.—A vertical groin incision is made to expose the femoral vein and, after administering heparin, an angioscope is introduced through the saphenous vein or 1 of its tributaries and advanced to the incompetent superficial femoral vein valve. The valve is repaired by placing 7-0 monofilament polypropylene sutures externally (Fig 16–17). The elongated valve leaflets are gradually shortened by placing sutures sequentially in the commissures, lateral to the insertion site of each leaflet (Fig 16–18). After removing the angioscope and reestablishing the

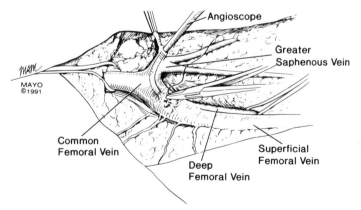

Fig 16–17.—The sequential placement of 3–4 sutures in each valve commissure usually is necessary. (Courtesy of Gloviczki P, Merrell SW, Bower TC: *J Vasc Surg* 14:645-648, 1991.)

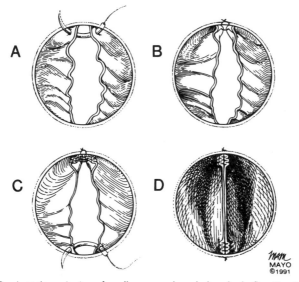

Fig 16–18.—**A,** angioscopic view of needle passage through the valve leaflets. **B,** valve leaflet redundancy may be reassessed after each suture is tied. **C,** sutures are usually required in both commissures to achieve complete valvular competence. **D,** final angioscopic appearance of a competent valve after repair. (Courtesy of Gloviczki P, Merrell SW, Bower TC: *J Vasc Surg* 14:645–648, 1991.)

circulation, a digital strip test is performed to confirm competence. A polytetrafluoroethylene cuff is then placed about the repair site.

Conclusion.—This method allows valve competence to be assured directly by angioscopy after placing each suture; 5 valves have been successfully repaired in 3 patients.

▶ The authors describe a clever method of angioscopically aided venous valve repair. The avoidance of a venotomy is theoretically attractive. If nothing else, the technique may provide an excuse to blow the dust off the angioscope every 4 or 5 years.—G.L. Moneta, M.D.

17 Portal Hypertension

Prophylactic Sclerotherapy for Esophageal Varices in Men With Alcoholic Liver Disease: A Randomized, Single-Blind, Multicenter Clinical Trial
VA Cooperative Variceal Sclerotherapy Group
N Engl J Med 324:1779–1784, 1991   17–1

Background.—The efficacy of sclerotherapy in preventing recurrent variceal bleeding suggests that it might also prevent initial bleeding in patients at risk. The Veterans Affairs cooperative study of prophylactic sclerotherapy, begun in 1985, enrolled only men with alcoholic liver disease. Control patients underwent both endoscopy and sham sclerotherapy.

Methods.—A prospective trial comparing prophylactic sclerotherapy with sham treatment included 281 men with alcoholic liver disease who had at least 3 variceal channels, but who had not bled. All of them underwent endoscopy, and 143 patients received sclerotherapy. The groups were well matched for the extent of liver disease, but other medi-

Primary Cause of Death During the Phase of Treatment With Sclerotherapy or Sham Therapy Among Men With Alcoholic Liver Disease and Esophageal Varices

CAUSE OF DEATH	SHAM THERAPY (N = 138)	SCLEROTHERAPY (N = 143)
	no. of patients	
Liver failure	6	12
Renal failure	1	0
Upper gastrointestinal bleeding	6	10
Respiratory failure	0	0
Cardiac failure	1	5
Infection	3	10
Other	7	7
Unknown	0	2
All causes (% of group)	24 (17.4)	46 (32.2)

(Courtesy of The Veterans Affairs Cooperative Variceal Sclerotherapy Group: N Engl J Med 324:1779–1784, 1991.)

cal illness was more frequent in patients assigned to receive sclerotherapy.

Results.—The study ended after 22.5 months, because all-cause mortality was significantly higher in the sclerotherapy group (32%) than among sham-treated patients (17%). The sclerotherapy patients did, however, have significantly fewer episodes of bleeding from esophageal varices. In sclerotherapy patients, complications were frequent, but they usually were not life-threatening. Excess mortality decreased after the trial ended. The primary causes of death during the phase of either treatment are seen in the table.

Conclusion.—Sclerotherapy should not be done in men with alcoholic liver disease until variceal bleeding occurs.

▶ This interesting Veterans Affairs cooperative study of the prophylactic use of sclerotherapy had to be cancelled after 22 months, because of the increased mortality in the sclerotherapy group compared with the randomized sham-treated patients. Curiously, the causes of death were quite varied and, in fact, the prophylactic sclerotherapy group had less bleeding than the sham-treated group. However, after the termination of the study, the excess mortality rate in the sclerotherapy group promptly decreased. This study has been widely accepted—probably rightly so, because of convincing evidence that prophylactic sclerotherapy is harmful.—J.M. Porter, M.D.

Endoscopic Variceal Sclerosis Does Not Increase the Risk of Portal Venous Thrombosis
Kawasaki S, Henderson JM, Riepe SP, Brooks WC, Hertzler G (Emory Univ, Atlanta)
Gastroenterology 102:206–215, 1992   17–2

Introduction.—The use of endoscopic sclerotherapy to treat bleeding esophageal varices has improved the outcome for patients with such lesions. Unfortunately for patients with chronic bleeding from the esophageal varices, the application of endoscopic sclerotherapy has not totally alleviated recurrent bleeding. In addition, thrombosis of the portal vein after sclerotherapy has been reported. Variceal sclerotherapy was compared with the distal splenorenal shunt procedure with the use of follow-up serial angiography assessments.

Methods.—Twenty-two patients with esophageal variceal bleeding were studied. All patients underwent angiography before the first sclerotherapy procedure, with expected follow-up angiography at 6 months, 1 year, and annually thereafter. All sclerotherapy was done with flexible endoscopy and either sodium morrhuate or sodium tetradecyl sulfate as the sclerosant.

Results.—The average time between the first and last angiography was 26.4 months in the 22 patients, who had had an average of 6.5 sclerotherapy procedures. Eight of the 24 patients randomized to sclerotherapy failed their treatment and required surgery during the study. Thrombosis did not occur in any of the major portal veins in any patient. The portal and splenic vein size did not change significantly throughout the therapy. Only minor alterations in the blood flow patterns were observed in 21 of the 22 patients. The results of histologic tests did not differ between patients undergoing sclerotherapy and normal controls.

Conclusion.—Chronic sclerotherapy does not seem to influence the thrombosis risk in patients with esophageal varices. The chronic use of sclerotherapy did not result in significant histologic changes of the splenic vein, other than those expected in patients with portal hypertension.

▶ Sclerotherapy continues to dominate the literature on portal hypertension. This study reaches the conclusion that sclerotherapy does not increase the risk of thrombosis in the portal venous system, and that the previously reported high incidence of this complication may be inaccurate.—J.M. Porter, M.D.

Portal Vein Thrombosis Complicating Endoscopic Variceal Sclerotherapy: Convincing Further Evidence
Korula J, Yellin A, Kanel GC, Nichols P (Univ of Southern California, Los Angeles)
Dig Dis Sci 36:1164–1167, 1991   17–3

Background.—Thrombosis of the portal and mesenteric veins after endoscopic variceal sclerotherapy (EVS) has been reported, but the evidence to date is not conclusive.

Case Report.—Man, 59, with quiescent alcoholic cirrhosis and portal hypertension was admitted with recurrent gastric variceal bleeding and underwent EVS. Portal vein thrombosis developed after obliteration of esophageal varices. The complication was apparent only at operation, when thrombectomy and endovenectomy were carried out before successful placement of a portocaval shunt. Amorphous material within the clot resembled the sclerosant that had been injected.

Conclusion.—There may be a substantial risk of portal vein thrombosis complicating EVS when the gastric varices are injected. The diagnosis may be made more often in the future with Doppler studies.

▶ Just in case you do not believe the information listed in Abstract 17–2, here is an alternate point of view. This case report and accompanying discussion suggest that there may be a considerable risk of portal vein thrombosis, especially when the gastric varices are injected.—J.M. Porter, M.D.

Propranolol in Prevention of Recurrent Bleeding From Severe Portal Hypertensive Gastropathy in Cirrhosis

Pérez-Ayuso RM, Piqué JM, Bosch JJ, Panés J, González A, Pérez R, Rigau J, Quintero E, Valderrama R, Viver J, Esteban R, Rodrigo L, Bordas JM, Rodés J (Hosp Clinic i Provincial, Univ of Barcelona; Hosp Mutua de Terrassa; Hosp General del Valle Hebrón, Univ Autónoma of Barcelona; Univ of Oviedo; Hosp General de Granollers, Spain)
Lancet 337:1431–1432, 1991

17–4

Introduction.—Gastrointestinal tract bleeding in patients with cirrhosis usually results from either esophageal varices or portal hypertensive gastropathy (PHG). Rebleeding from varices can be prevented with β-blockers such as propranolol.

Methods.—The effects of propranolol on rebleeding from severe PHG were evaluated in a controlled trial of 57 patients. The patients were randomly assigned to 2 groups, independently of the manifestation of bleeding from severe PHG and within a month of the diagnosis. In 1 group, 26 patients received propranolol twice daily by mouth. In the second group, 31 patients received no treatment, except iron when necessary. The frequency of clinical events in the 2 groups was compared.

Results.—The propranolol-treated group had a higher actuarial percentage of patients free of rebleeding from PHG at 12 months (65% vs. 38%), and the patients had fewer episodes of acute bleeding than did the controls. Propranolol treatment reduced the frequency of rebleeding from PHG independently of the initial manifestation or acute or chronic bleeding. The absence of propranolol treatment was the only predictive variable for rebleeding.

Conclusion.—Long-term propranolol treatment effectively reduces the incidence of rebleeding from PHG, and it may improve the prognosis of patients with cirrhosis. Propranolol prevented acute bleeding episodes whether the initial bleeding manifestation was acute or chronic. The absence of propranolol treatment was the only independent variable predicting rebleeding.

▶ This prospective, randomized trial concludes that propranolol is quite effective in reducing the incidence of rebleeding from portal hypertension in patients with cirrhosis. It appears that the role of this drug in the treatment of this condition is becoming much better established.—J.M. Porter, M.D.

Fasting and Post-Prandial Splanchnic Blood Flow Is Reduced by a Somatostatin Analogue (Octreotide) in Man

Cooper AM, Braatvedt GD, Qamar MI, Brown H, Thomas DM, Halliwell M, Read AE, Corrall RJM (Bristol Royal Infirmary, Bristol, England; Univ of Wales

College of Medicine, Cardiff, Wales)
Clin Sci 81:169–175, 1991   17–5

Introduction.—Somatostatin, a peptide found in the upper gastrointestinal tract, pancreatic islets, and CNS, exerts mainly inhibitory actions on the secretion of many hormones and can reduce portal venous pressure and splanchnic blood flow. The effects of octreotide, a long-acting somatostatin analogue, on splanchnic blood flow responses to a mixed solid meal were investigated in 8 individuals.

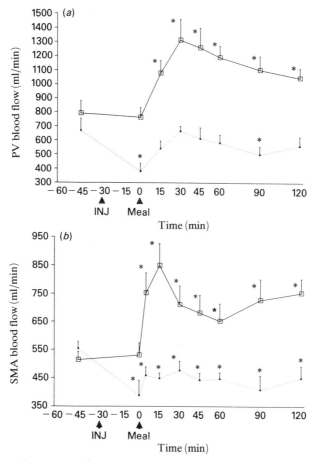

Fig. 17–1.—Splanchnic blood flow in response to feeding in 8 persons after administration of saline (*open squares*) or octreotide (50 μg; *solid squares*) subcutaneously. **Top,** portal venous (PV) blood flow. **Bottom,** superior mesenteric artery (SMA) blood flow. The values are means, with *bars* indicating SEM. Statistical significance; *asterisk* indicates $P < .05$ compared with baseline values. *INJ* indicates subcutaneous injection of saline or octreotide. The meal was consumed over 10 minutes. (Courtesy of Cooper AM, Braatvedt GD, Qamar MI, et al: *Clin Sci* 81:169–175, 1991.)

Overall Summary Statistic (Area Under the Curve Divided by 120 Minutes, i.e. Mean Change) and 95% Confidence Intervals for Responses

	Control	Octreotide	Mean difference (control minus octreotide)	P value for the difference between groups
Glucose (mmol/l)	0.80	2.41	−1.6	0.06
	(0.06 to 1.65)	(1.18 to 3.63)	(−2.04 to −1.20)	
Insulin (m-units/l)	21.4	4.3	18.2	<0.001
	(16.9 to 25.9)	(0.8 to 7.7)	(15.6 to 19.7)	
Glucagon (ng/l)	13.8	−10.0	29.3	<0.006
	(−0.04 to 27.5)	(−32.4 to −12.4)	(15.6 to 31.9)	
Pancreatic polypeptide (ng/l)	123	−6.3	127	<0.004
	(59 to 187)	(−24.5 to 11.9)	(111 to 148)	
Gastrin (ng/l)	10.7	29.8	−17	0.02
	(1.7 to 19.8)	(16.1 to 43.5)	(−23.7 to −14.5)	

The responses are of blood levels of glucose and plasma levels of insulin, glucagon, pancreatic polypeptide, and gastrin to a mixed solid meal in 8 individuals when saline (control) or octreotide (50 μg) was injected subcutaneously before the meal.
(Courtesy of Cooper AM, Braatvedt GD, Qamar MI, et al: *Clin Sci* 81:169-175, 1991.)

Methods.—The healthy, nonobese subjects were studied unblinded at least a week apart, after receiving either octreotide 50 μg, or a placebo, given subcutaneously before the standard meal. Splanchnic blood flow was measured by transcutaneous Doppler ultrasonography using arterial area multiplied by flow velocity.

Results.—Octreotide reduced fasting blood flow in the superior mesenteric artery and portal vein by at least half, and it also blunted the expected postprandial increase in flow (Fig 17-1). Neither meal ingestion nor octreotide injection altered the pulse or blood pressure significantly. Octreotide inhibited the postprandial release of insulin, glucagon, and pancreatic polypeptide (table), and it led to postprandial hyperglycemia.

Conclusion.—Inhibition of splanchnic blood flow and reduction of portal venous pressure by octreotide may prove useful in treating bleeding varices. Effective doses do not alter hemodynamics significantly.

▶ Is there anything for which octreotide is not good? Everything from intimal hyperplasia to migraine headache appears to be affected favorably by this agent. The current enthusiasm for this drug is reminiscent of the early days of dimethylsulfoxide (DMSO), which was initially reported to be a major advance against most of the world's ills, just as octreotide appears to be.—J.M. Porter, M.D.

Subject Index

A

Abdomen
  (*See also* Intraabdominal)
  ultrasound (*see* Ultrasound, abdominal)
  venous thrombosis, MRI in diagnosis of, 102
  vessels, MR angiography of, 103
Abuse
  cannabis, and carotid artery disease, in young adults, 279
  cocaine, and cerebral vasculitis, 141
  drug, causing femoral pseudoaneurysm, 134
  Mandrax, and carotid artery disease, in young adults, 279
Acetylsalicylic acid (*see* Aspirin)
Adventitial cystic disease
  popliteal artery, recurrence after percutaneous aspiration, 135
Age
  aortic aneurysm rupture and, 182
  aortic diameter and, 176
  coronary artery surgery results and, 153
  venous ulcers and, 381
Aging
  anticoagulant response to warfarin therapy and, 377
Alcohol
  consumption and coronary disease, 34
Alcoholic
  liver disease, prophylactic sclerotherapy for esophageal varices in, 405
Adlosterone
  plasma, effect of heparin on, 14
Allograft
  replacement, aortic, of abdominal aorta in aortic dissection, 193
  saphenous vein, cryopreserved
    biologic fate of, 320
    in infected fields, 321
Amputation
  lower limb
    after arterial embolectomy, 239
    for ischemia, 261
    for ischemia, severe acute, 240
    in peripheral vascular disease, 247
Anastomosis
  end-to-end, between prosthesis and vein of different diameters, 310
  paraanastomotic intraabdominal aneurysm after aortic bypass, 314
  sites, intimal hyperplasia at (in dog), 21
  technique, new prosthetic venous collar, 307
  vein patch in, in PTFE bypass grafting, 305
Ancrod

in heparin-induced thrombocytopenia, 364
Anesthesia
  for abdominal aortic surgery, 155
  for infrainguinal arterial reconstruction, 160
Aneurysm
  aortic
    abdominal (*see below*)
    rupture, age-standardized incidence of, 182
    thoracic, acute traumatic, 344
  aortic, abdominal
    aneurysmectomy, infrarenal, thoracoabdominal aneurysm resection after, 169
    in cardiac transplant patient, 178
    false, in Behçet's disease, 124
    graft for, aortic tube, late iliac artery aneurysm and occlusive disease after, 188
    graft for, transfemoral intraluminal, 189
    hernia and, inguinal, 179
    as incidental finding in abdominal ultrasound, 180
    infected, and HIV, 197
    inflammatory, CT of, 195
    leaking, causing testicular pain, 191
    natural history of, 186
    in occlusive peripheral vascular disease, 177
    prevalence of, increasing, 181
    after *Salmonella* infection, 194
    in screened patients, 198
    size, evaluation of new methods expressing, 175
    small, selective management, 184
    surgery for, 186
  arterial, in Behçet's disease, 122
  carotid artery, extracranial internal, due to fibromuscular dysplasia, 300
  false, infected, after iliac angioplasty, 55
  iliac artery, after aortic tube graft for abdominal aortic aneurysm, 188
  intraabdominal paraanastomotic, after aortic bypass, 314
  intracranial, saccular
    in cervical artery dissection, spontaneous, angiographic frequency of, 294
    familial association with cervical artery dissections, 293
  pseudoaneurysm (*see* Pseudoaneurysm)
  splenic artery, after liver transplant, 218
  thoracoabdominal, resection after previous infrarenal abdominal aortic aneurysmectomy, 169

Author Index

A Simple, Once-a-Year Dose!

Review the partial list of titles below. And then request your own FREE 30-day preview. When you subscribe to a Year Book, we'll also send you an automatic notice of future volumes about two months before they publish.

This system was designed for your convenience and to take up as little of your time as possible. If you do not want the Year Book, the advance notice makes it easy for you to let us know. And if you elect to receive the new Year Book, you need do nothing. We will send it on publication.

No worry. No wasted motion. And, of course, every Year Book is yours to examine FREE of charge for thirty days.

Year Book of **Anesthesia**® (22141)
Year Book of **Cardiology**® (22640)
Year Book of **Critical Care Medicine**® (22639)
Year Book of **Dermatology**® (22645)
Year Book of **Dermatologic Surgery**® (21171)
Year Book of **Diagnostic Radiology**® (22613)
Year Book of **Digestive Diseases**® (22625)
Year Book of **Drug Therapy**® (22630)
Year Book of **Emergency Medicine**® (22080)
Year Book of **Endocrinology**® (21174)
Year Book of **Family Practice**® (22124)
Year Book of **Geriatrics and Gerontology** (22611)
Year Book of **Hand Surgery**® (22618)
Year Book of **Hematology**® (22646)
Year Book of **Health Care Management**® (21177)
Year Book of **Infectious Diseases**® (22650)
Year Book of **Infertility** (22637)
Year Book of **Medicine**® (22638)
Year Book of **Neonatal-Perinatal Medicine** (22629)
Year Book of **Nephrology** (21175)
Year Book of **Neurology and Neurosurgery**® (22616)
Year Book of **Neuroradiology**® (21849)
Year Book of **Nuclear Medicine**® (22627)
Year Book of **Obstetrics and Gynecology**® (22636)
Year Book of **Occupational and Environmental Medicine** (22619)
Year Book of **Oncology** (22651)
Year Book of **Ophthalmology**® (22133)
Year Book of **Orthopedics**® (22644)
Year Book of **Otolaryngology – Head and Neck Surgery**® (22609)
Year Book of **Pathology and Clinical Pathology**® (21176)
Year Book of **Pediatrics**® (22130)
Year Book of **Plastic and Reconstructive Surgery**® (22635)
Year Book of **Psychiatry and Applied Mental Health**® (22649)
Year Book of **Pulmonary Disease**® (22624)
Year Book of **Sports Medicine**® (22111)
Year Book of **Surgery**® (22641)
Year Book of **Transplantation**® (21854)
Year Book of **Ultrasound** (21169)
Year Book of **Urology**® (22621)
Year Book of **Vascular Surgery**® (22612)

Mosby-Year Book, Inc. • 11830 Westline Industrial Drive • St. Louis, MO 63146